Re-defining Mineral Nutrition

D1766859

Re-defining Mineral Nutrition

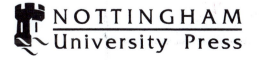
Nottingham University Press

Nottingham University Press
Manor Farm, Main Street, Thrumpton
Nottingham, NG11 0AX, United Kingdom

NOTTINGHAM

First published 2005
© The several contributors names in the list of contents

British Library Cataloguing in Publication Data
Redefining Mineral Nutrition
I. Tucker, L.A., II. Taylor-Pickard, J.A.

ISBN 1-904761-30-5

Disclaimer

Every reasonable effort has been made to ensure that the material in this book is true,
correct, complete and appropriate at the time of writing. Nevertheless, the publishers and
authors do not accept responsibility for any omission or error, or for any injury, damage,
loss or financial consequences arising from the use of the book.

Typeset by Nottingham University Press, Nottingham
Printed and bound by Hobbs the Printers, Hampshire, England

CONTENTS

Prof Bo Pehrson
*Department of Animal Environment and Health, Swedish
University of Agricultural Sciences, S-53223 Skara,
Sweden*

Prof David E Beever
Ruminations Ltd., Marlow, Bucks

Introduction

The field of mineral nutrition is one that has received scant attention from researchers since the 1970's. Data generated during the last decade has been indirect, via the development and understanding of phytase enzymes for example. Since the mid 1990's there has been increasing concern regarding pollution from intensive farming, particularly in densely polluted countries in, for example, Northern Europe or areas where geological conditions increase the potential for ground water contamination. Such concerns have forced animal producers to look at how they affect pollution. This began with changes in phosphorous and nitrogen delivery and is now expanding into other micronutrients and trace elements such as zinc and copper.

Analysis of the available literature shows that basic inorganic requirements for farm animals were devised, in some cases, half a century ago. The animals used then were of a completely different genetic character, with low growth potential, reared under radically different welfare and management systems, and fed diets that bear little resemblance to those used today. The low cost of inorganic minerals used in premixes and complete diets has resulted in limited investment into trace element research. With these points in mind, it seems that the feed industry is ill-prepared to make important changes to the way minerals are supplied to breeding and growing animals, allowing pollution targets to be met. It is therefore timely that the current state of mineral nutrition of farmed species is examined in closer detail, and put into commercial context. It is also necessary to identify and compare innovations in mineral supply via feed, to minimise excretion without compromising performance.

To give nutritionists, veterinarians and producers a concise and focussed review of the current and future state of mineral nutrition in farmed species, seminars hosted by Alltech, were run covering poultry, pigs and ruminants in October 2004. The key objectives of the seminars were to examine how and why minerals are fed, commercial requirements and constraints for in-feed minerals, the increasing regulations governing current and future disposal of excreted minerals, and new approaches to supplying minerals in lower dosed, more natural and less wasteful forms. This latter point gave rise to the concept of "redefining mineral nutrition".

To have such a complete coverage of a topic available is of great value to modern-day nutritionists and veterinarians. The opportunity to devote a single day at a dedicated species seminar is a highly useful and efficient way of reviewing existing information, and transferring novel concepts regarding these subjects, and enables informed decisions to be made regarding key issues such as improving performance or limiting pollution.

As part of an expanding series of specialist nutrition-focussed seminars, sponsored by Alltech, the topics covered have generated great interest amongst the many delegates from a spectrum of animal health and production operations from different parts of the world. We trust that readers of the papers will also find them as stimulating.

Dr Julie Taylor-Pickard
Dr Lucy Tucker
December 2004

Setting the NRC standards for minerals – were we right?

Gary L. Cromwell[1] and Charlotte Kirk Baer[2]
[1]*Department of Animal Sciences, University of Kentucky, Lexington, KY 40546, USA;* [2]*Board on Agriculture and Natural Resources, National Academy of Science, National Research Council, Suite 686 500 Fifth Street NW, Washington, DC 20001, USA*

Energy and essential nutrients such as amino acids, minerals, and vitamins are required by animals for the various processes of life, including maintenance, growth, reproduction, lactation, and work. Having accurate estimates of dietary nutrient requirements of animals is important. Deficiencies of even a single nutrient in a diet will limit an animal's performance and well-being, and diets with excessive nutrients are expensive and contribute to environmental pollution.

The National Research Council (NRC) plays an important role in establishing nutrient requirements for animals. Whether the nutrient requirements are accurate or not is often a subject of debate among nutritionists in academia and the feed industry. Before addressing the question of whether the nutrient requirement standards are, or are not, accurate, let's review what the NRC is and how this body goes about establishing nutrient requirements of animals raised to produce food and fiber and for work and recreation.

Background of the National Research Council

Contrary to what some people believe, the NRC is not part of the federal government. Instead, the NRC is a private, nonprofit organization with a long history. The NRC was established in 1916 to provide advice to the U.S. Federal Government on issues of science and technology. The NRC is the "working arm" of The National Academies, which includes the National Academy of Sciences (NAS), an honorary society instituted 141 years ago (in 1863) by President Abraham Lincoln through an act of Congress. Members are elected to the Academy based on their contributions to science. The NRC has ten major units, one of which is the Board on Agriculture and Natural Resources (BANR). The Committee on Animal Nutrition (CAN) has been the longest standing committee of the BANR and the NRC. Dating back to the establishment of the

NRC itself, CAN has addressed issues of animal feeding since 1917. It's series of publications on nutrient requirements, written by subcommittees and overseen by CAN, covers nearly 30 species of food, companion, and laboratory animals. These reports have been translated into seven languages and are used worldwide. Reviews of the history of CAN and the NRC were recently published (CAN, 1998; Ullrey, 2001).[1]

The first of the nutrient requirement publications, *Recommended Nutrient Allowances for Swine* and *Recommended Nutrient Allowances for Poultry* were published in 1944 (NRC, 1944a; b). These were concise documents (the swine publication was 10 pages) that identified the nutrients known at that time to be essential for pigs and poultry and that listed dietary requirements for some of these nutrients. The following year, similar publications were released for beef cattle, dairy cattle, and sheep (NCR, 1945a; b; c). The first publication of this type for horses was published four years later (NRC, 1949).

In 1953, the titles of the NRC publications were changed from "Recommended Nutrient Allowances" to "Nutrient Requirements." This was a major philosophical change in how nutrient standards were established by NRC. Prior to 1953, recommended allowances included subjectively established safety factors and were intended to ensure that minimal nutrient requirements would be met under any circumstances. In some cases, recommended allowances were based on practical experience. Since 1953, NRC requirements have been considered as the minimal dietary concentration of a nutrient required to support normal performance for the most demanding function.

Process of producing the NRC's nutrient requirement publications

The process by which nutrient requirement publications are prepared is relatively simple, but it is thorough, rigorous, and somewhat time-consuming. Once the study proposal has been approved, and an understanding exists between the sponsor and BANR, the study may commence. Studies may have one or several sponsors from government or the private sector, or both. Because

[1] The Committee on Animal Nutrition was dissolved at the end of 2003 due to inadequate support to maintain it as a standing activity of the National Academies. To improve efficiency of the animal nutrition operating program and to address needs for operating support, the program has been restructured and the responsibilities of CAN, including the nutrient requirement series, have been assumed by the Board on Agriculture and Natural Resources.

the NRC offers a one-of-a-kind service, not duplicated by other organizations, it does not compete for federal contracts. The NRC provides a public service, which is supported by the users of its products. In the case of nutrient requirement publications, the reports are produced by the non-profit NRC and are published and disseminated throughout the world by the non-profit National Academy Press. It is through the dedicated work of volunteer experts and the financial support of end-users that the reports are made widely available for use in the industry, government, research, and teaching communities.

Staff with input and oversight from the relevant boards initiates the search for candidates for subcommittee membership. In defining the areas of expertise that should be represented on a subcommittee and identifying individuals qualified to serve, the staff reviews scholarly literature and consults widely with members of the National Academies, BANR, knowledgeable authorities, and professional associations. Sponsors may offer suggestions but are not responsible for selecting subcommittee members. Subcommittee members are chosen on the basis of their experience in the various areas of nutrition, and after careful review by BANR, they are appointed by the chair of the NRC, who also is president of the NAS. Subcommittee members serve as individuals, not as representatives of organizations or interest groups. Members are sought with background and experience in academia, government, and industry. Each person is selected on the basis of his or her expertise and good judgment, and is expected to contribute accordingly to the study. Potential sources of bias and conflict of interest are significant issues that are taken into consideration in the selection of subcommittee members.

A successful report is the result of a dynamic group process, requiring that subcommittee members be open to new ideas and innovative solutions, and be willing to learn from one another and from other individuals who provide input. Subcommittees are expected to be even-handed and to examine all evidence dispassionately. The subcommittees review the world's literature, particularly research published since the last edition. Although all interested parties should be heard and their views given serious consideration, one of the subcommittee's primary roles is to separate fact from opinion, and analysis from advocacy. Scientific standards are essential in evaluating all arguments and alternatives. Experience suggests that completing the consensus process and writing a report that clearly represents the subcommittee's findings is the most difficult, frustrating, yet rewarding aspect of serving on a study subcommittee. Many audiences such as regulatory, research, and industry, to name a few, use the report. For this reason, the report must be of the highest quality. Although each subcommittee may approach the drafting of its report differently, every report is the collective product of a group process.

Like all good science, reports should be based on fact and rigorous analysis. All reports must undergo an independent review by anonymous expert panels of reviewers. Review is a multi-tiered process, which ensures the highest level of quality that sets the NRC apart from any other organization. While the report is reviewed by expert scientists, a review coordinator and monitor, as well as the NRC's report review subcommittee oversee the entire process.

Upon completion of the report, the National Academy Press publishes it. The Press prints and sells the report at cost, and strives to make the report widely available to users on a global scale.

Setting requirements for swine

The process for establishing nutrient requirements is similar for the various species of animals; however, this paper will specifically address the process of setting the requirements in the most recent edition of *Nutrient Requirements of Swine* (1998). The swine subcommittee was appointed in 1994 and consisted of the following members:

Dr. David H. Baker, University of Illinois
Dr. Richard C. Ewan, Iowa State University
Dr. E. T. Kornegay, Virginia Polytechnic Institute and State University
Dr. Austin J. Lewis, University of Nebraska
Dr. James E. Pettigrew, Pettigrew Consulting International, University of Illinois
Dr. Norman C. Steele, U.S. Department of Agriculture – Agricultural Research Service
Dr. Philip A. Thacker, University of Saskatchewan
Dr. Gary L. Cromwell, University of Kentucky (Chair)

The subcommittee initially met in 1994 and was given their charge by the Program Director of CAN, Charlotte Kirk Baer. The initial meeting included the chair of the Nutrition Council Swine Committee of the American Feed Industry Association, Dr. Kevin Halpin. He provided suggestions from nutritionists at feed companies and ingredient suppliers who were involved in servicing the swine feed industry that assisted the subcommittee in setting goals and establishing direction for the revised publication. He indicated that nutritionists from the feed industry were willing to provide data on feed composition and nutrient requirement studies if requested by the subcommittee.

At their initial meeting, the subcommittee decided to use a modelling approach to assist in establishing nutrient requirements. Realizing that this was a new area that would take an exceptional amount of time, it was decided to use this approach only in establishing energy and amino acid requirements. The subcommittee divided up their responsibilities, and then over the next several months, they conducted a thorough review of the literature regarding nutrient requirement studies in North America as well as throughout the world. Particular attention was paid to research reported since the previous edition was published. The subcommittee met several times over the following two years to share information and prepare the report. Both empirical data as well as mathematical relationships for the model were used in establishing nutrient requirements.

The swine models – a new approach to estimating requirements

Several subcommittees have used a modelling approach to more precisely estimate nutrient requirements. The beef subcommittees utilized models in their 1996 publication (NRC, 1996, 2000) and the dairy subcommittee has since utilized models to estimate requirements of dairy cattle (NRC, 2001). The horse subcommittee is currently revising their publication and plans to include models.

To illustrate the value of models in estimating nutrient requirements, let's review some of the background that went into the development of the swine models. In all previous editions of the swine publication, requirement estimates for growth were based mainly on weight classes of pigs and single estimates were made for pregnant and lactating sows without consideration for genetic differences among pigs. Environmental factors that are now known to have a profound influence on the pig's nutrient requirements also were not considered. Simply put, the committee agreed that a "one size fits all" approach to defining nutrient requirements was no longer acceptable in the current highly technical arena of swine nutrition.

Models (a series of integrated mathematical equations) were needed for the new edition to account for the many factors that are now known to influence nutrient requirements. A growth model was needed that would more accurately estimate nutrient requirements taking into consideration not only the pig's body weight, but also it's accretion rate of lean (protein) tissue, gender, and various environmental factors. Gestating and lactating sow models were needed that would, along with body weight, consider weight gain during gestation, weight loss during lactation, number of pigs in the litter, weight gain of the litter (a reflection of milk yield), and certain environmental factors.

Unfortunately, no models were available that met the needs for the task at hand. While there were a number of commercial models used in the swine industry, the equations are tightly guarded for proprietary reasons. Also, most simulation models predict animal performance as an output when certain levels of nutrients and various environmental factors were given as inputs. The NRC models are just the opposite; they predict the levels of nutrients (model outputs) needed to achieve a certain level of production under a given set of environmental conditions (model inputs). Therefore, it was necessary for the subcommittee to develop its own models.

Five principles guided the NRC swine subcommittee in developing the models. The principles were: (1) made for easy use by people with varying levels of nutritional expertise and with limited information; (2) developed for continued relevance for several years to come (*i.e.*, until the next edition will be published); (3) intended to be structurally simple, so they can be understood easily by users; (4) developed to be transparent so that all of the equations are available to the user; and (5) firmly anchored to empirical data at the whole-animal level rather than being simply based on theoretical values.

The tedious task of building the models from scratch and testing them took the subcommittee over two years. As the models were developed, they were tested with previously established requirements and with data sets from recently conducted research. The models were modified and refined to ensure that the requirement estimates produced were supported by empirical data. Finally, the models were validated with independent data from experiments that had not been used in the construction of the models. To allow nutritionists to understand the inner workings of the models, all of the equations are presented in the publication.

Three independent models were developed: a growth model, a gestation model, and a lactation model. The growth model estimates amino acid requirements of pigs from weaning to market weight, and the gestation and lactation models estimate energy and amino acid requirements of gestating and lactating sows. Along with energy and amino acid requirements, the software also allows the user to estimate mineral and vitamin requirements. The models are included in commercially produced, user-friendly software on a compact disk (CD-ROM) that accompanies the NRC publication.

Swine growth model

Although this paper deals with mineral requirements, a brief
description of the swine models is appropriate. The growth model
estimates the amino acid requirements of pigs over the range of 20
to 120 kg of body weight. The model estimates requirements on an
available amino acid basis, which is based on true absorption of
amino acids at the terminal ileum. The amino acid requirements
are estimated on a daily (grams/day) basis. The estimates are the
sum of the pig's daily requirements for (1) maintenance and (2)
deposition of whole-body protein.

Lysine is the first limiting amino acid in essentially all practical
swine diets, so it is estimated first. The daily lysine requirement for
maintenance is related to metabolic body weight (kilograms of
weight raised to the ¾ power) and is considered as 0.036 g of
lysine per kg of $BW^{0.75}$. The daily lysine requirement for protein
deposition is considered as 0.12 g of true ileal digestible lysine per
gram of whole-body protein accreted. The value of 0.12 involves
two components: the lysine content of whole-body protein
($\sim 7.0\%$), and the partial efficiency of incorporation of digestible
lysine into whole-body protein ($\sim 58\%$) (*i.e.*, 7.0/0.58 = 0.12).

To use this information, the daily rate at which pigs deposit protein
in the body tissues must be known. This can be calculated if one
knows the rate at which pigs deposit lean tissue in the carcass,
which can be determined from equations utilizing data from packing
plant kill sheets or from an equation based on hot carcass weight,
backfat, and loin eye area (NPPC, 2000).[2] In the model, whole-
body protein is calculated from carcass fat-free lean, using a
conversion factor of 2.55. This relationship is based on data from
studies in which carcass lean and whole-body protein were both
measured in the same experiment. Carcass lean is divided by 2.55
to obtain whole-body protein. Thus, a pig having 325 g/day of
carcass lean gain is predicted to have a whole-body protein gain of
127 g/day (325/2.55=127).

The user inputs mean daily lean gain (lean gain per day averaged
over the period from 20 to 120 kg of body weight), and the model
calculates the daily protein accretion at any given weight. This
calculation is based on the overall mean lean gain per day along
with an assumed shape to the lean gain (protein accretion) curve.

---

[2] Carcass fat-free lean, % = 100 x [3.899 + (0.465 x hot carcass weight, kg) – (3.914 x
10th rib backfat, cm) + (0.21146 x longissimus muscle area, cm²)] / hot carcass weight,
kg

The model uses a default curve (Figure 1) to make this calculation. The shape assumes that daily protein accretion rate accelerates during early growth, reaches a plateau, then the rate declines during the finishing period. Pigs with different lean growth rates have the same general pattern of protein accretion but the heights of the curves will differ (Figure 2). The software allows the user to input different shaped curves, if desired.

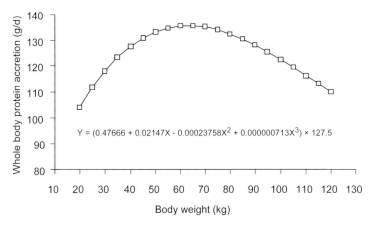

Figure inset equation:

$$Y = (0.47666 + 0.02147X - 0.00023758X^2 + 0.000000713X^3) \times 127.5$$

Figure 1. Potential whole-body protein accretion rate of pigs of high-medium lean growth rate with a carcass fat-free lean gain averaging 325 g/day from 20 to 120 kg of body weight using the NRC (1998) growth model. The lean growth rate of 325 g/day is converted to a mean whole-body protein accretion rate of 127.5 g/day (325/2.55 = 127.5).

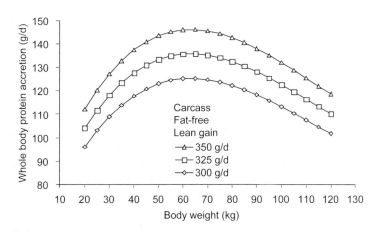

Figure 2. Whole-body protein accretion rates of pigs of medium, high-medium, and high lean growth rates with carcass fat- free lean gains averaging 300, 325, and 350 g/day from 20 to 120 kg of body weight as estimated by the NRC (1998) growth model.

After the daily lysine requirement is determined, the requirements for the other amino acids are estimated using blends of amino acids patterns. The "ideal protein" concept is used, which assumes that there is an ideal pattern of amino acids for maintenance and an ideal pattern for body protein accretion. These two patterns are blended depending on the proportion of lysine being used for maintenance and protein accretion in a given situation. Requirements are then converted to a percentage basis by dividing the daily amino acid requirements by the daily feed intake. Daily feed intake is predicted from body weight using a digestible energy (DE) intake equation in the model (Figure 3). Alternatively, feed intake can be entered by the user.

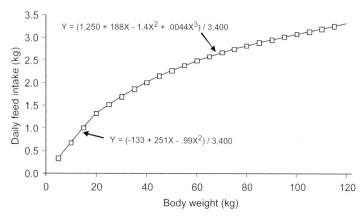

$$Y = (1{,}250 + 188X - 1.4X^2 + .0044X^3) / 3{,}400$$

$$Y = (-133 + 251X - .99X^2) / 3{,}400$$

Figure 3. Estimated feed intake of a diet containing 3,400 kcal of DE/kg of pigs from 3 to 120 kg of body weight as estimated by the NRC (1998) growth model.

The dietary percentage requirements of amino acids differ depending upon the gender of the pig (females and males require higher percentages of amino acids than castrates), environmental temperature, space allowance, and energy density of the diet. These factors, which are user inputs, affect energy intake, which, in turn, affects the requirements on a percentage basis. From the true ileal digestible amino acid requirements, apparent ileal digestible and total amino acid requirements are then calculated from equations. All three sets of requirements are presented to the user.

The growth model effectively estimates amino acid requirements of pigs based on their genetic ability to deposit lean tissue. Figure 4 illustrates the dietary lysine requirements, expressed as a percentage of the diet, from 20 to 120 kg body weight in pigs (1:1 mix of females and castrates) with medium, high-medium, and high lean growth rates (300, 325, and 350 g/day of carcass fat-free lean) under standard conditions. The model adjusts the lysine requirements if changes are made in the gender ratio, energy density of the diet, environmental temperature, animal space, or other factors.

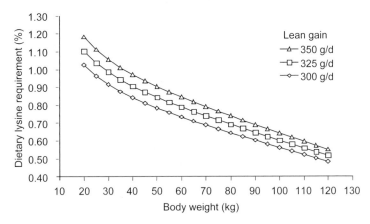

Figure 4. Dietary lysine requirements (%) of pigs of medium, high-medium, and high lean growth rates with carcass fat-free lean gains averaging 300, 325, and 350 g/day from 20 to 120 kg of body weight as estimated by the NRC (1998) growth model. The requirements are for total lysine, assuming a corn-soybean meal mixture.

The amino acid requirements for the young pig (3 to 20 kg) are estimated strictly from empirical data, due to a lack of information needed to model the requirements in the same manner as for growing-finishing pigs. The model uses an equation that fits a curvilinear regression line across estimated lysine requirements for several weight categories. The other amino acids are then handled by blending ideal patterns for maintenance and protein accretion.

Swine gestation and lactation models

These two models operate much like the growth model in terms of the amino acid requirements. Daily amino acid requirements of gestating sows are based on maintenance and the estimated protein accretion in the sow's body and in the products of conception (uterus, fetuses, placental tissues and fluids, etc.), which are calculated based on user inputs of breeding weight, gestational weight gain, and assumed litter size. Similarly, daily amino acid requirements of lactating sows are based on maintenance, body protein gain or loss during lactation, and milk production of the sow. These are calculated by the model from user inputs of the sow's postpartum weight and projected lactation weight change, lactation length, number of pigs nursed, and daily weight gain of the nursing pigs.

As with the growing pig, lysine is estimated first, then blends of ideal ratios of amino acids for maintenance, protein accretion, milk synthesis, and body protein breakdown are used to estimate requirements for the other amino acids. Daily energy requirements and feed intake are estimated by the model and the percentage requirements then are calculated. The user also has the option of entering daily energy intake; in that case, gestation weight gain or lactation weight loss (or gain) is then calculated by the model.

Mineral requirements – how were they estimated

The subcommittee did not use a modelling approach to estimate the mineral requirements due mainly to the fact that it was felt that there was not sufficient data available in the literature to develop an accurate model. As a result, all of the estimates were based on empirical data from research studies. Estimates were made for six weight classes of pigs (Table 1) and for sows during gestation and lactation (Table 2).

Table 1. Mineral requirements of weanling, growing, and finishing pigs allowed feed ad libitum (90% dry matter)[b] NRC (1998).

| Item | Body weight (kg) | | | | | |
	3-5	5-10	10-20	20-50	50-80	80-120
Average weight in range, kg	4	7.5	15	35	65	100
Estimated DE intake, kcal/kg	855	1,690	3,400	6,305	8,760	10,450
Estimated feed intake, g/day[c]	250	500	1,000	1,855	2,575	3,075
Requirements of major minerals			%			
Calcium[d]	0.90	0.80	0.70	0.60	0.50	0.45
Phosphorus[d]	0.70	0.65	0.60	0.50	0.45	0.40
Phosphorus, available[d]	0.55	0.40	0.32	0.23	0.19	0.15
Sodium	0.25	0.20	0.15	0.10	0.10	0.10
Chlorine	0.25	0.20	0.15	0.08	0.08	0.08
Magnesium	0.04	0.04	0.04	0.04	0.04	0.04
Potassium	0.30	0.28	0.26	0.23	0.19	0.17
Requirements of trace minerals[e]			ppm			
Copper	6.0	6.0	5.0	4.0	3.5	3.0
Iodine	0.14	0.14	0.14	0.14	0.14	0.14
Iron	100	100	80	60	50	40
Manganese	4.0	4.0	3.0	2.0	2.0	2.0
Selenium	0.30	0.30	0.25	0.15	0.15	0.15
Zinc	100	100	80	60	50	50

[b]Pigs of mixed gender (1:1 ratio of barrows to gilts). The requirements of certain minerals may be slightly higher for pigs having high lean growth rates (> 325 g/day of carcass fat-free lean), but no distinction is made.
[c]Assumes the diet contains 3,400 kcal of DE/kg.
[d]The percentages of calcium, phosphorus, and available phosphorus should be increased by 0.05 to 0.10 percentage points for developing boars and replacement gilts from 50 to 120 kg body weight.
[e]Chromium is recognized as an essential nutrient, but a requirement has not been established.

11

Table 2.
Mineral
requirements of
gestating and
lactating sows (90%
dry matter)[b] NRC
(1998).

	Dietary requirements		Daily requirements	
	Gestation	*Lactation*	*Gestation*	*Lactation*
Estimated DE intake, Mcal/kg	6.29	17.85	6.29	17.85
Estimated feed intake, kg/day[c]	1.85	5.25	1.85	5.25
Requirements of major minerals	%		g/day	
Calcium	0.75	0.75	13.9	39.4
Phosphorus	0.60	0.60	11.1	31.5
Phosphorus, available	0.35	0.35	6.5	18.4
Sodium	0.15	0.20	2.8	10.5
Chlorine	0.12	0.16	2.2	8.4
Magnesium	0.04	0.04	0.7	2.1
Potassium	0.20	0.20	3.7	10.5
Requirements of trace minerals[d]	ppm		mg/day	
Copper	5.00	5.00	9.3	26.3
Iodine	0.14	0.14	0.3	0.7
Iron	80	80	148	420
Manganese	20	20	37	105
Selenium	0.15	0.15	0.3	0.8
Zinc	50	50	93	263

[b]The requirements are based on the daily consumption of 1.85 and 5.25 kg of feed for gestation and lactation, respectively. If lower amounts of feed are consumed, the dietary percentages of some minerals, particularly calcium and phosphorus, may need to be increased.
[c]Assumes the diet contains 3.40 Mcal of DE/kg.
[d]Chromium is recognized as an essential nutrient, but a requirement has not been established.

In every case, the estimates were made on the basis of dietary concentration of minerals. The daily requirements were determined by multiplying the dietary concentration by the daily amount of feed consumed. Feed consumption, in turn, was estimated from the model-predicted energy consumption divided by the energy concentration of the diet.

Mathematical equations were utilized in order to estimate the dietary mineral requirements of weanling, growing, and finishing pigs at all body weights between 3 and 120 kg. This was accomplished by using generalized exponential equations for those minerals in which the dietary concentration decreased as pigs increased in body weight. The equations took the general form of $Y = e^z$, where $z = a + b(Ln\ X) + c(Ln\ X)^2$. The equations were based on the estimated requirements at the mean pig weight of each body weight classification. Figure 5 shows such an equation for the calcium requirement of pigs from 3 to 120 kg body weight.

There was an abundant amount of research data to draw upon in estimating requirements for certain minerals such as calcium and

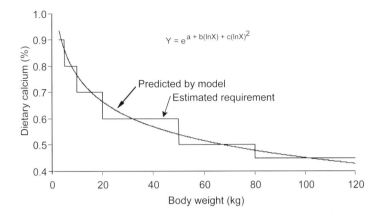

Figure 5. Dietary calcium requirement (%) of pigs from 3 to 120 kg of body weight using the generalized exponential equation in the NRC (1998) growth model.

phosphorus. Less, but adequate, information was available on other minerals such as sodium, copper, iron, zinc, and selenium. Other minerals such as chlorine, magnesium, potassium, manganese, and iodine have been researched less extensively and requirement estimates were more difficult to establish. Chromium was recognized as being an essential mineral, but the subcommittee did not estimate a requirement for this mineral due to insufficient research information.

Possibility of modelling mineral requirements

Very little research information is presently available that would allow one to model the requirements for the various minerals such as the NRC swine subcommittee did for amino acids and energy. Recently, we conducted several studies at the University of Kentucky to generate data that would allow us to model the phosphorus requirements of growing-finishing pigs. Several balance studies were conducted to estimate the maintenance requirements for phosphorus (Pettey *et al.*, 2003a; 2004a). Another series of experiments were conducted to assess the accretion rates of whole-body phosphorus (Pettey *et al.*, 2003b; 2004b; c). Figure 6 shows the results of these studies. The data indicate that our estimates of the phosphorus requirements, based on the sum of the requirements for maintenance and for deposition of phosphorus in body tissues, were similar to the bioavailable phosphorus requirements of NRC (1998), especially in the mid-weight range. The two sets of estimates differed some in the lighter- and heavier-weight pigs, in which case our estimates were less than those of NRC (1998). This study was done with a single genotype, and additional work of this type needs to be done with other genotypes of pigs to determine the effects, if any, that lean growth rate or perhaps other factors may influence phosphorus requirements.

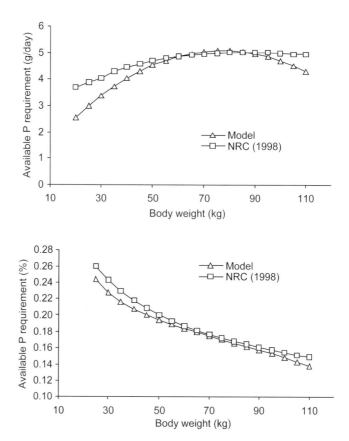

Figure 6. Model-predicted phosphorus requirement (g/day on top, % of diet on bottom) of pigs from 20 to 110 kg body weight based on the phosphorus required for maintenance and whole-body phosphorus accretion compared with the available phosphorus requirement of NRC (1998). Pettey *et al.* (2004a; c), University of Kentucky.

So are the mineral requirements accurate?

In some ways, this question (the title of this paper) is easy to answer depending on who is addressing the question. The subcommittee, including myself, would be tempted to answer "Why yes, of course they are accurate!" That answer would be based on the many hours spent by the subcommittee in conducting an extensive review of the literature (there are 533 mineral publications cited on 13 pages) followed by the laborious task of reaching consensus (sometimes it was a compromise), then setting the requirement. On the other hand, a better answer is that the estimates are only as accurate as the amount and scientific quality of the research data upon which they are based. Unfortunately, for some minerals, requirement studies were scarce or non-existent. In some of those studies, the results may have been confusing and interpretation may have been difficult. For sows, the data for some minerals were even sparser. In some cases (e.g., iodine), the estimates for sows were based on data from growing pigs.

Some important points that should be remembered as one deliberates an answer for this question are as follows:

- Remember that the NRC requirements are estimates of minimal nutrient requirements required to support normal performance. They are without safety factors designed to account for the variability that exists in the nutrient content of feed ingredients or the variability that exists among animals. They are not intended to necessarily be levels that are recommended for feeding pigs or sows. Instead, they are simply guidelines that nutritionists in industry and academia can use as a starting point to establish recommended allowances for animals. This is true, not only for minerals, but also for other nutrients.

- In most cases, the requirements are based on the amount of a nutrient that will result in optimal growth and efficiency of feed utilization or optimal reproductive and lactational performance. While it is well recognized that higher than NRC levels of calcium and phosphorus will increase bone mineralization and strength (which may improve long-term productivity), this was not included in the requirement estimates for calcium and phosphorus.

- Animals do change (genetics, health, etc.), so mineral requirements of pigs 20 years ago may be different from those of pigs today or of pigs 20 years in the future. What was accurate then might not be accurate now. But if research studies are not available with modern pigs, we have to use whatever data are available to make requirement estimates.

- Estimates of requirements change as new data become available. A good example is the manganese requirement of sows. In the 1988 NRC publication, the requirement was listed as 10 ppm; in the 1998 publication, the requirement was 20 ppm. Certainly the sow's requirement did not double during the 10-year period from 1988 to 1998. The higher estimate in 1998 was simply due to a study that was conducted during that 10-year interim that shed new light on the requirement.

- The NRC mineral requirements are based on dietary concentrations, not daily amounts of minerals. Daily requirements are simply calculated amounts based on estimated feed intakes. However, in some instances, animals may not consume as much feed as predicted from the NRC model such as high-producing lactating sows kept in a hot environment. In such cases, higher percentages of dietary calcium and phosphorus would be needed to meet their daily calcium and phosphorus needs for milk production.

- Very high levels of certain minerals such as copper (100-250 ppm copper as copper sulfate or copper chloride) and zinc (1,500- 3,000 ppm zinc as zinc oxide) will consistently produce a significant growth response in young pigs, but these responses are considered to be a pharmaceutical effect and are not included in the estimates of the copper and zinc requirements.

- The NRC mineral requirements, for the most part, do not take into consideration the bioavailability of minerals. The only exception is phosphorus in which case the NRC gives a requirement for total and available phosphorus along with estimates of the bioavailability of phosphorus in feedstuffs. For other minerals, the estimates are for total mineral levels. It is generally recognized that organic forms of minerals are more bioavailable than inorganic forms, such as in Alltech's selenized yeast (Sel-Plex®) versus sodium selenite, but this is not addressed in the nutrient requirements. A higher bioavailability of organic forms of several other minerals is also recognized (such as the minerals in Alltech's Bioplex™).

- Finally, we are recognizing more and more that certain minerals have an impact on the immune function in animals. For some time, it has been known that long-term deficiencies of almost any of the minerals can compromise the immune function in animals. But more recently, scientists have found that certain trace minerals such as copper, zinc, selenium, and chromium, bolster the immune status in pigs and other animals when fed at high levels and perhaps in a more bioavailable (organic) form. This type of response was recognized but not considered in the establishment of the mineral requirements.

So are the NRC mineral requirements really accurate? The answer likely will depend on who is answering the question. While some of the requirements may not be totally accurate, they were established based on the scientific knowledge at the time of publication and the best judgment of a distinguished group of swine nutritionists. Will some of the requirements change in the next publication? Probably so, because present and future research will generate new information in some areas that will allow the next subcommittee to better estimate the requirements of certain nutrients. Should the requirements be followed by every nutritionist in every situation? Probably not. They will require adjustment based on the understanding and experience of the nutritionist for the particular situation.

Summary

The NRC plays an important role in establishing nutrient requirements of animals used for food, service, recreation, companionship, and other purposes. The process of how nutrient requirements are estimated is important to understand in order to appreciate the fact that they are the best estimates of nutrient needs at the time of publication. Requirements will obviously change as genetic improvements are made in animals and as more research becomes available that clarify the animal's nutrient needs under differing environmental and health conditions.

Sidebar

The NRC publication, *Nutrient Requirements of Swine* and the compact disk containing the model programs, can be purchased from: National Academy Press, 2101 Constitution Avenue N.W., Lockbox 285, Washington, DC 20055 or on the internet at the National Academy Press web site, www.nap.edu. The publication and model as well as some of the other NRC publications can be downloaded free of charge from the web site by clicking on "Reading Room." For more information, contact Board on Agriculture and Natural Resources, National Research Council, Suite 686, 500 Fifth Street N.W., Washington, DC 20001.

References

CAN (1998) The First 70 Years, 1928-1998. Committee on Animal Nutrition, National Research Council. National Academy Press, Washington, DC.

NPPC (2000) Pork Composition and Quality Assessment Procedures. National Pork Producers Council. Des Moines, IA.

NRC (1944a) Recommended Nutrient Allowances for Swine. National Research Council, National Academy of Sciences, Washington, DC.

NRC (1944b) Recommended Nutrient Allowances for Poultry. National Research Council, National Academy of Sciences, Washington, DC.

NRC (1945a) Recommended Nutrient Allowances for Beef Cattle. National Research Council, National Academy of Sciences, Washington, DC.

NRC (1945b) Recommended Nutrient Allowances for Dairy Cattle. National Research Council, National Academy of Sciences, Washington, DC.

NRC (1945c) Recommended Nutrient Allowances for Sheep. National Research Council, National Academy of Sciences, Washington, DC.

NRC (1949) Recommended Nutrient Allowances for Horses. National Research Council, National Academy of Sciences, Washington, DC.

NRC (1988) Nutrient Requirements of Swine. Ninth Revised Edition. National Research Council, National Academy Press, Washington, DC.

NRC (1994) Nutrient Requirements of Poultry. Ninth Revised Edition. National Research Council, National Academy Press, Washington, DC.

NRC (1996) Nutrient Requirements of Beef Cattle. Seventh Revised Edition. National Research Council, National Academy Press, Washington, DC.

NRC (1998) Nutrient Requirements of Swine. Tenth Revised Edition. National Research Council, National Academy Press, Washington, DC.

NRC (2000) Nutrient Requirements of Beef Cattle. Update 2000. National Research Council, National Academy Press, Washington, DC.

NRC (2001) Nutrient Requirements of Dairy Cattle. Seventh Revised Edition. National Research Council, National Academy Press, Washington, DC.

Petty, Lee Allen (2004) The Factorial Estimation of Dietary Phosphorus Requirements for Growing and Finishing Pigs. Ph.D. Dissertation, University of Kentucky. Lexington.

Pettey, L. A., Cromwell, G. L., and Lindemann, M. D. (2003a) Phosphorus balance in growing pigs fed semi-purified diets adequate or low in dietary phosphorus. *Journal of Animal Science* **81**(Suppl. 2): 61.

Pettey, L. A., Cromwell, G. L., and Lindemann, M. D. (2003b) Whole body composition and phosphorus accretion in growing pigs. *Journal of Animal Science* **81**(Suppl. 2): 61.

Pettey, L. A., Cromwell, G. L., and Lindemann, M. D. (2004a) Estimation of endogenous phosphorus loss in growing-finishing pigs. Abstract 179 of the *Midwestern Section Meeting of the American Society of Animal Science*, Des Moines, IA, March 15-17, 2004. American Society of Animal Science, Savoy, IL.

Pettey, L. A., Cromwell, G. L., and Lindemann, M. D. (2004b)

Prediction of phosphorus requirements utilizing phosphorus accretion in whole empty body of growing-finishing pigs. Abstract 179 of the *Midwestern Section Meeting of the American Society of Animal Science*, Des Moines, IA, March 15-17, 2004. American Society of Animal Science, Savoy, IL.

Pettey, L. A., Cromwell, G. L., and Lindemann, M. D. (2004c) Estimation of Ca and P retention in bone, fat-free soft tissue, and other whole body and carcass components in growing-finishing pigs from 18 to 109 kg. *Journal of Animal Science* **82**(Suppl. 1): 254.

Ullrey, D. E. (2001) Scientific advances in animal nutrition. *Proceedings of a Symposium - Promise for a New Century*, December 9, Washington DC. pp. 7-12. National Academy Press, Washington DC.

Trace minerals: what text books don't tell you

G.G. Mateos, R. Lázaro, J.R. Astillero and M. Perez Serrano
Departamento de Producción Animal, Universidad Politécnica de Madrid

Introduction

Trace minerals are needed for efficient pig production but the requirements vary according to animal type, state of production and objectives. Furthermore, most of the research related to mineral requirements was carried out more than 30 years ago and may not apply to modern pigs. Until recently, trace minerals were added to diets to control nutritional deficiencies such as anaemia for iron (Fe), rough hair coat for zinc (Zn) and goiter for iodine (I). However, numerous researchers in the last two decades have demonstrated the positive effects of additional quantities of trace minerals on other aspects of animal production independent of classical signs of deficiencies. In this respect, supra-nutritional levels of Zn and selenium (Se) have been shown to improve immunity and resistance to disease, and chromium (Cr) and manganese (Mn) to increase carcass leanness. Furthermore, many piglet diets include pharmacological levels of copper (Cu) and Zn in order to reduce the incidence of digestive troubles and improve productive performance. Therefore, many trace minerals are currently included in the diet for purposes other than to meet traditional nutritional requirements and their recommended level of use are beyond ARC (1981), INRA (1989) or NRC (1998) recommendations.

In the last decade increased regulatory pressure has been imposed to minimise environmental contamination from animal production. The majority of trace minerals ingested by domestic animals (up to 99%) are not retained and appear in faeces and urine (Nys, 2001). Emission of trace minerals to the environment poses environmental pollution risks, specially for Cu and Zn, a problem that can be reduced by judicious inclusion of the mineral in the feed (Ferket *et al.*, 2002; Jondreville *et al.*, 2002; Revy *et al.*, 2003). The objectives of this review are to better understand the needs and use of trace minerals by pigs, as well as the potential interactions between minerals and other nutrients. This information will help to determine the composition of the trace mineral premix for pigs under practical production systems.

Trace minerals included in pigs diets

Fe, Cu, Zn, Mn, Se, and I are routinely included in trace mineral premixes for swine diets. Many premixes also include cobalt (Co) and occasionally Cr and molybdenum (Mo) are also added. The recommendations for trace mineral composition for piglets, growing pigs and lactating sows of different research institutions are shown in tables 1, 2, and 3, respectively, and the composition of premixes currently used in the Iberian peninsula for piglets, growing-finishing pigs and sows are shown in tables 4, 5 and 6, respectively. The data correspond to a total of 32 premixes, of which fourteen belong to premix manufacturers, ten to pig integrators and eight to private feed mills (approximately 55% of total pig production of the Iberian Peninsula). In general, the trace minerals had higher mineral contents than recommended by research institutions. The biggest differences are observed for Cu and Mn in sows and for Co and I in all type of pigs. A comparison between the composition of trace mineral premixes in 1986 (Mateos, 1987) and the beginning of 2004 (Mateos *et al.*, 2004) in the Iberian Peninsula is shown in table 7. In general, trace mineral content in pig diets has increased for Zn, and Se and has decreased for I and Co in the last two decades.

Table 1. Recommendations for trace mineral composition in mg/kg of diet for piglets

	INRA 1989	NRC 1998[1]	Hypor 1999	NSU 2000[1,2]	Rostagno 2000	KSU 2003[3]	BSAS 2003[5]	Mateos et al. 2004
Fe	100	100	80	90-150	100	150	120	90
Cu	10	6	10	6-15	10	15	6	8
Zn	100	100	70	90-150	100	+[4]	100	120
Mn	40	4	40	3-30	30	36	30	40
Se	0.3	0.30	0.30	0.3	0.3	0.27	0.2	0.3
I	0.6	0.14	0.50	0.15-0.5	1	0.27	0.2	0.6
Co	0.3	-	0.25	-	0.2	-	0.2	-

[1] 5 to 10 kg BW; [2] Nebraska and South Dakota State University; [3] Kansas State University; [4] 2700 ppm as Zn oxide; [5] 10 to 30 kg BW

Table 2. Recommendation for trace mineral composition in mg/kg of feed of premixes for growing pigs

	INRA 1989	KSU 1995[1]	NRC 1998[2]	Hypor 1999	Rostagno 2000	NSU 2000[1,3]	BSAS 2003[4]	Mateos et al. 2004
Fe	80	150	60	60	100	70-150	80	75
Cu	10	15	4	10	10	4-15	6	6
Zn	100	150	60	60	100	70-150	100	110
Mn	40	36	2	30	30	3-30	30	25
Se	0.1	0.09	0.15	0.2	0.3	0.3	0.2	0.3
I	0.2	0.27	0.14	0.50	1	0.15-0.5	0.2	0.4
Co	0.1	-	-	0.20	0.2	-	0.2	-

[1] Kansas State University; [2] 20 to 50 kg BW; [3] Nebraska and South Dakota State University; [4] 30 to 60 kg BW

	INRA 1989	KSU 1997[1]	NRC 1998	Hypor 1999	NSU 2000[2]	Rostagno 2000	BSAS 2003	Mateos et al. 2004
Fe	80	150	80	80	80-150	100	80	70
Cu	10	15	5	10	5-15	10	6	10
Zn	100	150	50	50	80-150	100	80	110
Mn	40	36	20	40	20-40	30	20	35
Se	0.1	0.27	0.15	0.2	0.3	0.3	0.25	0.3
I	0.6	0.27	0.14	0.75	0.15-0.5	1	0.2	0.7
Co	0.1	-	-	0.15	-	0.2	0.2	-

Table 3.
Recommendations for trace mineral in mg/kg of feed for lactating sows

[1] Kansas State University; [2] Nebraska and South Dakota State University

	Mean[1]	Mode[1]	CV,%[1]	NRC 1998	BSAS 2003
Fe	103	100	32.9	100	120
Cu	131[2]	150[2]	36.3	6	6
Zn	123	100	39.7	100	100
Mn	51	50	15.4	4	30
Se	0.20	0.20	38.2	0.30	0.20
I	0.97	1.00	48.1	0.14	0.20
Co	0.34	0.40	60.3	-	0.20

Table 4.
Composition of trace mineral premixes in mg/kg of feed for piglets in the Iberian Peninsula (Mateos et al., 2004)

[1] Iberian Peninsula; [2] As a growth promoter

	Mean[1]	Mode[1]	CV,%[1]	NRC 1998[2]	BSAS 2003[3]
Fe	94	80	35.4	60	80
Cu	99	90	46.7	4	6
Zn	109	110	29.6	60	100
Mn	46	50	18.3	2	30
Se	0.19	0.10	46.9	0.15	0.20
I	0.77	1.00	44.2	0.14	0.20
Co	0.27	0.40	61.5	-	0.20

Table 5.
Composition of trace mineral premixes in mg/kg of feed for growing-finishing pigs in the Iberian Peninsula (Mateos et al., 2004)

[1] Iberian Peninsula (Cu used as a growth promoter); [2] 20 to 50 kg; [3] 30 to 60 kg

	Mean[1]	Mode[1]	CV, %[1]	NRC 1998[1]	BSAS 2003[2]
Fe	82	100	27,1	80	80
Cu	16	10	63.6	5	6
Zn	105	100	21.2	50	80
Mn	55	50	25	20	20
Se	0.22	0.2	47	0.15	0.25
I	0.95	1	34.9	0.14	0.2
Co	0.41	0.5	60.9	-	0.2

Table 6.
Composition of trace mineral premixes in mg/kg of feed for sows in the Iberian Peninsula (Mateos et al., 2004)

[1] Iberian Peninsula; [2] Lactation diets

| | Piglets | | Growing-finishing | | Sows | |
	1986	2004	1986	2004	1986	2004
Fe	90	103	85	94	95	82
Cu	175	131	125	99	19	16
Zn	100	123	90	109	100	105
Mn	40	51	50	46	60	55
Se	0.18	0.20	0.16	0.19	0.19	0.22
I	1.3	0.97	1	0.77	0.90	0.95
Co	0.36	0.34	0.30	0.27	0.50	0.41
Vitamin E	15	44	10	17	12	32

[1] 12 sources for 1986 (Mateos, 1987) and 32 sources for 2004 (Mateos
et al., 2004)

Iron

Iron (Fe) is the most abundant trace element in the animal body
where approximately 60% is present as haemoglobin. Fe is required
for key biochemical functions such as DNA synthesis and O_2
transport and metabolism. The ease of oxidation and reduction of
Fe makes it a unique trace element for many cellular redox reactions.
Prolonged Fe deprivation is characterised by anaemia, loss of
appetite, lethargy, increased respiration rate and mortality. Fe
deficiency is the most common of the deficiency diseases in humans
worldwide. However, dietary Fe-supplementation has not improved
pig performance in many trials, indicating that supplies are generally
higher than requirements. For example, lactating animals are very
demanding of nutrients, but the extra need for Fe is limited because
of the low Fe content of milk. Plant materials used in pig rations
contain large amounts of Fe, although the concentration varies
according to plant species and type of soil and degree of soil
contamination. Cereal grains contain 30 to 60 ppm Fe, leguminous
seeds 60 to 100 ppm and oil-seed meals 200 to 400 ppm and even
more in the case of palm kernel meal (table 8). Also, animal
ingredients, except milk products, are good sources of Fe. Estimated
relative bioavailability of Fe in feeds with respect to iron sulfate for
pigs are not available, but in rats and chickens have ranged from
about 30 to 70% for forages, and somewhat higher for soybeans
and grains. Finally, calcium (Ca) and phosphorus (P) are routinely
added to pig diets as calcium carbonate and dicalcium phosphate
or monocalcium phosphate. The Fe content of these products range
from 600 to 800 ppm for the Ca source, and from 1,500 to 8,000
ppm for the P sources (NRC, 1998; Fedna, 2003; Mateos *et al.*,
2004). Ammerman *et al.* (1993) in a trial with chicks, found relative
bioavailabilities of Fe with respect to feed grade ferrous sulfate of
71% for dicalcium phosphate, and 50% for tricalcium phosphate.

Therefore, confined young pigs fed on milk diets or diets based on milk products might need more Fe supplementation than fattening pigs.

Table 8.
Iron content of selected ingredients (mg/kg)

	NRC 1998	INRA-AFZ 2002	CVB 2002	FEDNA 2003
Cereals				
Corn	29	32	29	35
Wheat	60	47	51	55
Barley	78	158	54	85
Leguminous and oil-seeds				
Peas	65	92	80	82
Lupins	54[1]	61[2,3]	52[2]	80[2]
Full fat soybean	80	143	230	100
Oil-seed meals				
Sunflower meal, 32 %	254	207	313	280
Soybean meal, 44 %	202	283	373	180
Palm kernel meal, 15%	–	534	611	480
Rapeseed meal, 34%	142	172	578	260
Animal proteins				
Fish meal, 66%	181[4]	351	359	300
Dried whey	130	10	4	1.5
Others				
Gluten feed	460	218	169	260
Wheat middlings	84	143	158	150
Manioc, 65% starch	18	15	635	280
Cane molasses	68	188	157	190
Alfalfa meal, 16%	333	312	712	300

[1] Lupin white (Lupinus albus)
[2] Lupin blue (Lupinus angustifolius)
[3] 24 ppm for Lupinus albus
[4] Herring meal

Neonatal pig tissues are Fe-deficient and many studies have been performed in which pregnant sows have been treated with exogenous Fe to improve reproductive performance. The results have been discouraging, especially when mineral, rather than organic sources of Fe were used (ARC, 1981). The reason is that Fe does not readily cross both the placental and mammary gland barriers, and consequently newborn piglets and sow's milk are very poor in this mineral. However, chelated Fe proteinates or amino acid-iron chelates given to sows during gestation and lactation at a dose of 60 mg/kg of diet increases the Fe content of the liver, and promotes haemoglobin formation and piglet growth (Ashmead, 1979). A possible explanation for this finding is that the piglets have access to sow faeces rich in Fe. Hence, not all the authors agree on the extra benefits of supplementing organic Fe to sow diets (Fox *et al.*, 1997).

A decreased resistance to infection with Fe deprivation has been described for rats and piglets. Iron-deficient pigs exhibit greater susceptibility to *Escherichia coli* endotoxins than healthy pigs (Osborne and Davis, 1968). However, Fe is essential for bacterial growth. An excess of iron intake increases the amount of Fe available in the gastrointestinal tract and the occurrence and severity of bacterial infections. Injection of Fe compounds reduces the survival rate of experimental animals infected with *Clostridium perfringens* or *Salmonella typhimurium* (Knight *et al.*, 1983). Therefore, large doses of Fe could stimulate bacterial growth and be detrimental to pig health. In practice, Fe contamination of water supplies (2 to 3 ppm) might contribute to maintain the persistency of *E. coli* infections. Therefore, when confronted with insidious *E. coli* problems, the level of Fe in the feed and it's concentration in the drinking water should be checked.

The importance of Fe in immunity was first recognised in the late 1960's and early 1970's and was associated with anaemia. More recently, numerous observations have found an association between Fe status and infection, and that some immune responses are altered by Fe deficiency (Kuvibidla and Surendra, 2002). Plasma Fe concentration changes during the acute phase response to immunological challenges and is reduced during inflammation, whereas the concentration of Cu is increased (Klasing, 1984). The reduction in Fe concentration during infection might be a defence mechanism to block Fe from uptake by certain bacterias.

Many trace mineral premixes for growing-finishing pigs of the Iberian Peninsula are high in Fe and do not consider the high content and relative good availability of the mineral sources and ingredients used in diets. There is evidence of a clear antagonism for absorption between Cu and Fe. Therefore, current European Union (EU-25) regulations that have reduced the level of Cu in feeds for finishing pigs will also decrease the need for additional Fe. Furthermore, body Fe, as a proportion of body weight (BW) decreases from 20 to 145 kg body weight (Mahan and Shields, 1998), indicating that Fe requirements decrease with age. Therefore, current inclusion levels of Fe for fatteners are not justified. The Fe content of selected ingredients used in pig diets is shown in table 8. The variation of Fe content observed is very high for gluten feed (169 ppm according to CVB, 2002 and 460 ppm according to NRC, 1998), soybean meal and full fat soybeans (202 and 80 ppm for NRC, 1998 and 373 and 230 ppm for CVB, 2002, respectively) and manioc (15 ppm according to INRA-AFZ, 2002 and 635 ppm according to CVB, 2002). For soy products, the differences found among sources might be due to the origin of the beans. In general, beans of South American origin (Brazil, especially) are higher in Fe content than beans of U.S. origin. For manioc, the variability in Fe content might be due to differences in soil contamination of the batches analysed.

Copper

Copper (Cu) is essential for proper bone growth and development and is required for numerous enzymes involved in Fe transport and metabolism, collagen formation, melanin production and integrity of the central nervous system. The concentrations of Cu needed to prevent physiological deficiencies are very low. In general, grasses contain less Cu than legumes, and grains more than leaves or stems. Cereal grains, legume seeds and milk products are poor sources of Cu (2 to 10 ppm), but oil-seed meals (15 to 30 ppm) are good sources (table 9). Furthermore, Cu of plant feedstuffs is only about 50% as available as that from animal ingredients, but Cu is up to ten times more available in cereal grains than in forages. Often overlooked, but of potential interest is the contribution that pipes can make to Cu intake from drinking water and equipment. Thus, a Cu deficiency is not frequent in animals reared under intensive production systems when fed 5 to 10 ppm extra Cu. Yet, British studies conducted in the 1960's estimated that Cu sulfate at 250 ppm improved daily gains by 8% and feed conversion by 5.5% in pigs compared to controls (Braude, 1980). Consequently, most pig producers throughout the world include pharmacological levels of Cu in the diet (125 to 250 ppm) to enhance health and growth (Barber et al., 1955, 1957; Davis et al., 2002).

The reasons for the effects of Cu on pig performance are not fully known, but Cu can contribute to intestinal health and growth by at least four different mechanisms: 1) acting as an antimicrobial agent; 2) improving nutrient digestibility; 3) improving immune function; and 4) protecting cells from free radical damage. Cu-stimulated growth is largely dependent on a simultaneous increase in feed intake that resembles the mode of action of in-feed growth promoters (Zhou et al., 1994a). High Cu levels are very efficacious in weanling pigs reared under poor management conditions, but the beneficial effects are very limited in healthy fattening pigs (Bradley et al., 1983). Intravenously injected Cu has been shown to stimulate pig growth (Zhou et al., 1994b), which suggests a systemic mode of action for Cu that could complement the more accepted antimicrobial hypothesis. The response of piglets and other monogastrics to pharmacological levels of Cu seems to be independent of the presence of antibiotics (Cromwell et al., 1998;

Trace minerals: what text books don't tell you

	NRC 1998	INRA-AFZ 2002	CVB 2002	FEDNA 2003
Cereals				
Corn	3	2	1	3
Wheat	7	5	3	6
Barley	7	9	4	7
Leguminous and oil-seeds				
Peas	9	7	7	8
Lupins (L. angustifolius)	6[1]	5[2]	5[2]	4[2]
Full fat soybean	16	34	12	17
Oil-seed meals				
Sunflower meal, 32 %	26	62	36	33
Soybean meal, 44 %	20	18	8	19
Palm kernel meal, 15%	-	21	23	28
Rapeseed meal, 34%	6	7	7	7
Animal proteins				
Fish meal, 66%	6	7	6	8
Dried whey	13	2	1	3
Others				
Gluten feed	48	5	5	8
Wheat middlings	10	17	10	13
Manioc, 65% starch	4	4	3	5
Cane molasses	17	29	6	19
Alfalfa meal, 16%	10	5	9	15

Table 9. Copper content of selected ingredients (mg/kg)

[1] Lupin white (Lupinus albus); [2] Lupin blue (Lupinus angustifolius)

Nys, 2001; Hill *et al.*, 2001) but it is lower or even absent in the presence of high levels of Zn in the diet (Hill *et al.*, 2000; Vieira and Shigueru, 2003). Data from Hill *et al.* (2000) indicate that both Cu at 250 ppm and Zn at 3,000 ppm reduce scours and improve piglet growth. However, a combination of Cu at 250 ppm as $CuSO_4$ and 3,000 ppm of Zn as ZnO does not improve piglet performance further (table 10). Cu as copper sulfate is used through water to control some fungal diseases, a practice that is more common in poultry than in swine production (Applegate *et al.*, 2004). Field studies have shown that high concentrations of Cu reduce (to variable degrees) the incidence of crop mycosis, and that Cu might also act similarly in the digestive tract of the pig. Furthermore, an additional benefit of high Cu diets is the improved odour characteristics of the faeces (Armstrong *et al.*, 2000) because of a better control of microbial populations in the pig intestine (McDowell, 2003). In addition, Dove (1995) observed that Cu supplementation to weanling pig diets improves the digestibility of animal fat from 75.6% to 85.1%.

	Diet				SEM
Zn, ppm	125	3125	125	3125	
Cu, ppm	12	12	262	262	
ADG, g/d[abc]	375	422	409	415	4.7
ADFI, g/d[ac]	637	690	671	681	7.9
Gain/feed, g/g[abc]	586	611	611	612	4.7

[1] From 22 to 50 d of age; [a] Main effect of Zn ($P < 0.01$); [b] Main effect of Cu ($P < 0.01$); [c] Zn x Cu interaction ($P < 0.01$)

Cu may protect body tissues from oxidative stress via two distinct pathways, one involving Fe metabolism and the other through the superoxide dismutase enzyme. The activity of catalase, an Fe-containing haem from the liver is reduced in situations of Cu deficiency. Elevated levels of ceruloplasmin, a Cu-containing enzyme, have been observed after infectious challenges with *Salmonella* spp, *E. coli* and other bacterias. Also, Cu through the superoxide dismutase, a Zn-, Mn- or Cu-dependent enzyme is involved in the phagocytosis system, and Cu metabolism affects neutrophils and macrophages. Therefore, adequate levels of Cu are essential to facilitate the response of the animal to immunological challenges. However, Kornegay et al. (1989) did not find any influence of 200 ppm Cu on the immune status of piglets.

Cu is a transition metal and as such is very effective in catalysing oxidation-reduction reactions. Ionised Cu favours oxidation of lipids and fat-soluble vitamins of the diet, which can have a negative impact on feed quality and palatability, ultimately reducing feed intake and performance. Vitamins are particularly susceptible to degradation in premixes during feed processing and storage. Supplementation of the diet with 250 ppm of Cu as copper sulfate increases the degradation rate of the tocopherol present in natural ingredients (Dove and Ewan, 1990), or added as acetate de-α-tocopherol (Dove and Ewan, 1991). In addition, finely ground Cu sulfate results in increased rates of fat oxidation in feed as compared to coarsely ground Cu sulfate (Miles et al., 1998). However, Cu in plasma is complexed to superoxide dismutase and ceruloplasmin, and protects polyunsaturated fatty acids found in cell membranes from harmful oxygen radicals. Therefore, the effects of Cu on oxidative reactions might be different dependent upon whether the Cu is free in the feed or organically bound inside the organism (Jondreville et al., 2002; Applegate et al., 2004).

High doses of Cu increase erosion to the lining of the gizzard (Poupolis and Jensen, 1976), inhibit the normal fermentation pattern in the caeca of the chick, and increase viscosity of faecal material and the stickness of the faeces in poultry (Leeson *et al.*, 1997). In addition, it has been observed that pharmacological levels of Cu reduce phosphorous retention in the chicken (Banks *et al.*, 2003), and accumulates in the liver and kidney. Jondreville *et al.* (2002) estimate that pigs fed diets containing 250 ppm of Cu during 100 to 150 d will increase Cu in liver tissue to levels of up to 400 to 500 ppm. Therefore, high levels of Cu in the diet may result in levels of Cu in pig meat and visceras above human needs (table 11). High levels of Cu may also affect the fatty acid profile of subcutaneous fat, increasing unsaturation of lard (Amer and Elliot, 1973). This observation might be important in the production of speciality pork meats such as Iberian and Parma ham where excessive unsaturation of the fat is undesirable. However, Bossi *et al.* (2000) did not find any influence of 175 ppm of Cu on fatty acid profile or meat quality in pigs destined to the Parma ham industry. The application of manure collected from pigs fed on diets containing pharmacological levels of Cu has serious environmental concerns; an excess of Cu results in undesirable effects on plant growth and will impair the activity of lagoon bacterias responsible for waste degradation.

Table 11.
Copper supply to human diets from pork products (adapted from Jondreville et al., 2002)

	Scenario	
	A	B
Cu in feed, ppm		
Piglets	30	175
Growing	15	175
Finishing	15	100
Daily supply from pork products, mg	1.5	3.6
Requirements for adults, mg/d	2-3	

The commercial premixes used in the Iberian Peninsula contain high levels of Cu for piglets and growing pigs up to 12 weeks of age (DOCE, 2003). Table 9 includes data from different sources concerning the Cu content of selected ingredients commonly used in pig diets. It is important to note that the wide range of values tabulated for gluten feed (5 ppm for INRA-AFZ, 2002 but 48 ppm for NRC, 1998), sunflower meal (26 ppm according to NRC, 1998 but 62 ppm according to INRA-AFZ, 2002) and soybean meal and full fat soybean (8 and 12 ppm for CVB, 2002 but 18 and 34 ppm for INRA-AFZ 2002, respectively). In some cases total Cu levels are close to legal EU-25 limits because the Cu content of the ingredients is not always determined in the laboratory by feed manufacturers (table 12). In this respect, it is of interest to analyse Mn and Zn sources for Cu content. Li *et al.* (2004) analysed twelve samples of organic Mn sources and found a Cu content that ranged from 20

G.G. Mateos et al.

ppm to 11,300 ppm. Also, Juarena and Danelon (2001) indicate that the average content of Cu in samples of ZnO for ruminants analysed in Argentina were close to 4%. Samples of ZnO analysed in Spain have shown a Cu content in the range of 200 to 700 ppm (Mateos et al., 2004).

Table 12.
Maximal levels of trace minerals in mg/kg allowed in pigs diets in the European Union-25 (DOCE, 2003, 2004)

Trace element	Before 2/2004	After 2/2004
Fe	1,250	750
Cu	35[1]	25[2]
Zn	250	150
Mn	250	150
Co	10	2
Se	0.5	0.5
I	10	10
Mo	2.5	2.5

[1,2]For piglets, has changed from 175 ppm up to 16 weeks of age to 170 up to 12 weeks of age. Values depend on age and European region considered

Zinc

The first clinical sign associated with a Zn deficiency, was growth retardation and abnormal hair coat in rats seventy years ago. In the 1950's Zn was recognised as an essential nutrient in pigs. Zn is critically involved in cell replication and in the development of cartilage and bone, and a deficiency results in severe growth retardation, dermatitis (parakeratosis), and impaired reproduction both in males and females. In addition, Zn is involved in the regulation of appetite, which may involve gene expression. In the absence of Zn, dietary carbohydrates are selectively rejected by the rat against proteins and fats (Kennedy et al., 1998). Zn requirements are quite high in piglets but decrease rapidly with age (table 13). However, Zn content of cereals and leguminous seeds is relatively low and between 20 to 30 ppm. In cereal grains the distribution of Zn is not homogenous, and the external components are richer than the internal parts. Consequently, cereal by-products such as wheat middlings and gluten feed are good sources of Zn (60 to 90 ppm). Finally, oil-seed meals (50 to 80 ppm) and animal proteins such as fishmeal are good sources of Zn, whereas sugars and oils are poor sources (table 14). Li et al. (2004) have found that the Zn content of twelve sources of organic Mn tested, varied from 82 ppm to 53,200 ppm. Analyses conducted in Spain (Romero; personal communication) have found a Zn content in selected dried whey samples of around 100 ppm. These

31

Table 13.
Requirements of
zinc by the pig
according to
plasma or bone
status (Revy et
al., 2003 and
NRC, 1998)[1]

BW kg	Estimated requirement	NRC 1998
6-15	80[2]	80-100
15-25	65[2]	60-80
25-50	50[2]	60
50-100	50[3]	50

[1] Total Zn supplied by ingredients and sulfate (mg/kg of diet); [2] Plasma status;
[3] Bone status

	NRC 1998	INRA-AFZ 2002	CVB 2002	FEDNA 2003
Cereals				
Corn	18	19	21	16
Wheat	28	27	22	23
Barley	25	30	23	27
Leguminous and oil-seeds				
Peas	23	32	31	30
Lupins	32[1]	31[2]	37[2]	30[2]
Full fat soybean	39	40	38	45
Oil-seed meals				
Sunflower meal, 32 %	66	69	100	75
Soybean meal, 44 %	50	47	50	51
Palm kernel meal, 15%	-	32	41	40
Rapeseed meal, 34%	69	65	62	65
Animal proteins				
Fish meal, 66%	132	85	83	83
Dried whey	10	20	18	25
Others				
Gluten feed	70	53	68	60
Wheat middlings	92	74	85	80
Manioc	10	15	8	11
Cane molasses	5	13	9	10
Alfalfa meal, 16%	24	19	22	21

Table 14.
Zinc content of
selected ingredients
(mg/kg)

[1] Lupin white (Lupinus albus); [2] Lupin blue (Lupinus angustifolius)

unexpected high values are probably due to contamination during milk and whey processing. Galvanised pipes might enrich the water supply with Zn, and in many instances prevent a deficiency in animals. Similar situations occur with sows because bars and cages are often rich sources of Zn. A Zn deficiency is more evident in high Ca, vegetable based diets, because Ca may induce the formation of a Zn-Ca-phytate complex in the upper gastrointestinal tract, as has been demonstrated by Davies and Olpin (1979) in the rat. Therefore, the use of exogenous phytase, and the reduction of the level of Ca in the diet might be beneficial for pig growth, especially with Zn deficient diets (Adeola et al., 1995; Ashida et al., 1999).

Recently, several researchers have found that Zn is involved in organic functions related to immunity and the development of phagocytic cells (Kidd et al., 1996), and that it also plays an essential role in gene expression and in mitosis of lymphoid cells (Prasad, 2002). Also, Zn participates in processes related to the production and regeneration of keratin, and has a direct effect on the integrity of the udder lining and the protection of the mammary gland. Therefore, even a mild deficiency of Zn impairs multiple mediators of host immunity, ranging from the physical barrier of the skin to acquired cellular and humoral immunity.

Feeding pharmacological levels of Zn to weanling pigs increases performance and reduces scouring due to E. coli. Early studies conducted in the 1990's demonstrated that 2,000 to 3,000 ppm of Zn either as zinc oxide (ZnO) or zinc sulfate improved performance in the early stages of life (Hahn and Baker, 1993). These results have been confirmed by many other reports (Hill et al., 2000; 2001) that also indicate that pharmacological levels of ZnO improved consistency, and altered the colour of the faeces. However, other studies have not found a consistent response to Zn supplementation on pig growth (Schell and Kornegay, 1996; Augspurger et al., 2004). In practical conditions, and in the absence of in-feed antibiotics, it is evident that ZnO at a dose of 2,500 ppm of Zn or higher, reduces the incidence of scours and improves consistency of faeces and piglet performance (Mateos, 2004). Therefore, ZnO is a potent and reliable growth-promoting agent in young pigs although it's beneficial effects disappear with age (Poulsen, 1995; Mavromichalis et al., 2000).

The Zn content of selected ingredients commonly used in swine diets is shown in table 14. The greatest differences among sources are observed for fishmeal (132 ppm for NRC, 1998 but 83 ppm for CVB, 2002). The trace mineral premixes marketed in the Iberian Peninsula have increased the level of Zn for piglets and fattening pigs by approximately 20% from 1986 to 2004 (table 7). On the bases of ingredient content and animal needs, it seems that the current Zn content of most Iberian premixes for swine (90 to 125 ppm) are appropriate.

Manganese

The nutritional importance of manganese (Mn) for pigs has been an area of active investigation. Mn is widely distributed in very low concentrations in body tissues, and is necessary for enzyme activity, bone growth, lipid and carbohydrate metabolism, and proper functioning of reproductive processes in both males and females. Seeds and seed products vary in Mn content depending upon the pH of the soil (lower content in the seed with increasing pH of the soil), but in general wheat and oats (30 to 45 ppm) are richer than maize (5 to 8 ppm). Mn concentrates in the outer layers of the grain, and wheat middlings are a very good source of Mn (100 to 130 ppm). The most striking difference in Mn content relates to lupin species; seeds of *Lupinus albus* analysed in Spain contain 925 to 1,026 ppm of Mn, or some 25 to 40 times more than other common lupin species such as *Lupinus angustifolius* growing on the same sites (Mateos *et al.*, 2004). The requirements of pigs (but not growing birds) for Mn are low. In fact, classical symptoms of deficiency are not observed in practical diets for fattening pigs even in the absence of exogenous sources. Pigs have been maintained on semipurified diets containing as little as 1.5 ppm from weaning to slaughter without any deficiency symptoms (Liebholz *et al.*, 1962). However, the Mn requirements for satisfactory reproduction are substantially higher than those needed for body growth.

Mn plays a role in immunological function, and an interaction of Mn with neutrophil and macrophage activity has been demonstrated. Severe Mn deprivation has been shown to impair immunity and central nervous system function (Underwood and Suttle, 2001). Additionally, Atherton (1993) has found that extra-supplementation of pig diets with Mn improves carcass leanness. Furthermore, Apple *et al.* (2004) observed that the inclusion of 320 to 350 ppm of an amino acid-Mn complex improved feed efficiency and meat quality in pigs. However, 700 ppm of the same complex did not elicit any response. Also, Kats *et al.* (1994) compared diets containing 24 or 88 ppm of Mn of either an inorganic or chelated source on growth performance and carcass characteristics of pigs. No beneficial effect of the extra-supplementation on growth performance, backfat thickness or longissimus muscle area were reported. Therefore, further research is needed in order to recommend this practice under commercial conditions.

The Mn concentration of most commercial Iberian trace mineral premixes has not changed much for the last two decades, and currently is higher than required. It is unlikely that supplementation at these rates are needed for piglets or growing-fattening pigs. The Mn content of selected ingredients according to different sources is offered in table 15. The greatest differences among sources are found for lupins, because of the different varieties included in the

study, for wheat 26 ppm for CVB, 2002 but 37 ppm for NRC, 1998)
and for fishmeal (8 ppm for NRC, 1998 but 18 ppm for CVB, 2002).

	NRC 1998	INRA-AFZ 2002	CVB 2002	FEDNA 2003
Cereals				
Corn	7	8	5	6
Wheat	37	34	26	30
Barley	18	16	16	15
Leguminous and oil-seeds				
Peas	23	9	16	11
Lupins	1,390 [1]	38 [2,3]	34 [2]	35 [2]
Full fat soybean	30	28	34	28
Oil-seed meals				
Sunflower meal, 32 %	41	48	56	45
Soybean meal, 44 %	29	38	50	35
Palm kernel meal, 15%	-	131	281	210
Rapeseed meal, 34%	49	52	47	49
Animal proteins				
Fish meal, 66%	8	13	18	8
Dried whey	3	3	0	1
Others				
Gluten feed	24	18	21	24
Wheat middlings	100	112	115	110
Manioc	28	26	26	26
Cane molasses	15	59	18	25
Alfalfa meal, 16%	32	49	38	40

Table 15. Manganese content of selected ingredients (mg/kg)

[1] Lupin white (Lupinus albus); [2] Lupin blue (Lupinus angustifolius); [3] 1,707 ppm for Lupinus albus

Selenium

Selenium (Se) is a constituent of selenoproteins and plays both
structural and enzymatic roles in pig nutrition. The history of Se as
a nutrient in animal diets has moved from prohibition as a toxic
element to recognition of the need of supplementation in the diet.
Originally, Se was recognised as a toxic mineral with carcinogenic
properties, and its utilisation in feeds was tightly controlled.
Paradoxically, it is now recognised that Se has powerful anti-cancer
properties. In the 1950's it becomes apparent that diets formulated
with corn and soybean meal cultivated in certain regions of the
world characterised for low pH soils needed additional Se for
optimal performance. In 1987, the Food and Drug Administration
(FDA) allowed an increase in permissible levels of Se in pig diets

from 0.1 to 0.3 ppm. However, in 1993 there was a case of high mortality in the waterfowl population of the Keterson Reservoir in the State of California that was attributed to Se contamination of the water, and the FDA reversed that decision to allow only 0.1 ppm. In 1994, 0.3 ppm was once more allowed. In the EU-25 the current maximum level authorised for pigs is 0.5 ppm (table 12). In the pig, both organic and inorganic Se sources are toxic when fed at 20 ppm or more (acute poisoning) or at 5 to 10 ppm for prolonged periods (chronic toxicity) (Kim and Mahan 2001 a; b; c).

While Se deficiency diseases have been recognised since 1954, evidence is mounting that less-overt deficiencies can cause adverse effects on animal health. Furthermore, it is believed that supra-nutritional levels of Se may give additional advantages protecting the animals from some diseases (Levander *et al.*, 1995). The immunomodulatory effects of Se occur through three principal mechanisms; 1) anti-inflammatory effects; 2) alteration of the redox state of the cell by acting as an antioxidant; and 3) generation of cytostatic and anticancer compounds (McKenzie *et al.*, 2002). Se intake is essential for both cell-mediated and humoral immunity and supra-nutritional levels may enhance the immune response and protect against certain viral infections conferring additional health benefits (Rayman, 2002; McKenzie *et al.*, 2002).

Beneficial effects of trace amounts of dietary Se were first observed in vitamin E-deficient rats and a strong metabolic interaction between these two micronutrients was apparent. Se and vitamin E tend to spare one another's requirement for the prevention of certain nutritional diseases such as liver necrosis and exudative diathesis, but the sparing effect is not found for other diseases (Levander *et al.*, 1995; Surai, 2003). Se is a key element in antioxidant defence and conditions associated with oxidative stress or inflammation, as occur at weaning, might be expected to be influenced by Se and vitamin E status. Many of the benefits of both micronutrients could be adequately explained by its antioxidant properties. Finally, it appears that certain forms of Se, such as Se-methionine are better adapted to avoid damage of tissues or to help in tissue repair than Se in the form of selenite (Surai, 2003).

Until recently it was considered that the main and almost unique role of Se was to be part of glutathione peroxidase (GSH-Px), an enzyme that maintains membrane integrity reducing the negative effects of peroxides. However, to date, more than fourteen mammalian selenoproteins have been characterised, some of them with enzymic-redox activity and others with structural and transport functions (Gladyser, 2001; McKenzie *et al.*, 2002). In fact, Se is the only trace mineral to be specified in the genetic code as Se-cysteine and it is now recognised as the 21st amino acid (Rayman, 2002). New nutritional functions of Se include the production and regulation of the level of active thyroid hormones from thyroxine and the stabilisation of proteins required for sperm maturation and fertility (Rayman, 2002). Se is incorporated into the developing spermatozoa of monogastric animals in much the same way as Zn. For spermatogenic development and boar semen quality the role of Se might be more important than the role of vitamin E (Marin-Guzman et al., 1997, 2000; Kolodziej and Jacyno, 2004). However, it is a common practice within the industry to heavily increase the levels of vitamin E of working boar diets whilst maintaining the Se levels constant.

There are certain difficulties in establishing Se bioavailability from feed ingredients, since different end points give different results. In fact, there is no universal criterion to assess Se bioavailability. Indeed, total Se content of a feed cannot be used as an indicator of its efficacy in animals. The bioavailability of Se sources of animal origin was believed to be low, at around 10 to 25%, while that in plant feedstuffs was around of 80% of that in sodium selenite. However, Henry and Ammerman (1995) indicate that in general Se in animal products is 60 to 90% as available as sodium selenite, while the Se in plant products averages 25% or less. Therefore, the bioavailability of Se in ingredients depends on the criterion used in the assessment with the greatest discrepancy occurring between sources containing Se as selenite or as Se-methionine. For example, most of the Se in grains and soybean meal is in the form of Se-methionine whereas in wheat straw it is in the form of selenate which is probably less active (Whanger, 2003). Se-methionine can be incorporated directly into body proteins and stored, thereby inflating bioavailability estimates based on body retention. On the other hand, Se reserves can be beneficial in stress conditions, Clearly, there is a need to improve our knowledge on the mode of action of different Se-containing compounds.

The average level of Se included in the premixes of the Iberian Peninsula for pigs are 0.20 ppm for piglets, 0.19 ppm for fatteners and 0.22 ppm for sows (tables 4, 5 and 6). These levels are only slightly higher than the levels used in 1986; 0.18, 0.16 and 0.19 ppm, respectively (table 7). However, the levels of vitamin E in the same period have increased from 15 ppm to 44 ppm for piglets, from 10 ppm to 17 ppm for fattening pigs and from 12 ppm to 32 ppm for sows. This information indicates that in general nutritionists have not taken into account in their formulation programs that Se and vitamin E might spare each other's requirement in many circumstances, and that to increase Se levels in the premix makes economic sense since this is cheaper than to add vitamin E.

However, an excess of Se leads to toxic effects and suppression of immunity and therefore, has to be avoided.

Iodine

Iodine (I) is required for the synthesis of thyroid hormones and the most obvious consequence of a deficiency is goiter, in which the thyroid gland enlarges as it tries to compensate for a lack of thyroid hormone production. In the pig, reproductive failure and weak, unusually larger, newborn piglets are the outstanding manifestations of I deficiency. The I content of animal feedstuffs is extremely variable. Plants grown in regions with I deficiency, such as lixiviated, granite soils in the inland of the continents are often deficient in I. Cereals and oil-seed meals are poor sources of I, whereas fishmeal is an excellent source. However, when iodised salt (3 g KI/kg) or marine salt is used as a source of Na, there is no need to use additional I.

Goiter might occur in pigs fed diets otherwise adequate in I content. Stability of the I-containing compounds is always a concern, especially when the mineral mixtures containing the I are stored under high moisture and heat conditions. Iodate form and sodium thiosulfate stabilises the mineral, reducing its vaporisation. Also, I deficiency can be associated with the presence of goitrogenic substances in the feed. Contamination with mustard seeds is quite frequent in rapeseed meal imported from developing countries such as India. Also, dried clover and other grasses might be rich in cyanogenetic compounds. In these cases, the control of the glucosinolate content of the meal and the extra-supplementation of the diet with I are good measures. Finally, a Se deficiency may produce goiter that cannot be reversed by I extra-supplementation (Underwood and Suttle, 2001).

The I content of the Iberian Peninsula premixes have been reduced over the last two decades, but still are higher than recommended by most research institutions. Therefore, I concentration could be reduced without jeopardising animal performance, particularly in growing-finishing pigs (table 5).

Chromium

For approximately 45 years chromium (Cr) has been considered by many nutritionists as an essential nutrient for humans and animals, but no need for exogenous supplementation was found. Cr is part of the glucose tolerance factor, which enhances sensitivity of tissues to insulin and facilitates glucose uptake and utilisation by cells. The biologically relevant form is the trivalent Cr^{3+} and is required for proper carbohydrate and lipid metabolism. Fortunately Cr deficiency is difficult to achieve and clinical symptoms have never been reported in intensive pig production. However, there is some evidence showing that additional dietary Cr might be beneficial for people undergoing physical or metabolic stress because stress and disease increase urinary excretion of Cr (NRC, 1997). In fact, in the last decade Cr has become popular as a nutritional supplement in urban populations to help humans to loose weight, and in athletes for muscle development. Among commercial mineral supplements for humans, products containing Cr are second in sales only to Ca-containing products (Nielsen, 1996).

In respect to pig production, several authors have shown that organic Cr at levels of 100 to 200 ppb of the diet improves nutrient digestibility (Kornegay et al., 1997), and increases muscling and decrease fatness in pigs (Page et al., 1993; Boleman et al., 1995; Southern 2001). In addition, other researchers have shown that organic Cr at levels of 200 ppb and beyond increases conception rate and number of pigs born alive (Lindeman et al., 1995; Lindeman et al., 2004) and might improve the immune status of stressed animals (Kegley and Spears, 1995). However, the beneficial effects of Cr are elusive and often are not observed in humans (Vincent, 2003, 2004), nor in pigs (Van Heugten and Spears, 1997; Savoini et al., 1998; Van de Ligt et al., 2002 a; b; c). In consequence of the variable response, the NRC (1998) does not make any recommendation on dietary Cr supplementation for swine. The NRC (1997) study found that when supplemental $CrCl_3$ or CrPicolinate was used, increases in carcass leanness were reported in 9 out of 24 experiments, and decreases in carcass fat in 11 out of 26 experiments. The NRC committee concludes that although the responses to supplemental Cr are inconsistent, Cr may favourably alter the metabolism of swine under some circumstances with resultant improvements in growth rate, carcass traits and reproductive performance. Thus, in practice it is recommended to carry out in-house studies on the potential benefits versus the cost of supplementation. Furthermore, the decision to use supplemental Cr in pig diets must be based on the confidence in the quality and characteristics of the Cr product used.

Cobalt

The only known function of Co is its participation in metabolism as a component of vitamin B_{12}. Evidence of Co deficiency distinct from vitamin B_{12} deficiency has never been described for the pig. Mammalian tissues lack the enzyme needed to incorporate Co as the prosthetic group of the vitamin, and only certain bacteria and algae have this capability. However, the capability of most monogastric species to synthesise vitamin B$_{12}$ in the lower portion of the intestinal tract is limited, and diets must supply Co in its active form. Therefore, the inclusion of Co in the trace mineral premix of the diet is only justified when the pig has free access to faeces as might occur in traditional pig production (free-range Iberian pigs). Consequently, the Co levels of most trace mineral premixes marketed in the Iberian Peninsula are not justified (tables 4 to 6).

Bioavailability of trace minerals

The term "bioavailability" is generally used to describe properties of absorption and utilisation of nutrients. Trace minerals either free or bound to low molecular weight ligands can be absorbed, and be present in body fluids and tissues, yet they might not be utilised. Determination of the concentration of trace minerals in feeds and animal tissues are usually performed with some accuracy through modern analytical techniques (table 16), but unfortunately such analyses do not provide information on mineral utilisation by animals (Ammerman *et al.*, 1995). Research has shown that the bioavailability of inorganic sources of minerals varies according to numerous factors including animal species, physiological state, previous nutrition, response criteria used, interactions among minerals and other nutrients, and chemical form and solubility of the source tested.

Table 16.
Permitted
analytical
variations (AV)
based on AAFCO
(1999) check
sample programs

Trace mineral	Method[1]	AV, %	Range
Fe	968.08	25	0.01-5%
Cu	968.08	25	0.03-1%
Zn	968.08	20	0.002-6%
Mn	968.08	30	0.01-17%
Se	969.06	25	ppm
I[2]	934.02	40	ppm
Co	968.08	25	0.01-0.16%

[1] AOAC (2000); [2] 935.14 and 925.56

Traditionally, trace mineral supplementation was achieved by the addition of simple inorganic salts such as chlorides, sulfates, carbonates and oxides. In general, chlorides and sulfates are considered to be more available than carbonates, with oxides having the lowest bioavailability. For example, pigs are more tolerant to pharmacological levels of Zn supplied as ZnO than from other sources such as ZnSO$_4$, indicating that Zn availability is lower for ZnO than for ZnSO$_4$ (Hahn and Baker, 1993). However, the range of bioavailability of ZnO sources is very high ranging from 41 to 97% with respect to the bioavailability of ZnSO$_4$ (table 17).

Table 17.
Bioavailability of
zinc of various
sources in chicks
(Edwards and
Baker, 1999)

Source	Supplemental Zn mg/kg[1]	Weight gain g	RBV[2] %
Control	0	104	-
$ZnSO_4 \cdot 7H_2O$	10.12	228	100[x]
ZnO (Source 1)	7.46	180	89[xy]
ZnO (Source 2)	7.75	187	97[x]
ZnO (Source 3)	8.23	139	41[z]
$ZnSO_4 \cdot H_2O$ (Source 1)	7.29	176	89[xy]
$ZnSO_4 \cdot H_2O$ (Source 2)	7.25	173	86[xy]
$ZnSO_4 \cdot H_2O$ (Source 3)	7.04	171	87[xy]
Zn metal dust	7.88	161	67[y]
Pooled SEM		6	8

[1] The basal diet contained 13.5 ppm of Zn; [2] Relative bioavailability of Zn with respect to $ZnSO_4 \cdot 7H_2O$; Different superscript letter in the same column means $P < 0.05$

Therefore, in some instances a ZnO source might be as bioavailable as a $ZnSO_4$ source. For Cu many reports indicate that cupric sulfate is the most available source of Cu for both domestic and laboratory animals. Cu as cupric oxide was absorbed to a lesser extent than that as cupric sulfate, and cupric carbonate was intermediate in response between the oxide and the sulfate forms. Cupric chloride has been shown to be more bioavailable than cupric sulfate in the chick (Miles and Henry, 1999). For Fe and Mn, a similar pattern for bioavailability of the different inorganic sources is observed (Baker and Halpin, 1987). Ferric iron as ferric oxide is very poorly utilised and considerable differences have been observed in Fe bioavailability in the form of ferrous carbonate. In spite of the lower bioavailability, oxides and carbonates are many times preferred to sulfates as a source of trace minerals because of the lower reactivity in the trace mineral premix. Also, ZnO is generally preferred to Zn sulfate when used at pharmacological levels to reduce the incidence of diarrhoea and to improve piglet performance (Kansas State University, 2003). Estimates of the bioavailability of inorganic trace mineral sources for pigs are shown in table 18 (NRC, 1998).

During recent years, many trials have found that using highly bioavailable sources of trace minerals has a positive effect on performance and health of pigs. Organic minerals can replace inorganic sources at a lower level while maintaining or even improving performance (Fremaut, 2003). Miles and Henry (1999) have listed the following perceived benefits for organic minerals as reported in the popular press:

- The ring structure protects the mineral from unwanted chemical reactions in the gastrointestinal tract.

Mineral element	Source	Formula	Content of element, %	RB, %[1]
Copper	Cupric acetate	$Cu(C_2H_3O_2)_2$	100	-
	Cupric carbonate	$CuCO_3 \cdot Cu(OH)_2$	50 to 55	60 to 100
	Cupric chloride[2]	$Cu_2(OH)_3Cl$	58	100
	Cupric oxide	CuO	75	0 to 10
	Cupric sulfate	$CuSO_4 \, 5H_2O$	25.2	100
Iodine	EEDI[3]	$NH_2CH_2CH_2NH_2 \cdot HI$	79.5	100
	Calcium iodate	$Ca(IO_3)_2$	64.0	100
	Potassium iodide	KI	68.8	100
Iron	Ferric Chloride	$FeCl_3 \cdot 6H_2O$	20.7	40 to 100
	Ferric oxide	Fe_2O_3	69.9	0
	Ferrous carbonate	$FeCO_3$	38	15 to 80
	Ferrous fumarate	$FeC_4H_2O_4$	32.5	95
	Ferrous oxide	FeO	77.8	Unkn.[4]
	Ferrous sulfate ($1H_2O$)	$FeSO_4 \cdot H_2O$	30	100
	Ferrous sulfate ($7H_2O$)	$FeSO_4 \cdot 7H_2O$	20	100
Manganese	Manganous dioxide	MnO_2	63.1	35 to 95
	Manganous carbonate	$MnCO_3$	46.4	30 to 100
	Manganous chloride	$MnCl_2 \cdot 4H_2O$	27.5	100
	Manganous oxide	MnO	60	70
	Manganous sulfate	$MnSO_4 \cdot H_2O$	29.5	100
Selenium	Sodium selenate	$Na_2 \, SeO_4 \cdot 10H_2O$	21.4	100
	Sodium selenite	Na_2SeO_3	45	100
Zinc	Zinc carbonate	$ZnCO_3$	56	100
	Zinc oxide	ZnO	72	50 to 80
	Zinc sulfate ($1H_2O$)	$ZnSO_4 \cdot H_2O$	35.5	100
	Zinc sulfate ($7H_2O$)	$ZnSO_4 \cdot 7H_2O$	22.3	100

Tabla 18.
Trace mineral sources and bioavailability for pigs (NRC, 1998)

[1] Relative bioavailability (values expressed in relation to the bioavailability in the most common source); [2] Tribasic; [3] Ethylenediamine dihydroiodiode; [4] Unknown but probably below 20%

- Chelates easily pass intact through the intestinal wall into the blood stream.

- Passive absorption is increased because of fewer interactions between the mineral and other nutrients.

- The mineral in a chelate is delivered in a form more similar to that found in the body.

- Chelates are absorbed by different routes than inorganic minerals.

- Each mineral in the chelate facilitates the absorption of other minerals in the chelate.

- Chelates carry a negative charge so they are absorbed and metabolised more efficiently.

- Chelation increases solubility and movement through cell membranes.

- Chelation increases passive absorption by increasing water and lipid solubility of the mineral.

- Chelation increases stability at low pH.

- Chelates can be absorbed by the amino acid transport system.

As the authors state, it remains to be seen how many of these perceived benefits will be validated experimentally.

There are many organically-bound compounds available on the market. All of them belong to one of these four categories: 1) metal amino acid chelate that is resultant from the reaction of a soluble metal salt with amino acids; 2) a metal amino acid complex which results from complexing a soluble metal salt with an amino acid(s); 3) a metal proteinate which is the product resulting from chelation of a soluble salt with partially hydrolysed protein; and 4) a metal polysaccharide complex which is the product resulting from the complexing of a soluble salt with a polysaccharide solution (AAFCO, 1997).

Hahn and Baker (1993) have found that plasma Zn concentrations in pigs fed $ZnSO_4$, Zn-lysine, or Zn-methionine were substantially higher than those in pigs fed ZnO. These results, that do not show any benefit of organic sources on productivity, have been corraborated by Wedekind et al. (1994a) and Revy et al. (2002; 2004). However, it has been suggested that poultry appear to benefit more from organic sources of minerals than swine (Wedekind et al., 1992; Cao et al., 2002). Spears (1989) indicated that in lambs more Zn was retained from Zn-methionine than from ZnO as a result of a lower urinary excretion of Zn. For Cu, the bioavailability of the organic sources has been evaluated using cupric sulfate as the standard (Baker et al., 1995). Baker and Ammerman (1995) reported that the bioavailability estimates of organic Cu sources ranged from 88% to 147% of the response to cupric sulfate in domestic species. In general, Cu-amino acids and Cu-proteinates show somewhat greater Cu absorption than cupric sulfate (Hahn and Baker, 1993). Coffey et al. (1994) and Zhou et al. (1994a) have found that growth performance was greater in pigs fed a Cu-lysine complex than in pigs fed $CuSO_4$. Also Eckhart et al. (1999) reported that Cu from a copper-proteinate source resulted in greater ceruloplasmin activity than Cu from copper sulfate.

The utilisation of Fe from organic sources including citrate, fumarate, and gluconate forms is essentially equal to that of ferrous sulphate heptahydrate. However, in pigs, Fe-proteinate and Fe-methionine are better utilised (Ammerman *et al.*, 1995). For example, in a farm trial, the addition of Fe-proteinate to a normal lactation diet fed seven days before farrowing and throughout a 26-day lactation improved sow feed intake, as well as weaning weight of the piglets (Close, 1999). The suggestion is that the organic Fe source crosses the placenta and is transferred into the foetuses with greater efficacy than inorganic Fe sources. Organic forms of Se such as Se-cystine, Se-methionine and properly produced seleno-yeast were about equal to sodium selenite on the basis of their ability to promote GSH-Px activity. However, when tissue deposition of body retention was used as the response, inflated relative bioavailability values were obtained (Mahan and Parret, 1996). Mahan (2004) has indicated that feeding organic Se from an enriched Se-yeast source to reproducing sows as compared with sodium selenite enhances the Se states of both the sow and the progeny because the organic Se form is more readily incorporated into colostrum and milk than the inorganic Se form. However, both products result in equivalent GSH-Px activities. Surai (2003) indicates that the transfer of organic Se from feed to the egg and embryonic tissues, and from feed to the foetus, colostrum or milk, is more efficient than the transfer of inorganic Se as selenite. The response is probably due to the metabolism and deposition of the Se as an integral part of the amino acid (Ammerman *et al.*, 1995). Kim and Mahan (2001) observed that both the organic (Se-enriched yeast) and inorganic (sodium selenite) sources were toxic for pigs when fed at 7 to 10 ppm (up to 20 times higher than EU legislation permits) for a prolonged period, but that organic Se affected more the reproductive performance, whereas inorganic Se was more detrimental during lactation suggesting metabolic differences in the utilisation of the Se contained in these two sources.

Many authors have not found any benefit regarding mineral availability or pig performance when replacing the inorganic source of Fe (Lewis *et al.*, 1995), Zn (Wedekind *et al.*, 1994a; Schell and Kornegay, 1996; Revy *et al.*, 2002), Cu (Baker and Ammerman, 1995) or Mn (Baker and Halpin, 1987; Scheideler, 1991) with different organic sources. Schell and Kornegay (1996) found that compared with the bioavailability of Zn in $ZnSO_4$, the bioavailability of Zn was lowest for ZnO and intermediate for Zn-lysine and Zn-methionine. Revy *et al.* (2002) reported that Zn sulfate and a Zn-methionine complex exhibited similar bioavailability in weanling pigs. Zn retained as measured by the balance technique was 27% of Zn intake, regardless of the Zn source tested. The reasons for the inconsistencies found in the literature are not known, but the technological processes used to obtain the commercial products might result in products with similar names (e.g. generic chelate), but containing variable concentrations of bioavailable minerals.

A summary of data on bioavailability of Cu sources is shown in table 19 (Jondreville et al., 2002). Similar data for Zn sources is shown in table 20 (Revy et al., 2003). There is a lack of a simple, standarised methodology for verification of the type and quality of commercial sources of organic minerals. Moreover, no industry methods are available to test the degree of chelation or bonding of a mineral element to an organic ligand or to relate the characteristics of the source to in vivo bioavailability. Recently, Li et al. (2004) have proposed a new method based on polarographic analysis that allows prediction of the relative bioavailability of organic Mn sources based on chemical characteristics with more accuracy than methods based on solubility. However, further work is needed in this respect. Therefore, caution is needed when evaluating sources of organic minerals available on the market.

Table 19. Bioavailability of copper sources in pigs (adapted from Jondreville et al., 2002)

Source	Growth	Feed to gain ratio	(Liver)	Number of studies
CuS	=	=	<	1
CuO	=	=	<	6
CuCO$_3$	=	>	=	2
Cu$_2$(OH)$_3$Cl	=	=	=	6
Chelate CuAA	=	=	=	2
Complex Cu-Lys	=>	=	=	11
Complex Cu-Met	=	=	=	2

Table 20. Bioavailability of zinc sources in pigs based on zinc plasma/serum values (adapted from Revy et al., 2003)

	Relative value	Number of studies
Zn sulfate	100	Control
Zn oxide	55-87	6
Chelate Zn-amino acids	100	1
Complex Zn-Met	77-120	5
Complex Zn-Lys	79-110	6

Interactions among trace minerals and between trace minerals and other nutrients

Hill and Matrone (1970) were the first to propose that elements with similar physical and chemical properties act antagonistically to each other in biological systems, and that the electronic configuration of the element can be used to predict possible interactions. The implication was that such metals could compete for binding sites on transport proteins or on enzymes requiring metals as co-factors. In this section we will describe briefly only those interactions that might have a significant impact in practical diets for pigs.

Chelating capacity of phytic acid and influence of calcium concentration

Phosphorus (P) is predominantly stored in mature seeds as myoinositol, a phytate complex. Phytin carries a strong negative charge, and has the ability to chelate di- and trivalent cations rendering the elements partially or totally unavailable to the pig. Thus, phytin not only reduces P availability, but also the availability of other mineral cations such as Ca, Co, Cu, Fe, Mg and Zn, and apparently, plant phytates have the highest binding affinity for Zn and Cu. It is well established from research in different species that phytic acid decreases the absorption of Zn, and that the inhibitory effect is more pronounced when Ca intake is high. The reason is the formation of insoluble Zn-Ca-phytate complexes in the lumen of the gastrointestinal tract (Lowe *et al.*, 2002). The solubility of the complex, and consequently the bioavailability of the mineral, depends on the pH, the molar ratio between Ca, phytate and Zn, and the presence of other minerals (Revy *et al.*, 2003). Therefore, phytase supplementation to the diet should improve the utilisation of Zn and Cu by the pig. In fact, Adeola *et al.* (1995) observed that apparent Zn retention in pigs was approximately 29% of Zn intake, regardless of dietary Zn level. However, when phytase was added to the diet, Zn retention increased to 43 and 48% of Zn intake for pigs fed diets containing 0 and 100 mg of supplemental Zn/kg of diet, respectively. The data indicate that phytase is effective in increasing Zn bioavailibility. Based on available information, Revy *et al.* (2003) estimate that 1,000 units of exogenous phytase per kg of feed is equivalent to the inclusion of 24 ppm of Zn as Zn sulfate in diets for 15 kg BW piglets.

Wedekind *et al.* (1992, 1994a) compared the bioavailability of Zn-methionine relative to that of zinc sulfate using a purified or a practical corn-soybean meal diet. The authors found that bioavailability estimates for Zn-methionine relative to Zn sulfate were 117 and 206%, respectively. The results clearly indicate that the higher phytate and fiber content of the commercial diet reduced the bioavailability of Zn from Zn sulfate but not from the organic form. Similarly, Wedekind *et al.* (1994b) reported that the bioavailability of zinc-methionine was 166% relative to zinc sulfate at a dietary Ca concentration of 0.60% and 292% at 0.74% Ca. On the other hand, Augspurger *et al.* (2004) demonstrated that pharmacological levels of Zn chelate the phytate complex, thereby decreasing the P releasing efficiency of phytase by 30%. Therefore, the Zn effect on the P-releasing efficacy of phytase could have significant implications in diets for early-post-weaned pigs. However, in this same report it was demonstrated that Cu (200 mg/ kg of diet) did not affect phytase efficacy.

Interaction among minerals

Mineral to mineral interactions can occur anywhere in the food chain but most of the important interactions take place in the gastrointestinal tract through several mechanisms including competition for mineral binding ligands and uptake, co-adaptation and influencing physiological variables (Fairweather-Tait, 1995). The mutual antagonism between Zn and Cu has been regarded as a prime example of competitive biological interactions between metals with similar chemical and physical properties. High Zn supply inhibits intestinal absorption, hepatic accumulation and placental transfer of Cu, as well as inducing clinical signs of Cu deficiency (Bremmer and Beattie, 1995). The reverse interaction, namely the effects of excess Cu on Zn metabolism are less clear, and there is not consistent evidence that an excess of Cu reduces Zn absorption. Bremmer and Beattie (1995) recommend supra-nutritional supplementation of Zn to reduce Cu accumulation in humans with high Cu intakes or those affected by genetic disturbances in Cu metabolism. However, care should be taken in the use of excess Zn when Cu status is suboptimal. In animal production, Zn supplements might help to alleviate toxicity in sheep fed high levels of Cu. Also the use of pharmacological levels of Zn in weaning diets might jeopardise the Cu status of the piglet.

High levels of Cu and Fe depress Zn absorption, and an excess of any of them tends to increase the requirement of the others (Fairweather-Tait, 1995). The presence of Cu and Fe in the chyme affect Zn absorption, but it is not clear whether both minerals actually interfere with the cellular uptake of Zn (competition for common transporters in the cell membrane or common cytosolic proteins involved in intracellular transport of Zn) or interact with Zn to form non-absorbable complexes within the lumen of the gut (Swinkels et al., 1994). In piglets, an excess of Cu in the diet reduces Fe reserves in the liver that may lead to anaemia. Therefore, when high levels of Cu are used in weaning diets, an excess of Fe (up to 250 ppm) in the feed is recommended (Bradley et al., 1983). Also, vitamins and minerals can interact with each other; a riboflavine deficiency impairs Fe absorption and increases the rate of gastrointestinal loss of endogenous Fe, which may increase the need for this trace mineral in recently weaned pigs (Powers, 1995).

An interesting interaction among minerals, particularly important in ruminants, is that of Cu, Mo and S (refer to MacKenzie's chapter in this publication). An excess of Mo reduces the retention of Cu in organs and the synthesis of ceruloplasmin. As a result, Cu excretion in urine increases. Additionally, incremental amounts of dietary S further exacerbate the primary interaction of Cu-Mo because of the formation of insoluble Cu-Mo-S complexes in the digestive tract. Therefore, in pigs fed pharmacological levels of Cu, or in sheep grazing pastures rich in Cu, it is convenient to include Mo and a source of additional S in the premix mixture. Also, in the presence of high concentrations of Mo in the diet, Cu in the chelated form would have an advantage over an inorganic form as it may escape the complexing that occurs in the digestive system among Mo, Cu and S.

Trace mineral nutrition and environmental contamination

Nutrient accumulation into ground and surface waters from livestock manure has generated environmental concerns. In current production conditions more than 95 to 99% of all trace minerals ingested appear in the faeces (Nys, 2001). The majority of the emphasis has been placed on nitrogen (N) and P pollution; however, many geographical regions are becoming sensitive to the build-up of Zn and Cu because of their use as therapeutical agents in pig production. Unlike excess land application of N and P, Zn and Cu remain bound to soil and do not migrate extensively to water supplies except during soil erosion (Ferket *et al.*, 2002). Therefore, unless they are removed via plant growth, accumulation will occur and eventually result in toxicity of crops. Williams *et al.* (1999) listed five basic strategies to reduce mineral burden from intensive animal production: 1) use wastes as fertiliser; 2) recycle wastes through animal feeds; 3) relocate wastes from production sites to nutrient deficient areas; 4) reduce the total amounts of the minerals in the feeds, minimising their concentration in the manure and 5) improve the efficiency of use of minerals by the animals. Clearly, the use of wastes as fertiliser and the reduction of trace mineral concentration in the feed are the best strategies.

An excess of Zn is toxic to plants, and when the Zn concentration in the soil is over 200 to 300 ppm, the activity of the soil microflora is reduced. The slurry produced by growing-finishing pigs fed diets with 100 and 250 ppm of Zn contains between 850 and 1,300 mg Zn/kg DM (Levasseur and Texier, 2001; Revy *et al.*, 2003). Paboeuf *et al.* (2001) found that a reduction of the Zn content of feeds from 150 ppm to 90 ppm reduced the content of Zn in faeces by 40%. Also, Revy *et al.* (2003) indicated that a reduction in the Zn content of piglet diets from 3,000 to 150 ppm, and of fattener diets from

100 to 60 ppm will reduce the concentration of Zn in the slurry from 1,860 to 450 mg/kg DM (table 21). Similarly, a study by Jondreville et al. (2002) demonstrated that a reduction of the Cu content from 175 ppm to 6 ppm in piglet feeds, and from 100 ppm to 4 ppm in fattener feeds will reduce the Cu content in the slurry from 911 to 31 mg/kg DM (table 22). In chickens, Dozier et al. (2003) have found that decreasing the Zn concentration in the diet from 120 to 40 mg/kg reduced Zn excretion by 50%, and that decreasing supplemental Cu from 12 to 4 mg reduced Cu excretion by 35%. These works clearly show the need to reduce the trace mineral content of current diets in order to decrease environment contamination. The trend towards reducing the trace mineral content of pig diets is expected to continue in the EU-25 (DOCE, 2003), a decision that might favour the use of phytases and organic sources of trace minerals.

Table 21. Estimation of soil contamination by zinc from pig slurry (adapted from Revy et al., 2003)

	Scenario		
	A	B	C
Zn in feed, ppm			
Piglets	100	2,000	3,000
Fatteners	60	100	150
Zn excreted			
g Zn/pig	14	36	60
mg Zn/kg DM slurry	450	1,120	1,860
Time needed to reach 300 mg Zn/kg DM of soil[1]			
Min, years	270	110	55
Max, years	1,100	390	190

[1] According to slurry processing practices

Conclusions

The information available concerning the requirements and bioavailability of commercial sources of trace minerals for pigs is scarce and incomplete. Not a single recommendation for trace mineral composition can be given because it will not fit all circumstances. In practical conditions it is a wise decision to recommend a range of supplementation levels, rather than a single value for each mineral. The lower values in the recommended range are better adapted for pig integrators with good control of the production chain and quick access to farms and to marketing needs. In this case, a good insurance in the form of an excess of minerals at a high cost is not always the best solution. Alternatively, the higher values in the recommended range might be more convenient for feeds destined to parent stock, or high producing pigs and farms under stress or poorly controlled conditions. Under these circumstances, a good insurance (extra-supplementation with trace minerals beyond research institution recommendations) might be a wise decision. The use of phytases and organic sources of trace elements is increasing, and might help to improve performance and reduce environmental contamination. However, further research is needed to evaluate their value for swine. In the meantime, special care is needed for better evaluation of organic sources of trace minerals available in the market.

Table 22. Estimation of soil contamination by copper from pig slurry (adapted from Jondreville *et al.*, 2002)

	Scenario		
	A	*B*	*C*
Cu in feed, ppm			
Piglets	6	175	175
Fatteners	4	35	100
Cu excreted			
g Cu/pig	1	14	29
mg Cu/kg DM slurry	31	443	911
Time needed to reach 100 mg Cu/kg DM of soil[1]			
Min, years	647	83	16
Max, years	16,024	289	56

[1] According to slurry processing practices

References

AAFCO. (1997). Official Publication. *Association of American Feed Control Officials.* Inc. St. Louis. MO.

AAFCO. (1999). Official Publication. *Association of American Feed Control Officials.* Inc. St. Louis. MO. pp 165 - 167.

Adeola, O., Lawrence, B.V., Sutton, A.L., and Cline, T.R. (1995). Phytase-induced changes in mineral utilization in zinc-supplemented diets for pigs. *Journal of Animal Science* **73:** 3384 - 3391.

Amer, M.A., and Elliot, J.I. (1973). Effects of level of copper supplement and removal of supplemental copper from the diet on the physical and chemical characteristics of porcine depot fat. *Canadian Journal of Animal Science* **53:** 139 - 145.

Ammerman, C.B., Henry, P.R., and Miles, R.D. (1993). Feed phosphates serve as source of iron for chicks. *Feedstuffs:* May 3; 14 - 21.

Ammerman, C.B., Baker, D.H., and Lewis, A.J. (1995). Bioavailability of Nutrients for Animals. Amino Acids, Minerals, and Vitamins. Academic Press, New York, USA.

AOAC. (2000). Official Methods of Analysis (17th ed.). AOAC, Gaithersburg, MD.

ARC. (1981). *The Nutrient Requirements of Pigs.* CAB. Farnham Royal. United Kingdom.

Apple, J.K., Roberts, W.J., Maxwell, C.V., Boger, C.B., Fakler, T.M., Friesen, K.G., and Johnson, Z.B. (2004). Effect of supplemental manganese on performance and carcass characteristics of growing-finishing pigs. *Journal of Animal Science* **82:** 3267 - 3276.

Applegate, T.J., Banks, K.M., and Pang, Y. (2004). Copper in Poultry Diets: Benefits and consequences. *Proceedings California Animal Nutrition Conference* Fresno, California. pp 246 - 252.

Armstrong, T.A., Williams, C.M., Spears, J.W., and Schiffman, S.S. (2000). High dietary copper improves odor characteristics of swine waste. *Journal of Animal Science* **78:** 859 - 864.

Ashida, K.Y., Tamura, A., Matsui, T., Yano, H., and Nakajima, T. (1999). Effect of dietary microbial phytase on zinc bioavailability in growing pigs. *Journal of Animal Science* **70:** 306 - 311.

Ashmead, D. (1979). The influence of chelated iron proteinate fed to sows with no iron supplementation to their baby pigs. *Journal of Animal Science* **49** (Supp. 1)**:** 235 (Abst.)

Atherton, D. (1993). A nutritional approach to maximizing carcass leanness. In: *The roles of amino acid chelates in animal nutrition.* (H.J.D. Ashmead (ed)). Thomas and Joseph Limited, Norwich, England.

Augspurger, N.R., Spencer, J.D., Webel, D.M., and Baker, D.H. (2004). Pharmacological zinc levels reduce the phosphorus-releasing efficacy of phytase in young pigs and chickens. *Journal of Animal Science* **82:** 1732 - 1739.

Baker, D.H., and Ammerman, C.B. (1995). Copper availability. In: *Bioavailability of Nutrients for Animals. Amino Acids, Minerals, and Vitamins.* C.B. Ammerman, D.H. Baker, and A.J. Lewis (eds). Academic Press. New York, U.S.A. pp 127 - 156.

Baker, D.H., and Halpin, K.M. (1987). Research note: Efficacy of a manganese-protein chelate compared with that of manganese sulfate for chicks. *Poultry Science* **66:** 1561 - 1563.

Banks, K.M., Thompson, K.L., Rush, J.K., and Applegate, T.J. (2003). The effects of copper source on performance and phosphorus retention in broiler chicks. *Poultry Science* **92** (Supp. 1)**:** 36 (Abst.).

Barber, R.S., Braude, R., and Mitchell, K.E. (1955). Antibiotic and copper supplements for fattening pigs. *British Journal of Nutrition* **9:** 378 - 381.

Barber, R.S., Braude, R., Mitchell, K.E., Rook, J.A.F., and Rowell, J.G. (1957). Further studies on antibiotic and copper supplements for fattening pigs. *British Journal of Nutrition* **11:** 70 - 79.

Boleman, S.L., Boleman, S.J., Bidner, T. D., Southern, L.L., Ward, T.L., Pontif, J.E., and Pike, M.M. (1995). Effect of chromium picolinate on growth, body composition, and tissue accretion in pigs. *Journal of Animal Science* **73:** 2033 - 2042.

Bossi, P., Cacciavillani, J.A., Casini, L., Fiego, D.P.L., Marchetti, M., and Mattuzzi, S. (2000). Effects of dietary high-oleic acid sunflower oil, copper and vitamin E levels on the fatty acid composition and the quality of dry cured Parma ham. *Meat Science* **54:** 119 - 126.

Bradley B.D, Graber, G., Condon, R.J., and Frobish, L.T. (1983). Effects of graded levels of dietary copper on copper and iron concentrations in swine tissues. *Journal of Animal Science* **56:** 625 - 630.

Braude, R. (1980). Twenty five years of widespread use of copper as an additive to diets of growing pigs. In: *Copper in animal wastes and sewage sludge.* P. L'Hermite, and J. Dehandtschutter (eds). Proceedings EEC Workshop, INRA Publisher. Bordeaux, France. pp 3 - 15.

Bremner, I., and Beattie, J.H. (1995). Copper and zinc metabolism in health and disease: speciation and interactions. *Proceedings of the Nutrition Society* **54:** 489 - 499.

BSAS. (2003). *Nutrient Requirement Standards for Pigs.* British Society of Animal Science. Penicuik, United Kingdom.

Cao, J., Henry, P.R., Davis, P.R., Cousins, R.J., Miles, R.D., Littell, R.C., and Ammerman, C.B. (2002). Relative bioavailability of organic zinc sources based on tissue and metallothionein in chicks fed conventional dietatary zinc concentrations. *Animal Feed Science and Technology* **101:** 161 - 170.

Close, W.H. (1999). Organic minerals for pigs: an update. In: *Nutritional Biotechnology in the Feed Industry.* T.P. Lyons. and K.A. Jacques (eds). Alltech 15th Annual Symposium. Nottingham University Press. Nottingham. U.K. pp 51 - 60.

Coffey, R.D., Cromwell, G.L., and Monegue, H.J. (1994). Efficacy of a copper-Lysine complex as a growth promotant for weanling pigs. *Journal of Animal Science* **72:** 2880 - 2886.

Cromwell, G.L., Lindemann, M.D., Monegue, H.J., Hall, D.D., and Orr, D.E. (1998). Tribasic copper chloride and copper sulfate as copper sources for weanling pig. *Journal of Animal Science* **76:** 118 - 123.

CVB. (2002). Veevoedertabel. Chemische samenstelling, verteerbaarheid en voederwaarde van voedermiddelen. Centraal Veevoederbureau. Lelystad. The Netherlands.

Davies, N.T., and Olpin, S.E. (1979). Studies on the phytate : zinc molar contents in diets as a determinant of Zn availability to young rats. *British Journal of Nutrition* **41:** 590 - 603.

Davis, M.E., Maxwell, C.V., Brown, D.C., de Rodas, B.Z., Johnson, Z.B., Kegley, E.B., Hellwig, D.H., and Dvorak, R.A. (2002). Effect of dietary mannan oligosaccharides and (or) pharmacological additions of copper sulfate on growth performance and immunocompetence of weanling and growing/finishing pigs. *Journal of Animal Science* **80:** 2887 - 2894.

DOCE. (2003). Reglamento (CE) N° 1334/2003 de la comisión por la que se modifican las condiciones para la autorización de una serie de aditivos en la alimentación animal pertenecientes al grupo de los oligoelementos. B.O.E., Madrid.

DOCE. (2004). Reglamento 2004/C 50/01 de la comisión. Listado de los aditivos autorizados en los piensos. Publicada conforme a lo dispuesto en la letra b) del artículo 9 unvicies de la Directiva 70/524/CEE del Consejo sobre aditivos en la alimentación animal. B.O.E., Madrid.

Dove, C.R. (1995). The effect of copper level on nutrient utilization of weanling pigs. *Journal of Animal Science* **73:** 166 - 171.

Dove, C.R., and Ewan, R.C. (1990). Effect of excess dietary copper, iron, or zinc on the tocopherol and selenium status of growing pigs. *Journal of Animal Science* **68:** 2407 - 2413.

Dove, C.R., and Ewan, R.C. (1991). Effect of trace minerals on the stability of vitamin E in swine grower diets. *Journal of Animal Science* **69:** 1994 - 2000.

Dozier, W.A., Davis, A.J., Freeman, M.E., and Ward, T.L. (2003). Early growth and environmental implications of dietary zinc and copper concentrations and sources of broiler chicks. *British Poultry Science* **44:** 726 - 731.

Eckhart, G.E., Greene, L.W., Carstens, G.E., and Ramsey, W.S. (1999). Copper status of ewes fed increasing amounts of copper from copper sulfate or copper proteinate. *Journal of Animal Science* **77:** 244 - 249.

Edwards, H.M., and Baker, D.H. (1999). Bioavailability of zinc in several sources of zinc oxide, zinc sulfate, and zinc metal. *Journal of Animal Science* **77:** 2730 - 2735.

Fairweather-Tait, S.J. (1995). Iron-zinc and calcium-Fe interactions in relation to Zn and Fe absorption. *Proceedings of the Nutrition Society* **54:** 465 - 473.

FEDNA. (2003). Tablas de composición y valor nutritivo de alimentos para la fabricación de piensos compuestos (2nd ed). C. De Blas, G.G. Mateos, and P.G. Rebollar. (eds). Fundación Española para el Desarrollo de la Nutrición Animal, Madrid.

Ferket, P.R., Van Heugten, E., van Kempen, T.A.T.G., and Angel, R. (2002). Nutritional strategies to reduce environmental emissions from nonruminants. *Journal of Animal Science* **80** (E. Suppl. 2): E168 - 182.

Fox, T.E., Eagles, J., and Fairweather-Tait, S.J. (1997). Bioavailabilty of an iron glycine chelate for use as a food fortificant compared with ferrous sulphate. In: *Trace Elements in Man and Animals* 9. Proceedings of the Ninth International Symposium. P.W.F. Fisher, M.R. L'Abbé, K.A. Cockell, and R.S. Gibson (eds). NRC

Research Press, Ottawa. pp. 460-462.

Fremaut, D. (2003). Trace mineral proteinates in modern pig production: reducing mineral excretion without sacrificing performance. In: *Nutritional Biotechnology in the Feed and Food Industries*. Lyons. T.P., and K.A. Jacques (eds). Alltech 19th Annual Symposium. Nottingham University Press. Nottingham. U.K. pp 171 - 178.

Gladyser, V.N. (2001). Identity, evolution and function af selenoproteins and selenoprotein genes. In: *Selenium: Its Molecular Biology and Role in Human Health*. D.L. Hatfield (ed). Kluwer Academic Publishers. Dordrecht, The Netherlands. pp. 99 - 104.

Hahn, J.D., and Baker, D.H. (1993). Growth and plasma zinc responses of young pigs fed pharmacological levels of zinc. *Journal of Animal Science* **71:** 3020 - 3024.

Henry, P.R., and Ammerman, C.B. (1995). Selenium availability. In: *Bioavailability of Nutrients for Animals*. C.B. Ammerman, D.H. Baker, and A.J. Lewis (eds). Academic Press, New York. pp 303 - 348.

Hill, C.H., and Matrone, G. (1970). Chemical parameters in the study of *in vivo* and *in vitro* interactions of transition elements. *Federation Proceedings* **29:** 1474 - 1481.

Hill, M.G., Mahan, D.C., Carter, S.D., Cromwell, G.L., Ewan, R.C., Harrold, R.L., Lewis, A.J., Miller, P.S., Shurson, G.C., and Veum, T.L. (2001). Effect of pharmacological concentrations of zinc oxide with or without the inclusion of an antibacterial agent on nursery pig performance. *Journal of Animal Science* **79:** 934 - 941.

Hill, M.G., Cromwell, G.L., Crenshaw, T.D., Dove, C.R., Ewan, R.C., Knabe, D.A., Lewis, A.J., Libal, G.W., Mahan, D.C., Shurson, G.C., Shurson, G.C., Southern, L.L., and Veum, T.L. (2000). Growth promotion effects and plasma changes from feeding high dietary concentrations of zinc and copper to weanling pigs (regional study). *Journal of Animal Science* **78:** 1010 - 1016.

INRA-AFZ. (2002). Tables de composition et de valeur nutritive des matières premières destinèes aux animaux d'élevage: Porcs, volailles, bovins, ovins, caprins, lapins, chevaux and poissons. D. Sauvant, J.M. Perez, and G. Tran (eds). INRA, Paris, France.

INRA. (1989). L´alimentation des animaux monogastriques: Porc, lapin, volailles (2ª ed). INRA, Paris, France.

Jondreville, C., Revy, P.S., Jaffrezic, A., and Dourmad, J.Y. (2002). Le cuivre dans l´alimentation du porc: oligoélément essential, facteur de croissance et risqué potential pour l´homme et l´environnement. *INRA Productions Animales* **15:** 247 - 265.

Juarena, G., and Danelon, J. (2001). Tablas de composición de alimentos para rumiantes de la región Pampeana Argentina. Hemisferio Sur, S.A. Buenos Aires, Argentina.

Kansas State University. (1995). *Swine Nutrition Guide*. Cooperative Extension Service. Manhattan, Kansas, U.S.A.

Kansas State University. (1997). *Swine Nutrition Guide*. Cooperative Extension Service. Manhattan, Kansas, U.S.A.

Kansas State University. (2003). *Starter pig and breeding herd recommendations*. Cooperative Extension Service. Manhattan, Kansas, U.S.A.

Kats, L.J., Nelssen, J.L., Goodband, R.D., Tokach, M.D., Friesen, K.G., Owen, K.Q., and Richert, B.T. (1994). Effect of manganese level and source on growth performance and carcass characteristics of finishing pigs. *Journal of Animal Science* **72** (Suppl. 1): 217(Abst.).

Kegley, E.B., and Spears, J.W. (1995). Immune response, glucose metabolism, and performance of stressed feeder calves fed inorganic or organic chromium. *Journal of Animal Science* **73:** 2721 - 2726.

Kennedy, K.J., Rains, T.M., and Shay, N.F. (1998). Zinc deficiency changes preferred macronutrient intake in subpopulations of Sprague-Dewley outbred rats and reduces hepatic pyruvate kinase gene expression. *Journal of Nutrition* **128:** 43 - 49.

Klasing, K. (1984). Effect of inflammatory agents and interleukin 1 on iron and zinc metabolism. *American Journal of Physiology* **247:** R901 - R904.

Kidd, M.T., Ferket, P.R., and Qureshi, M.A. (1996). Zinc metabolism with special reference to its role in immunity. *World's Poultry Science Journal* **52:** 309 - 324.

Kim, Y.Y., and Mahan, D.C. (2001a). Effect of dietary selenium source, level and pig hair color on various selenium indices. *Journal of Animal Science* **79:** 949 - 955.

Kim, Y.Y., and Mahan, D.C. (2001b). Prolonged feeding of high dietary levels of organic and inorganic selenium to gilts from 25 kg to body weight through one parity. *Journal of Animal Science* **79:** 956 - 966.

Kim, Y.Y., and Mahan, D.C. (2001c). Comparative effects of dietary levels of organic and inorganic selenium on selenium toxicity of growing-finishing pigs. *Journal of Animal Science* **79:** 942 - 948.

Knight, C.D., Klasing, K.C., and Forsyth, D.M. (1983). *E. Coli* growth in serum of iron dextran-supplemented pigs. *Journal of Animal Science* **57:** 387 - 395.

Kolodziej, A., and Jacyno, E. (2004). Effect of dietary selenium and vitamin E supplementation in reproductive performance of young boars. *Electronic Journal of Polish Agricultural Universities* **7:** 102 - 107.

Kornegay, E.T., Heugten, P.H.G., Lindemann, M.D., and Blodgett, D.J. (1989). Effects of biotin and high copper levels on performance and immune response of weanling pigs. *Journal of Animal Science* **67**: 1471 - 1477.

Kornegay, E.T., Wang, Z., Wood, C.M., and Lindemann, M.D. (1997). Supplemental chromium picolinate influences nitrogen balance, dry matter digestibility, and carcass traits in growing-finishing pigs. *Journal of Animal Science* **75**: 1319 - 1323.

Kuvibidla, S., and Surendra, B. (2002). Role of iron in immunity and infection. In: *Nutrition and Immune Function*. P.C. Calder, C.J. Field and H.S. Gill, (eds). CABI Publishing. Wallingford. United Kingdom. pp. 209 - 228.

Leeson, S., Zubair, A.K., Squires, E.J., and Forsberg, C. (1997). Influence of dietary levels of fat, fiber and copper sulfate and fat rancidity on cecal activity in the growing turkey. *Poultry Science* **76**: 59 - 66.

Levander, O.A., Ager Jr, A.L., and Beck, M.A. (1995). Vitamin E and selenium: contrasting and interacting nutritional determinants of host resistance to parasitic and viral infections. *Proceedings of the Nutrition Society* **54**: 475 - 487.

Levasseur P., and Texier, C. (2001). Teneurs en éléments trace métalliques des aliments et des lisiers de porcs à l'engrais, de truies et de porcelets. *Journées Rech. Porcine en France* **33**: 57 - 62.

Lewis, A.J., Miller, P.S., and Wolverton, C. K. (1995). Bioavailability of iron in iron methionine for weanling pigs. *Journal of Animal Science* **73** (Suppl. 1): 172 (Abstr.).

Li, S., Luo, X., Liu, B., Crenshaw, T.D., Kuang, X., Shao, G., and Yu, S. (2004). Use of chemical characteristics to predict the relative bioavailability of supplemental organic manganese sources for broilers. *Journal of Animal Science* **82**: 2352 - 2363.

Liebholz, J.M., Speer, V.C., and Hays, V.W. (1962). Effect of dietary manganese on baby pig performance and tissue manganese levels. *Journal of Animal Science* **21**: 772 - 776.

Lindemann, M.D., Wood, C.M., Harper, A.F., Kornegay, E.T., and Anderson, R.A. (1995). Dietary chromium picolinate additions improve gain:feed and carcass characteristics in growing-finishing pigs and increase litter size in reproducing sows. *Journal of Animal Science* **73**: 457 - 465.

Lindemann, M.D., Carter, S.D., Chiba, L.I., Dove, C.R., LeMieux, F.M., and Southern, L.L. (2004). A regional evaluation of chromium tripicolinate supplementation of diets fed to reproducing sows. *Journal of Animal Science* **82**: 2972 - 2977.

Lowe, N.M., Fraser, W.D., and Jackson, M.J. (2002). Is there a potential therapeutic value of copper and zinc for osteoporosis? *Proceedings of the Nutrition Society* **61**: 181 - 185.

Mahan, D.C., and Parrett, N.A. (1996). Evaluating the efficacy of selenium-enriched yeast and sodium selenite on tissue selenium retention and serum glutathione peroxidase activity in grower and finisher swine. *Journal of Animal Science* **74:** 2967 - 2974.

Mahan, D.C., and Shields, R.G. (1998). Macro- and micromineral composition of pigs from birth to 145 kilograms of body weight. *Journal of Animal Science* **76:** 506 - 512.

Mahan, D. (2004). The role of selenium and Sel-Plex® in sow reproduction. In: *Nutritional Biotechnology in the Feed and Food Industries.* T.P. Lyons. and K.A. Jacques (eds). Alltech 20th Annual Symposium. Nottingham University Press. Nottingham. U.K. pp 131-139.

Marin-Guzman, J., Mahan, D.C., Chung, Y.K., Pate, J.L., and Pope, W.F. (1997). Effects of dietary selenium and vitamin E on boar performance and tissue responses, semen quality, and subsequent fertilization rates in mature gilts. *Journal of Animal Science* **75:** 2994 – 3003.

Marin-Guzman, J., Mahan, D.C., and Pate, J.L. (2000). Effect of dietary selenium and vitamin E on spermatogenic development in boars. *Journal of Animal Science* **78:** 1537-1543.

Mateos, G.G., García Valencia, D., and Jiménez Moreno, E. (2004). Microminerals in diets for monogastrics: technical and legal aspects (in Spanish). Cursos de especialización FEDNA. De Blas, C., G.G. Mateos, and P. García (eds). *FEDNA* **20:** 210 - 265.

Mateos, G.G. (2004). Óxido de zinc y sulfato de cobre. *Suis* **10:** 3 - 4.

Mateos, G.G. (1987). Alimentación de porcino. In: *Nutrición y Alimentación del Ganado.* C. De Blas, G.G. Mateos and A. Argamenteria, (eds). Mundi-Prensa. Madrid. pp 337 - 356.

Mavromichalis, I., Peter, C.M., Parr, T.M., Ganessunker, D., and Baker, D.H. (2000). Growth-promoting efficacy in young pigs of two sources of zinc oxide having either high or low bioavailability of zinc. *Journal of Animal Science* **78:** 2896 - 2902.

McKenzie, R.C., Arthur, J.R., Miller, S.M., Rafferty, T.S., and Beckett, G.J. (2002). Selenium and the immune system. In: *Nutrition and immune function.* P.C. Calder, C.J. Field and H.S. Gill (eds). CABI Publishing. Wallingford. United Kingdom. pp. 239 - 250.

McDowell, L. R. (2003). *Minerals in Animal and Human Nutrition.* (2nd ed). Elsevier. The Netherlands.

Miles, R.D., and Henry, P.R. (1999). Relative trace mineral bioavailability. *Proceedings of California Animal Nutrition Conference,* Fresno, CA. pp. 1- 24.

NRC. (1997). *The role of chromium in animal nutrition.* National Academic Science, Washington DC. USA

NRC. (1998). *Nutrient Requirements of Swine*. 10th rev. National Academic Science, Washington DC. USA

Nebraska and South Dakota State University. (2000). *Swine Nutrition Guide*. Nebraska Cooperative Extension. EC 95-273-C, Lincoln Nebraska, U.S.A.

Nielsen, F. (1996). Controversial chromium: does the superstar mineral of the mountebanks receive appropriate attention from clinicians and nutritionists? *Nutrition Today* **31:** 226 - 233.

Nys. Y. (2001). Oligo-éléments, croissance et santé du poulet de chair. *INRA Productions Animales* **14:** 171 - 180.

Osborne, J.C., and Davis, J.W. (1968). Increased susceptibility to bacterial endotoxin of pigs with iron-deficiency anaemia. *Journal of American Veterinary Medical Society Association* **152:** 1630 - 1632.

Paboeuf, F., Calvar, C., Landrain, B., and Roy, H. (2001). Impact de la reduction des niveaux alimentaires en matières azotée totale, en phosphore, en cuivre et en zinc sur les performances et les rejets des porcs charcutiers. *Journal Recherche Porcine en France* **33:** 49 - 56.

Page, T.G., Southern, L.L., Ward, T.L., and Thompson Jr., D.L. (1993). Effect of chromium picolinate on growth and serum and carcass traits of growing-finishing pigs. *Journal of Animal Science* **71:** 656 - 662.

Poulsen, H.D. (1995). Zinc oxide for weanling piglets. *Acta Agric. Scand. Section A. Animal Science* **45:** 159 - 167.

Poupoulis, C., and Jensen, L.S. (1976). Effects of high dietary copper on gizzard integrity of the chick. *Poultry Science* **54:** 113 - 121.

Powers, H.J. (1995). Riboflavine-iron interactions with particular emphasis on the gastrointestinal tract. *Proceedings of the Nutrition Society* **57:** 509 - 517.

Prasad, A.S. (2002). Zinc, infection and immune function. In: *Nutrition and immune function*. P.C. Calder, C.J. Field and H.S. Gill (eds). CABI Publishing. Wallingford. UK. pp 193 - 207.

Rayman, M.P. (2002). The argument for increasing selenium intake. *Proceedings of the Nutrition Society* **61:** 203 - 215.

Revy, P.S., Jondreville, C., Dourmad, J.Y., and Nys, Y. (2004). Effect of zinc supplemented as either an organic or an inorganic source and of microbial phytase on zinc and other minerals utilisation by weanling pigs. *Animal Feed Science and Technology* **116:** 93 - 112.

Revy, P.S., Jondreville, C., Dourmad, J.Y., and Nys, Y. (2003). Le zinc dans l'alimentation du porc: oligoélément essential et risque potential pour l'environnement. *INRA Productions Animales* **16:** 3 - 18.

Revy, P.S., Jondreville, C., Dourmad, J.Y., Guinotte, F., and Nys, Y. (2002). Bioavailability of two sources of zinc in weanling pigs. *Animal Research* **51:** 315 - 326.

Rostagno, H.S. (2000). Tabelas brasileiras para aves e suinos. Universidad Federal de Viçosa. Viçosa, Brazil.

Savoini, G., Cheli, F., Bontempo, V., Baldi, A., Fantuz, F., Politis, I., and Dell´Orto, V. (1998). Effect of chromium yeast supplementation on performance, reproduction and immune function in pigs. *Annales de Zootechnie* **47:** 273 - 278.

Scheideler, S.E. (1991). Interaction of dietary calcium, manganese and manganese source (manganese oxide or manganese methionine chelate) on chick performance and manganese utilization. *Biological Trace Element Research* **29:** 217 - 223.

Schell, T.C., and Kornegay, E.T. (1996). Zinc concentration in tissues and performance of weanling pigs fed pharmacological levels of zinc from ZnO, Zn-Methionine, Zn-Lysine, or ZnSO4. *Journal of Animal Science* **74:** 1584 - 1593.

Smith, J.W, Tokach, M.D., Goodband, R.D., Nelssen, J.L., and Richert, B.T. (1997). Effects of the interrelationship between zinc oxide and copper sulfate on growth performance of early-weaned pigs. *Journal of Animal Science* **75:** 1861 - 1866.

Smith, M.O., Sherman, I.L., Miller, L.C., and Robbins, K.R. (1995). Relative biological availability of manganese from manganese proteinate, manganese sulfate, and manganese monoxide in broilers reared at elevated temperatures. *Poultry Science* **74:** 702 - 707.

Southern, L.L. (2001). Increasing profit by optimizing nutrition-chromium. *Advances in Pork Production* **12:** 153 - 158.

Spears, J.W. (1989). Zinc methionine for ruminants: Relative bioavailability of zinc in lambs and effects on growth and performance of growing heifers. *Journal of Animal Science* **67:** 835 - 843.

Surai, P.F. (2003). Selenium - Vitamin E interactions: does 1 + 1 equal more than 2?. In: *Nutritional Biotechnology in the Feed and Food Industries*. T.P. Lyons. and K.A. Jacques (eds). Alltech 19th Annual Symposium. Nottingham University Press. Nottingham. U.K. pp 51 - 58.

Swinkels, J.W., Kornegay, E.T., and Verstegen, M.W.A. (1994). Biology of zinc and biological value of dietary organic zinc complexes and chelates. *Nutrition Research Reviews* **7:** 129 - 149.

Underwood E.J., and Suttle, N.F. (2001). *The Mineral Nutrition of Livestock*. (3rd ed). CABI Publishing. Wallingford. United Kingdom.

Van de Ligt, C.P.A., Lindemann, M.D., and Cromwell, G.L. (2002a). Assessment of chromium tripicolinate supplementation and dietary protein level on growth, carcass, and blood criteria in growing pigs. *Journal of Animal Science* **80:** 2412 - 2419.

Van de Ligt, C.P.A., Lindemann, M.D., and Cromwell, G.L. (2002b). Assessment of chromium tripicolinate supplementation and dietary energy level and source on growth, carcass, and blood criteria in growing pigs. *Journal of Animal Science* **80:** 483 - 493.

Van de Ligt, C.P.A., Lindemann, M.D., Harmon, R.J., Monegue, H.J., and Cromwell, G.L. (2002c). Effect of chromium tripicolinate supplementation on porcine immune response during the postweaning period. *Journal of Animal Science* **80:** 449 - 455

Van Heugten, E., and Spears, J.W. (1997). Immune response and growth of stressed weanling pigs fed diets supplemented with organic or inorganic forms of chromium. *Journal of Animal Science* **75:** 409 - 416.

Vieira, I.A., and Shigueru, V. (2003). Cobre orgânico e inorgânico como promotores do crescimento de leitoes recém-desmamados. *R. Bras. Zootec.* **32:** 1657 - 1662.

Vincent, J.B. (2003). The potential value and potential toxicity of chromium picolinate as a nutritional supplement, weight loss agent, and muscle development agent. *Sports Medicine* **33:** 213 - 230.

Vincent, J.B. (2004). Recent advances in the nutritional biochemistry of trivalent chromium. *Proceedings of the Nutrition Society* **63:** 41 - 47.

Wedekind, K.J., Hortin, D.E., and Baker, D.H. (1992). Methodology for assessing zinc bioavailability: efficacy estimates for zinc-methionine, zinc sulfate and zinc oxide. *Journal of Animal Science* **70:** 178 - 187.

Wedekind, K.J., Lewis, A.J., Giesemann, M.A., and Miller, P.S. (1994a). Bioavailability of zinc from inorganic and organic sources for pigs fed corn-soybean meal diets. *Journal of Animal Science* **72:** 2681 - 2689.

Wedekind, K.J., Collings, G., Hancock, J., and Titgemeyer, E. (1994b). The bioavailability of zinc-methionine relative to zinc sulfate is affected by calcium level. *Poultry Science* **73** (Suppl. 1)**:** 114 (Abst.).

Whanger, P.D. (2003). Metabolic pathways of selenium in plants and animals and their nutritional significance. In: *Nutritional Biotechnology in the Feed and Food Industries.* T.P. Lyons. and K.A. Jacques (eds). Alltech 19th Annual Symposium. Nottingham University Press. Nottingham. U.K. pp 51 - 58.

Williams, C.M., Barker, J.C., and Sims, J.T. (1999). Management and utilization of poultry wastes. *Environmental Contamination and Toxicology* **162:** 105 - 157.

Zhou, W., Kornegay, E.T., van Laar, H., Swinkels, J.W., Wong, E.A., and Lindemann, M.D. (1994a). The role of feed consumption and feed efficiency in copper-stimulated growth. *Journal of Animal Science* **72:** 2385 - 2394.

Zhou, W., Kornegay, E.T., Lindemann, M.D., Swinkels, J.W.,

Welten, M.K., and Wong, E.A. (1994b). Stimulation of growth by intravenous injection of copper in weanling pigs. *Journal of Animal Science* **72:** 2395 - 2403.

Feeding the sow and piglet to achieve maximum antioxidant and immunity protection

Don Mahan

Professor, Animal Sciences, The Ohio State University, Columbus, Ohio USA

Summary

With the introduction of modern swine genotypes capable of rapid lean growth rates and high reproductive performance, there are concurrent problems associated with this type of pig. One of the encountered problems is high mortality in both weaned pigs and sows. Longevity of sows in the sow herd is of major concern in most commercial swine herds. It appears that the highest producing and fastest growing animals seem to be more affected by this malady and that "sudden deaths" are commonly encountered in both the breeding herd and weanling pigs. Our studies suggest that the antioxidant capability of weaned pigs and sows is at its lowest with the sudden death occurrence. Trace minerals added to the diet at higher "insurance levels" may contribute to higher oxidative states in the animals and when the animal is stressed sudden death occurs. High mineral levels have been shown to reduce reproductive performance, reduce sow longevity in the herd, and increases free radical formation. In addition, inorganic trace minerals may increase the incidences of splay legged and stillborn pigs. Vitamin E, Se, and Zn methionine may be influential in improving the sows udder health and overall reproductive health. The results to date suggest that organic minerals may be important as a source of trace minerals for preventing free radical accumulation, and in enhancing sow reproductive performance.

Introduction

Natural defense systems exist and guard the body against disease and stress, and both are affected by the other. It is generally considered that uncontrolled oxidation reactions caused by various stressors can not only lead to poor animal performance, but may impair the animal's immune status and in severe cases even cause death. Various environmental, genetic, and physiological stressor agents can exacerbate the breakdown of these defense systems in both animals and humans. Many of the recognized diseases that commonly afflict humans (e.g. Parkinson's disease, Alzheimer's disease, amyotrophic lateral sclerosis (ALS) or Lou Gehrig disease, diabetes, auto immune disease, cancer, etc.) are thought to be influenced by genetic factors, but recent evident suggests that they may also be directly linked to the inability of the cell and neuron to handle oxidative end products or free radicals (Markesbery et al., 2001). Increasingly evidence suggests that at least some of the common maladies that affect animals (i.e. high sow mortality, sudden death of pigs, etc) may also result from oxidative free radical damage occurring at an increased rate once stressors are imposed on high producing animals.

An increase in oxidative reactions within the cell or at the site of the cell membrane produces free radicals or activated molecules which subsequently can damage cellular functions, cellular membranes, and the subsequent destruction of the cell. Oxidation-reduction reactions occur in the body under normal metabolic processes, but it is when the reactions are uncontrolled and the end products of the oxidation reaction accumulate (i.e., free radicals) when tissue damage occurs. These free radicals are often denoted as activated O_2^*, O^*, OH^*, NO^* or from $C-C=C-C$, the former four occurring in the cytoplasm of the cell, while the latter occur in the lipoprotein layer of the cell membrane and fat body components. In the process of protection, the cell attempts to prevent the accumulation of free radicals by the action of several antioxidants present in the body (Table 1).

Table 1. Antioxidants present in body tissue (Markesbery et al., 2001).

Enzymatic	Nonenzymatic
Cu-Zn superoxide dismutase	Ascorbic acid
Mn superoxide dismutase	Ceruloplasmin
Catalase	Uric acid
Glutathione peroxidase	Bilirubin
Glutathione reductase	Melatonin
Alpha and gama tocopherol	Isoflavone
	Glutathione
	Methionine

Various factors cause the accumulation of free radicals resulting in the breakdown of cellular tissue, but it is generally the additional stressors (high temperatures or other environmental factors, high physiological demands, etc.) that cause the cell to work harder, whereupon the effects frequently result in the death of animal. Animals that are stress prone, those under stress at farrowing, and animals with rapid growth rates have been shown to frequently encounter the "sudden death" syndrome. Each of these conditions is thought to contribute to an excessive accumulation of free radicals that cannot be handled by the animal. Obviously, if the antioxidant(s) that prevents the build-up of free radicals are absent, antioxidants are preset at a low level in the cell, or if they are not present at the precise place within the cell where free radicals are formed, damage can occur.

Deficient or excessive nutrient supply to tissue

We all understand that when cells do not receive adequate nourishment, cellular components cannot perform their metabolic function and poor performance results, but when nutritional excesses are provided the tissue must either rid itself of these excesses, or store the nutrient in tissue. If the nutrient has oxidative properties tissue damage may result with death often ensuing.

One example of a common malady of commercial swine production is the sudden death of pigs during the post-weaning period. In this situation it is common for the largest, fastest growing pigs to suddenly die from no apparent cause. The pig at this stage is just beginning to synthesize vitamin C, and vitamin E and Se are generally declining; thus the animal's antioxidant status is poor. These animals do not display any signs of a deficiency or disease, but are suddenly found dead. When one considers that these pigs are probably also consuming the largest amount of feed (hence the rapid growth rate and larger size), they are also metabolizing more nutrients and producing more free radicals from metabolic activity. Not only do they have a higher nutrient requirement, but they also have a higher requirement for the antioxidants that are used to prevent the accumulation of the free radicals. It seems that when an additional stress is imposed (e.g., disease challenge, fighting for dominance, etc.) the additional metabolic activity is thought to result in the build up of free radicals and if not controlled the animal could die. The high rate of metabolism of carbohydrates and the excitation of the animal yields activated O_2^*, OH*, and NO* which accumulates, thus potentially causing the death of the animal. Necropsy signs of such animals sometimes show evidence of fluid accumulation in the pericardial sac, mulberry heart, and in some cases degenerative liver and ceroid pigment in body fat, which are all indicators of accumulated free radicals.

The role of trace minerals

Some trace minerals have high oxidative capacity, namely Fe, Cu, Se, and to a lesser extent Zn. Coincidently, these minerals are capable of changing their chemical valence in the body thus causing them to be less reactive when the valence is in a reduced state, but more reactive when in the oxidative state. In nature and in the body, these organic minerals are bound to proteins where their chemical reactivity is kept in check. The mineral elements are also components of antioxidants (e.g. Fe in catalase; Zn and Cu in superoxide dismutase; Se in glutathione peroxidase) and thus are required by the body. The NRC (1998) recommends dietary levels without a "safety factor" added. However, most nutritionists generally suggest such safety factors in their recommendations. The questions posed are; what is the effect of some of these trace minerals when added at higher dietary levels on animal performance, and what is the effect of providing an organic source of these minerals rather than the more reactive inorganic source?

Preliminary research by Peters and Mahan (2004) indicated that when conventional dietary levels of trace minerals (generally recommended by university and industry nutritionists) were fed to reproducing gilts and sows and compared to dietary trace mineral levels suggested by NRC (1998) (Table 2), the reproductive performance of animals was less when the "industry average levels" were provided (Figure 1).

Table 2.
NRC mineral levels and those recommended by industry and university nutritionists.

Mineral	NRC (1998) (ppm)	Industry and University practices (ppm)
Cu	5	10 - 20
I	0.14	0.15 - 0.20
Fe	80	100 - 200
Mn	20	40 - 80
Se	0.15	0.2 - 0.5
Zn	50	100 - 150

Figure 1.
Effect of dietary trace mineral level (NRC and industry standard) and source (inorganic or organic) fed to reproducing sows on reproductive performance (2 parities) (Peters and Mahan, 2004)

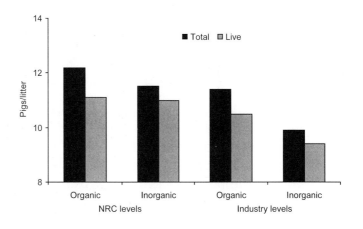

66

Ascorbic acid is an excellent water-soluble antioxidant but exists in two forms in the body (oxidized and reduced form). It is the reduced form that is biologically active as an antioxidant. When the ratio of oxidized to reduced ascorbic acid was evaluated in these reproducing sows (Figure 2), the amount of oxidized ascorbic acid was higher (*i.e.*, both organic and inorganic) when the dietary levels of trace minerals were elevated in the sows diet. Because ascorbic acid is an excellent antioxidant used by the body, the ratio obtained in this study suggests that the amount of the antioxidant used by the sow to reduce the amount of free radicals formed is greater.

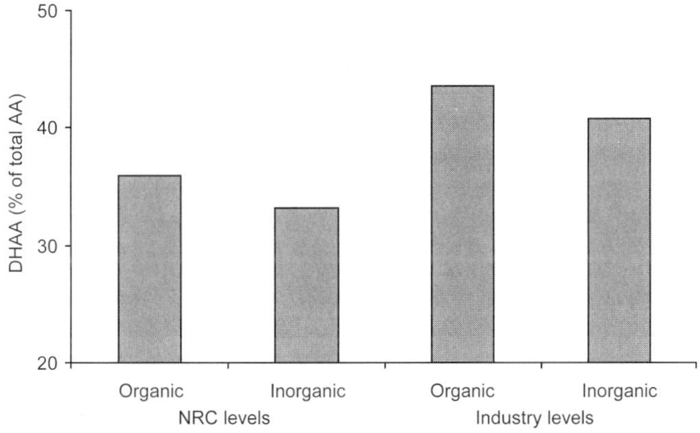

Figure 2. Ratio of oxidized to reduced ascorbic acid in sow when fed trace mineral sources (inorganic or organic) at two dietary levels (NRC standards or industry standards). Mahan and Peters (unpublished). DHAA = dehydroascorbic acid (oxidized form of vitamin C).

Another study by Mahan and Peters (2004) indicated that more sows completed a 4-parity study when evaluating the dietary levels of inorganic or organic Se at NRC (1998) of 0.15 ppm or 0.30 ppm Se levels compared to a basal (unsupplemented) ration. The results demonstrated a reproductive benefit to the organic Se source, but when the dietary Se level (both the organic and inorganic sources) was increased to 0.30 ppm, fewer sows completed the 4-parity study (Figure 3).

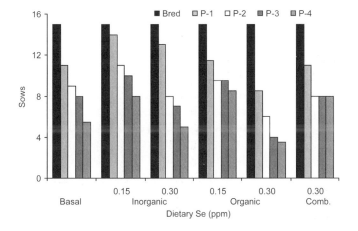

Figure 3. Effect of sows remaining on trial over a 4-parity period when fed organic (Sel-Plex™) or inorganic (selenite) Se sources at various levels (P = parity). Mahan and Peters (2004)

Interestingly, the number of stillborn pigs (P < 0.05; Figure 4), and the number of splay legged pigs were greater (Figure 5) when the inorganic Se source was compared to the organic Se (*i.e.*, Sel-Plex™) treatment groups. Both of these studies suggest that high dietary trace mineral levels may be detrimental to sow health and longevity.

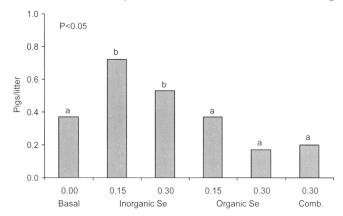

Figure 4. Stillborn pigs from sows fed organic (Sel-Plex™) or inorganic (selenite) Se at various levels. Mahan and Peters (2004)

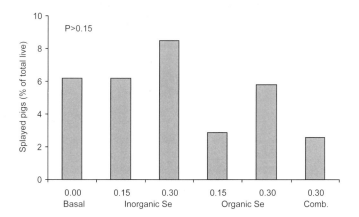

Figure 5. Percentage of splay legged pigs (severe) when sows are fed organic (Sel-Plex™) or inorganic (selenite) Se sources at various levels (over a 4-parity period). Mahan and Peters (2004)

The role of trace minerals and vitamins in immunological responses

The role of vitamin E and Se in the immunological process in the pig has been investigated for the past few years. The early work of Peplowski *et al.* (1981) demonstrated that when either Se or vitamin E were injected into young pigs at weaning or when provided in the diet, the antibody titer response to an antigen improved, but the combination of both nutrients further enhanced the hemagglutination response (Figure 6).

D. Mahan

Figure 6.
Effect of Se or
Vitamin E or their
combination
(injected or diet) on
hemagglutination
titers in weanling
pigs. Peplowski *et
al.* (1981)

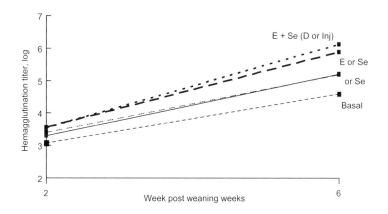

Hayek *et al.* (1989) demonstrated that the immunological level of
IgM and IgG was increased in sow colostrum with vitamin E and
Se injections (Table 3). This suggests that the health status of pigs
at weaning would be improved when the sow was administered
adequate levels of both nutrients. Wuryastuti *et al.* (1993)
demonstrated that the colostrum and milk of sows fed vitamin E
and Se had greater phagocytic activity in colostrum and milk than
animals fed diets without these nutrients (Table 4).

Table 3.
Immunoglobulin
concentration in sow
colostrum.

| | | | Treatment[b] | | |
| | | | | Vitamin E | |
Immunoglobulin	Control	Vitamin E	Selenium	+ Se	SEM
IgA	13.8	12.7	14.5	12.4	1.9
IgM	8.4	9.8	10.0	9.6	0.8[c]
IgG	54.0	63.9	64.3	64.1	7.0

[b]Treatments were intramuscularly administered at 100 day of pregnancy; Control
= 1 ml saline; Vit E = 100 IU α-tocopherol; Se = 5 mg; [c] Se vs Control (P <
0.05). (Hayek *et al.*, 1989).

Table 4.
Phagocytic and
microbicidal
activities of
polymorphonuclear
(PMN) cells of
colostrum and milk
from control sows
and sows fed vitamin
E-and (or) selenium-
depleted diets
between conception
and 4 days
postpartum.
Wuryastuti *et al.*
(1993).

| | Phagocytic activity[a] | | Microbicidal activity[b] | |
Diet	Colostrum	Milk	Colostrum	Milk
Neg. control (no E/Se)	35.2±0.9[d]	21.2±2.5	3.2±2.7[d]	1.2±0.10[d]
Control (+E/Se) (-E)	50.2±5.4	27.5±3.0	6.2±0.8	2.7±0.2
	43.6±3.2	23.7±1.5	3.6±0.6[d]	2.2±0.5
Control (+E/Se) (-Se)	44.6±8.3	30.2±5.0	6.2±1.0	2.4±0.1
	33.4±5.1	19.9±3.4	2.6±0.60[d]	1.6±0.4

[a] Percentage of PMN cells containing two or more yeast particles.
[b] Percentage of PMN cells containing two or more dead yeast particles.
[c] Control diets were fortified with vitamin E (IU/kg) and Se (0.3 ppm) while
treatment diets deleted one or both nutrients.
[d] Significantly (P < 0.05) different from respective control.

The health status of sows with a Se and vitamin E deficiency under certain feeding practices was demonstrated by Whitehair *et al.* (1983). The results presented in Table 5 demonstrated that clinical signs of Mastitis, Metritis, Aglactia (MMA) occurred when sows were fed a basal diet, but when the diet was fortified with Se and vitamin E, the MMA syndrome was eliminated. In addition to improved udder health, milk production was increased as evidenced by larger litter gains and higher weaning percentages.

Table 5. Responsiveness of gilts to vitamin E-selenium supplementation on various postpartum measurements. Whitehair *et al.* (1983).

| | High moisture corn | | |
| | Basal | Basal | |
Item		+ Se + E	SEM (PM)
Gilts, no.	10	9	-
Clinical MMA, no.	5	0	-
Litter			
Pigs born, no.	8.8	10.9	0.7
Weight, birth	11.2	15.2	0.9 (0.02)
Weight, 21 day	31.4	45.1	3.4 (0.05)
Weaning, %	80.2	86.8	5.7
Litter gain (9 to 21 day)	20.2	29.9	
Pig gain (0 to 21 day)	3.4	3.7	

That Se or vitamin E and their combination enhanced immunological responses was further demonstrated by Larsen and Tollersud (1981). Their results demonstrated that phytohaemagglution of the blood cell was improved with dietary Se and vitamin E and further improved with their combination (Table 6). Further research reported by Wuryastuti *et al.* (1993) demonstrated that lymphocyte blastogenesis and blood polymorphonuclear immune responses were improved with vitamin E and Se fortification during the reproductive cycle of the gilt (Table 7).

Table 6. Effect of dietary vitamin E and selenium on pig lymphocyte response to phytohaemagglutinin (PHA). Larsen and Tollersud (1981).

| Dietary treatments | | PHA response |
Se (ppm)	Vitamin E mg/day	(log)
0.0	0	0.97
0.0	40	1.88
0.05	0	1.65
0.05	40	2.16
0.10	0	1.31
0.10	40	1.68

Table 7.
Effect of Vitamin E and Selenium Deficiency on Blood Lymphocyte Blastogenesis, Blood Polymorphonuclear cell (PMN) phagocytic activity and PMN microbicidal activity. Wuryastuti et al. (1993).

	Vitamin E[b]					Selenium[c]				
	Day 90 gest.		Parturition			Day 90 gest.		Parturition		
Item	+E	-E	+E	-E	SEM	+Se	-Se	+Se	-Se	SEM
Lymphocyte blastogenesis										
PHAa	4.90	4.54*	5.13	3.93*	0.22	5.19	5.20	5.32	4.50	0.21
PWa	5.19	4.64*	5.17	3.79*	0.20	5.28	5.18	5.31	4.67	0.23
Blood polymorphonuclear immune response										
Phagocytic,%	90.7	86.2*	90.1	83.8*	2.3	92.9	80.5*	90.2	72.2*	3.2
Microbicidal	57.6	48.7*	58.1	40.6*	2.6	53.1	38.4*	56.3	34.3*	2.9

[a] The immunoresponsiveness of the lymphocytes was accessed by measuring their responses to phytohemagglutin (PHA) and pokeweed (PW) mitogens.
[b] Fortified diets contained vitamin E at 60 IU/kg.
[c] Fortified diets contained Se at .3 ppm.

Although organic Zn has been previously suggested to improve animal health, a review of research with dairy cows demonstrates that milk yield increased and udder health improved when Zn methionine top-dressed their diet. It has been demonstrated that the somatic cell count (SCC) was reduced when Zn methionine was added to the diets. This study was conducted in several locations with all studies showing the same general response (Table 8). The application to the swine industry is obvious. Because many high producing sows produce as much milk as a dairy cow, when expressed on a body weight basis, udder health and milk yield is extremely important. These results suggest that organic Zn may be an important factor in maintaining the health and longevity of sows in the reproducing herd.

Table 8.
Effect of Zinc methionine on somatic cell count (SCC) in a regional dairy study. Kellogg et al. (2004).

	Diets	
Item	Control[a]	Zinc methionine[b]
No. cows	363	368
Milk yield, kg/d	29.7	31.2
SCC (x103/mL)	282	184

[a] Inorganic Zn supplemented to the diet
[b] Supplemented the control diet with the addition of 180 to 400 mg Zn/day from zinc methionine

Conclusions

Historically the research performed with trace minerals has largely been conducted with inorganic sources with most efforts being directed towards determining the animal's requirement and their subsequent bioavailability from various mineral sources. Certain minerals are highly reactive chemically in nature and within the body. When trace minerals are supplied in excess, recent research is beginning to suggest that they may produce detrimental effects in animals, particularly in the reproducing herd. Two major points need to be made from the research presented. The first is that high dietary levels of trace minerals or those normally recommended by university and feed industry personnel, may not be beneficial to reproducing animals, and secondly the use of organic minerals may have a more beneficial role in animal feed formulations than previously considered. Future research will be necessary to resolve these issues.

Literature cited

Hayek, M. G., Mitchell, G. E. Jr., Harmon, R. J., Stahly, T. S., Cromwell, G. L., Tucker, R. E., and Barker, K. B. (1989) Porcine immunoglobulin transfer after preparatum treatment with selenium or vitmin E. *Journal of Animal Science* **67:**1299.

Kellogg, D. W., Tomlinson, D. J., Socha, M. T., and Johnson, A. B. (2004) Review: Effects of zinc methionine complex on milk production and somatic cell count of dairy cows: Twelve-trial summary. *Professional Animal Scientist* **20:** 295-301.

Larsen, H. J., and Tollersud, S. (1981) Effect of dietary vitamin E and selenium on the phytohaemagglutinin response of pig lymphocytes. *Research in Veterinary Science* **31:** 301.

Mahan, D. C., and Peters, J. C. (2004) Long-term effects of dietary organic and inorganic selenium sources and levels on reproducing sows and their progeny. *Journal of Animal Science* **82:**1343-1358.

Markesbery, W. R., Montine, T. J., and Lovell, M. A. (2001) Oxidative alterations in neurodegenerative diseases. In: *Pathogenesis Disorders* (ed. M. P. Mattson) Humans Press Inc. Totowa, NJ.

NRC. (1998) *Nutrient Requirement of Swine* (10th Ed.). National Academy Press. Washington, DC.

Peplowski, M. A., Mahan, D. C., Murray, F. A., Moxon, A. L., Cantor, A. H., and Ekstrom, K. E. (1981) Effect of dietary and injectable vitamin E and selenium in weanling swine antigenically challenged with sheep red blood cells. *Journal of Animal Science* **51:** 344-351.

Peters, J. C., and Mahan, D. C. (2004) Sow and litter responses to dietary trace mineral source and level over two parities *Journal of Animal Science* (Abstr.), pg 52.

Whitehair, C. K., and Miller, E. R. (1985) Vitamin E and selenium in swine production. In: *Selenium Responsive Diseases in Food Animals*. West States Veterinary Conference pg. 11.

D. Mahan

Wuryastuti, H., Stowe, H. D., Bull, R.W., and Miller, E. R. (1993) Effects of vitamin E and selenium on immune responses of peripheral blood, colostrum, and milk leukocytes of sows. *Journal of Animal Science* **71:** 2464.

Piglet diets: can we manage without zinc oxide and copper sulfate?

Marcia Carlson Shannon
University of Missouri, Columbia, MO

Since the first scientific report stating that the dietary additions of inorganic zinc and copper to nursery pig diets enhanced growth performance post-weaning, the global pig industry has routinely added, in combination or individually, high concentrations of inorganic Zn oxide (2,000 to 3,000 ppm Zn) or Cu sulfate (125 to 250 ppm Cu). These dietary concentrations are much greater than the established requirements of Zn (100 ppm) and Cu (6 ppm) for the nursery pig (NRC, 1998). However it is noteworthy that, supplementing high concentrations of one trace mineral for an extended period could have detrimental effects on pig performance due to trace mineral interactions (O'Dell, 1989).

With heightened concern regarding environmental sustainability, there has been increasing interest in feeding lower dietary concentrations of Zn and Cu in nursery pig diets that adhere to new legislation without compromising pig performance. Organic trace mineral complexes were developed based on the theory that they are more bioavailable, or more similar to naturally-occurring forms in the body than inorganic trace minerals and exhibit improved metabolic utilization resulting in enhanced performance responses and less nutrient excretion (Wedekind *et al.*, 1994). The type of ligands used to form a mineral complex or chelate varies, but in most organic products, the trace mineral of interest is bound to an amino acid(s), hydrolyzed protein, or a polysaccharide (Spears, 1993). All organic trace minerals are not the same and the nature of the ligand may affect the degree of improvement or otherwise in growth performance. However, there may be some biological difference in the nursery pig, based on the type of ligand binding, which causes inconclusive research results. This paper is an effort to summarize current research results focussing on Zn and Cu supplementation of nursery pig diets and aims to provide applicable conclusions.

The Zn Story

The commercial practice of feeding high concentrations of Zn to nursery pigs initiated from European reports (Poulsen, 1995) that suggested supplemental ZnO decreased the incidence of non-specific post-weaning scours, but more importantly *Escherichia coli* proliferation which accounts for a majority of the death loss in the pig industry. In addition, reports from the United States have shown that the addition of high concentrations of Zn in the form of ZnO can promote growth performance of the newly-weaned pig (Table 1). The summary indicates that high Zn supplementation either as inorganic or organic sources in nursery pig diets shows a clear response in increasing growth performance. Several unreported or uncontrollable conditions such as environmental housing (commercial or university), trace mineral status of the pig, level of mineral antagonists (Zn, Fe, Cu, or Ca), other dietary factors (phytate), molecular size of the organic trace mineral, or health status of the pig could affect the magnitude of the growth performance response. The average improvement in growth performance (ADG) observed from these studies shows an increase of 7.85 % for early (< 21 d) weaned pigs or 8.3 % for traditionally (> 22 d) weaned pigs fed high concentrations of Zn for a minimum of 2 wks immediately post-weaning (Table 1). Research from Smith *et al.* (1997) and Hill *et al.* (2001) reported a greater improvement in ADG for earlier (< 21 d) weaned pigs fed supplemental Zn; however, Carlson *et al.* (1999) and Case and Carlson (2002) observed better ADG response in nursery pigs weaned after d 21. The majority of these studies fed supplemental Zn for 4 wks post-weaning, but no additive effect was observed after 2 wks post-weaning. Carlson *et al.* (1999) reported that the greatest response in growth performance associated with supplemental Zn fed to nursery pigs occurs during the first 2 wks post-weaning. In addition, these studies fed a wide range of dietary Zn concentrations (80 to 3,000 ppm). A North Central Region Swine Nutrition study (Hill *et al.*, 2001) has shown that 2,000 ppm Zn is just as efficacious as 3,000 ppm Zn as ZnO in improving growth performance in nursery pigs post-weaning. Additional research has shown that the inorganic ZnO inclusion rate could be lowered to 1,000 ppm when dietary phytase (500 FTU/kg) is included in the nursery diet (Martinez *et al.*, 2004). Overall, the relative bioavailability of the ZnO source used in these studies more than likely would not affect the growth performance response in nursery pigs (Mavromichalis *et al.*, 2000).

The summarization of organic Zn supplementation in nursery pig diets post-weaning indicates that the ligand binding or source has little effect on improvement in growth performance with an average

M. Carlson Shannon

Table 1. Summarization of several nursery pig Zn supplementation studies effect on growth performance (ADG) compared to pigs fed NRC requirements.

Reference [a]	Zn source	Level feed (ppm)	Study length (d)	Initial pig age (d)	Initial pig wt. (kg)	Overall ADG % increase
Carlson et al., 1999	Oxide	3000	28	11.5	3.8	9.1
	Oxide	3000	28	24.5	7.2	19.0
Case & Carlson, 2002	Amino acid	500	28	24	6.45	5.4
	Polysaccharide	500				20.5
	Oxide	500				7.9
	Oxide	3000				23.9
	Amino acid	500	28	18	5.47	-6.2
	Polysaccharide	500				8.6
	Oxide	500				3.0
	Oxide	3000				20.0
Carlson et al., 2004	Polysaccharide	125	42	17	5.14	2.0
	Oxide	2000				4.3
	Proteinate	100	28	17	5.27	5.7
	Oxide	2000				8.0
Cheng et al., 1998	Sulfate	100	28	20.5	7.25	2.85
	Lysine	100				4.1
Davis et al., 2004	Oxide	2500	10	19	6.2	21.3
	Oxide	2500	38	19	4.6	19.3 (d1-10)
						6.0 (d1-38)
	Oxide	500	35	19	5.6	-1.4
	Oxide	2500				1.1
de Rodas et al., 1999 [b]	Amino acid	100	52	19.5	6.1	- simple diet + complex diet
Hahn & Baker, 1993	Oxide	3000	21	35	8.33	12.6
	Sulfate	3000				14.3
	Oxide	3000	14	28	7.93	11.0
	Sulfate	3000				-7.0
	Methionine	3000				-1.8
Hill et al., 2000	Oxide	3000	28	22	6.55	11.1
	Oxide + CuSO$_4$	3000				9.6
Hill et al., 2001	Oxide	500	28	12.8	4.15	11.2
	Oxide	1000				11.2
	Oxide	2000				22.8
	Oxide	3000				15.8
	Oxide	500	28	22.7	7.09	-0.8
	Oxide	1000				4.9
	Oxide	2000				9.2
	Oxide	3000				7.0
Mavromichalis, 2000	Oxide (HS)	1500	21	28	6.5	20.4
	Oxide (HS)	3000				34.1
	Oxide (W)	1500	21	28	6.1	19.5
	Oxide (HS)	1500				25.5
	Oxide (W)	1500	17	21	5.4	21.0
	Oxide (HS)	1500				19.6

Piget diets: can we manage without zinc oxide and copper sulphate?

Reference[a]	Zn source	Level feed (ppm)	Study length (d)	Initial pig age (d)	Initial pig wt. (kg)	Overall ADG % increase
McCalla et al., 1999[b]	Oxide	2000	35	18	NR	10.0
	Amino acid	100				-
	Amino acid	200				-
	Amino acid	300				-
	Amino acid	400				-
Mullan et al., 2002	Oxide	1500	21	21	8.0	26.0
	Oxide	2500				34.0
	Oxide	3500				2.0
	Oxide	2000	39	21	6.58	5.7
	Proteinate	100				9.4
	Proteinate	250				14.1
Schell & Kornegay, 1996	Oxide	3000	14	28	7.5	13.3
	Methionine	3000				7.7
	Lysine	3000				NC
	Sulfate	3000				-25.0
	Oxide	2000	14	26	7.1	NC
	Methionine	2000				-13.3
	Lysine	2000				NC
	Sulfate	2000				16.7
	Oxide	1000	14	23	5.3	-13.3
	Methionine	1000				-6.7
	Lysine	1000				6.7
	Sulfate	1000				NC
Smith et al., 1997	Oxide	3000	28	17	4.95	-2.9
	Oxide	3000	28	21	5.67	-1.1
	Oxide	3000	28	15	4.45	21.4
	Oxide+CuSO$_4$	3000				16.8
	Oxide	3000	28	12	4.17	4.2
	Oxide+CuSO$_4$	3000				-6.3
van Heugten et al., 2003	Sulfate	80	35	21	6.45	-1.3
	Methionine	80				5.7
	Lysine	80				-3.8
	Met+Lys	40+40				-2.0
Ward et al., 1996	Oxide	2000	33	19	6.5	5.5
	Methionine	250				4.8
	Oxide	2000	38	19	6.0	4.0
	Methionine	250				4.5
Woodworth et al., 1999[b]	Amino acid	100	34	12	4.25	-
	Amino acid	200				-
	Amino acid	300				-
	Amino acid	400				-
	Amino acid	500				-
	Oxide	3000				+

Table 1.
Contd.

[a] Studies vary in design setup such as number pigs per pen, duration of feeding Zn, commercial or university facilities, diet formulation, nutrient concentrations, and antibiotic inclusion (NC = no change).
[b] Studies did not report actual data, but indicated either an improvement (+) or no improvement (-) in growth performance.

increase of 3.1 %. Numerous researchers have shown that pigs fed lower concentrations of organic Zn forms have similar growth stimulation as pigs fed 3,000 ppm Zn as ZnO (Ward et al., 1996; de Rodas et al., 1999; Case and Carlson, 2002; Mullan et al., 2002). Conversely, Woodworth et al. (1999) and McCalla et al. (1999) reported that lower concentrations of organic Zn from a Zn amino acid complex did not support the same growth performance as nursery pigs fed 3,000 ppm Zn as ZnO up to 34-d post-weaning. The growth performance response does seem dependent on the complexity of the overall diet formulation for the nursery pigs (de Rodas et al., 1999). Overall, the response in ADG observed in nursery pigs post-weaning appears to not be as large when feeding lower concentrations of an organic Zn source compared to pigs fed 2,000 to 3,000 ppm Zn as inorganic ZnO post-weaning, but there is still a boost in growth performance.

The Cu Story

In 1955, Barber et al. first reported an enhancement in growth performance of pigs fed 250 ppm Cu in the form of Cu sulfate ($CuSO_4$). A summary of research studies that have evaluated the response of nursery pigs fed high concentrations of Cu in the diet is shown in Table 2. Several unreported or uncontrollable conditions could affect the growth performance response similarly to the discussion with Zn. The summary of Cu studies had supplemental Cu concentrations ranging from 15 to 250 ppm (independent of source) that were fed for at least 28 d post-weaning, resulting in an average increase in growth performance (ADG) of 5.2 % for nursery pigs (Table 2). The supplementation of Cu appears to have a greater affect on ADG (14.5 % vs. 7.1%) when pigs are weaned at an age greater than 22 d compared to studies with early-weaned pigs (< 21 d). These results are similar to the Zn studies except that the supplementation of Cu appears to generate a greater growth response when fed for at least 28 d post-weaning. Similarly to Zn supplementation studies, the inclusion of a feed-grade antibiotic does not enhance the growth performance response observed when feeding supplemental Cu to nursery pigs (Stahly et al., 1980 and Roof and Mahan, 1982).

A majority of the research supports that organic Cu complexes appear to have equal effectiveness to $CuSO_4$ in improving growth performance of the nursery pig. The summarization of studies conducted show that the organic Cu complexes improved growth performance in nursery pigs (Coffey et al., 1994; Zhou et al., 1994a; b; deRodas et al., 1999; Veum et al., 2004) with an average increase in ADG of 10.7 % compared to 10.5% for pigs fed diets supplemented with various concentrations of $CuSO_4$.

Table 2. Summarization of several nursery pig Cu supplementation studies effect on growth performance (ADG) compared to pigs fed NRC (1998) requirements.

Reference [a]	Cu source	Level feed (ppm)	Study length (d)	Initial pig age (d)	Initial pig wt. (kg)	Overall ADG % increase
Apgar et al., 1995	Sulfate	100	35	31	8.3	23.8
	Sulfate	150				17.9
	Sulfate	200				26.6
	Lysine	100				20.2
	Lysine	150				18.3
	Lysine	200				29.6
Armstrong et al., 2004	Sulfate	62	45	17	4.99	1.7
	Sulfate	125				10.8
	Sulfate	250				10.8
	Citrate	15				2.9
	Citrate	31				5.5
	Citrate	62				4.6
	Citrate	125				9.2
Coffey et al., 1994	Lysine	50-200	28-35	30	7.4	16.8
	Sulfate	50-200				11.5
Cromwell et al., 1998	Chloride	100	28	29	13.7	5.5
	Chloride	200				7.0
	Sulfate	200				9.0
Davis et al., 2002	Sulfate	175	38	18	6	50.9 (d1-10)
						13.7 (d1-38)
Dove, 1995	Sulfate	250	21	26	6.8	20.7
Dove, 1993	Sulfate	125	28	25	6.6	8.2
	Sulfate	250				13.7
Dove & Haydon, 1992	Sulfate	250	28	26	6.9	15.0
Hill et al., 2000	Sulfate	250	28	22	6.55	8.3
	Sulfate + ZnO	250				9.6
Roof & Mahan, 1982	Sulfate	125	33	28	6.8	5.7
	Sulfate	250				2.9
	Sulfate	375				2.9
	Sulfate	500				-9.1
Smith et al., 1997	Sulfate	250	28	15	4.45	11.8
	Sulfate + ZnO	250				16.8
	Sulfate	250	28	12	4.17	-4.7
	Sulfate + ZnO	250				-6.3
Stahly et al., 1980	Sulfate	250	28	28	6.4	8.3
	Sulfate	62.5	28	28	6.3	5.4
	Sulfate	125				13.1
	Sulfate	250				11.4
Stansbury et al., 1990	Sulfate	125	28	28	6.4	5.0
	Organic	31.25				2.6
	Organic	62.5				7.3
	Organic	125				5.0

Reference [a]	Cu source	Level feed (ppm)	Study length (d)	Initial pig age (d)	Initial pig wt. (kg)	Overall ADG % increase
Veum et al., 2004	Proteinate	25	28	19	6.3	5.2
	Proteinate	50				10.1
	Proteinate	100				8.8
	Proteinate	200				2.3
	Sulfate	250				NC

Table 2. Contd.

[a] Studies vary in design setup such as number pigs per pen, duration of feeding Cu, commercial or university facilities, diet formulation, nutrient concentrations, and antibiotic inclusion (NC = no change).

The concentration of Cu in the diet does not appear to enhance the growth performance response observed when nursery pigs are fed supplemental Zn. Hill et al. (2000) and Smith et al. (1997) observed an average reduction in ADG of 3 % when Zn and Cu supplementation are added in combination compared to just Zn supplementation during the first 4 wks post-weaning.

Possible mechanism for the growth response

The hypothesized mechanism behind the growth response of feeding 2,000 to 3,000 ppm Zn as ZnO, or 125 to 250 ppm Cu as $CuSO_4$ is that these trace minerals act as an antimicrobial agent or enterically on the intestinal microflora by reducing turnover of the intestinal cells and leaving more nutrients available for absorption (Fuller et al., 1960). Carlson et al. (1998) reported that feeding pharmacological concentrations of Zn (3,000 ppm Zn as ZnO) altered duodenal morphology (deeper crypts and greater total thickness), and increased intestinal metallothionein concentrations, which indicates that high concentrations of Zn may have an enteric effect on the growing pig. Research that is more recent has shown that ZnO can be used to control post-weaning scours caused by Escherichia coli bacteria (Owusu-Asiedu et al., 2003). Other research has indicated that ZnO may protect intestinal cells from E. coli infections by inhibiting the adhesion and internalization of bacteria, preventing the disruption of barrier integrity, and modulating cytokine gene expression, but not by a direct antibacterial effect (Roselli et al., 2003). Therefore, the research reported by Roselli et al. (2003) possibly explains the reason why most of the research does not show an additive response in ADG when both supplemental Zn or Cu and (or) a feed-grade antibiotic are fed to nursery pigs post-weaning (Hill et al., 2001).

Other researchers have reported that Cu enhances growth through a systemic effect within the body rather than an antimicrobial effect in the intestinal tract (Zhou *et al.,* 1994a; b). The concept that supplemental Cu may be acting systemically is supported by the wide variety of biological systemic functions, which are related to growth. If a systemic effect is the more likely mode of action, nutritionists and the feed industry need to develop ways to improve the efficacy of delivering Cu into circulation. This may be accomplished more readily by feeding organic trace minerals to growing pigs.

It has been reported that Cu and Zn retention is affected by the mineral status of the pig as well as the dietary Cu and Zn concentrations. Previous research has found that faecal Zn excretion increases and percent retention decreases with increasing dietary Zn concentrations (Poulsen and Larsen, 1995). Pigs fed 2,000 ppm Zn as ZnO excreted the largest quantity of faecal and urinary Zn, but also retained the most Zn due to the higher daily Zn intake (Carlson *et al.,* 2004). Pigs fed 400 ppm Zn as organic Zn or 2,000 ppm Zn as ZnO had higher Zn absorption and retention compared to pigs fed 200 ppm Zn as organic Zn or the basal diet (Carlson *et al.,* 2004). This indicates that elevated dietary Zn concentrations may increase Zn retention rates. Poulsen and Larson (1995) reported that Zn retention in growing pigs increased linearly as supplemental ZnO increased up to 0.30 g/d.

Pigs fed diets supplemented with either the organic Cu complex or inorganic $CuSO_4$ above their nutrient requirement excreted greater quantities of Cu in faeces and urine, but have higher retention rates similarly to Zn supplementation (Veum *et al.,* 2004). Pigs fed 50 or 100 ppm Cu as organic Cu with normal concentrations of inorganic Zn (150 ppm Zn) had a higher Zn retention and absorption and lower faecal Zn concentrations (Veum *et al.,* 2004), possibly due to nutrient interaction (O'Dell, 1989) and the higher bioavailability of the organic complex (Wedekind *et al.,* 1994). Apgar *et al.* (1996) reported that 71 kg barrows excreted 6.9 times more Cu when pigs were fed 250 versus 36 ppm Cu as $CuSO_4$. The bottom line is that, as Cu and Zn concentrations increase in the diet, urinary and faecal Cu and Zn excretion increase, as well as retention and absorption rates.

Conclusion

The summary of existing research publications strongly supports the feeding of high supplemental concentrations of Zn or Cu to nursery pigs at least 2 wks post-weaning resulting in improved growth performance. In addition, these results indicate that the decision to use high concentrations of Zn or Cu in nursery diets should be made on a case-by-case basis (under veterinary supervision), especially since there appears to be no specific conditions for when supplementation should occur. It is important to monitor the pigs and determine if positive responses to Zn or Cu are occurring. Otherwise, the practice of feeding supplemental Zn or Cu should be stopped because producers may be taking unnecessary risk (environmental and nutrient interactions), and possibly causing performance to decline. However, the replacement of an inorganic trace mineral source with an organic trace mineral source is a viable approach, as the organic trace mineral sources are more bioavailable than the inorganic trace mineral sources presently used. As a result of increased bioavailability of organic trace minerals, digestion and absorption rates in the intestinal tract are enhanced; therefore, less is needed in the diet to meet the pig's requirements. Current EU legislation states a maximum total mineral level in feedstuffs of 150mg/kg Zn, 170 mg/kg Cu up to 12 weeks of age and 25 mg/kg thereafter. Evidence suggests that feeding the lower concentrations of organic Zn or Cu (satisfying EU legislation), instead of high inorganic sources of Cu and Zn will result in adequate growth performance with substantially less nutrients being excreted into the environment.

References

Apgar, G. A., Kornegay, E. T., Lindemann, M. D., and Notter, D. R. (1995) Evaluation of copper sulfate and a copper lysine complex as growth promoters for weanling swine. *Journal of Animal Science* **73:** 2640-2646.

Apgar, G. A., and Kornegay, E. T. (1996) Mineral balance of finishing pigs fed copper sulfate or copper-lysine complex at growth-stimulating levels. *Journal of Animal Science* **74:** 1594-1600.

Armstrong, T. A., Cook, D. R., Ward, M. M., Williams, C. M., and Spears, J. W. (2004) Effect of dietary copper source (cupric citrate and cupric sulfate) and concentration on growth performance and fecal copper excretion in weanling pigs. *Journal of Animal Science* **82:** 1234-1240.

Barber, R. S., Braude, R., and Mitchell, K. G. (1955) Antibiotic and copper supplements for fattening pigs. *British Journal of Nutrition* **9:** 378-382.

Carlson, M. S., Hoover, S. L., Hill, G. M., Link, J. E., and Turk, J. R. (1998) Effect of pharmacological zinc on intestinal metallothionein concentration and morphology in nursery pigs. *Journal of Animal Science* **76** (Suppl. 1)**:** 57 (Abstr.).

Carlson, M. S., Hill G. M., and Link, J. E. (1999) Early- and traditionally weaned nursery pigs benefit from phase-feeding pharmacological concentrations of zinc oxide: Effect on metallothionein and mineral concentrations. *Journal of Animal Science* **77:** 1199-1207.

Carlson, M. S., Boren, C. A., Wu, C., Huntington, C. E., Bollinger, D. W., and Veum, T. L. (2004) Evaluation of various inclusion rates of organic zinc either as polysaccharide or proteinate complex on the growth performance, plasma, and excretion of nursery pigs. *Journal of Animal Science* **82:** 1359-1366.

Case, C. L., and Carlson, M. S. (2002) Effect of feeding organic and inorganic sources of additional zinc on growth performance and zinc balance in nursery pigs. *Journal of Animal Science* **80:** 1917-1924.

Cheng, J., Kornegay, E. T., and Schell, T. (1998) Influence of dietary lysine on the utilization of zinc from zinc sulfate and a zinc-lysine complex by young pigs. *Journal of Animal Science* **76:** 1064-1074.

Coffey, R. D., Cromwell, G. L., and Monegue, H. J. (1994) Efficacy of copper-lysine complex as a growth promotant for weanling pigs. *Journal of Animal Science* **72:** 2880-2886.

Cromwell, G. L., Stahly, T. S., and Monegue, H. J. (1989) Effects of source and level of copper on performance and liver copper stores in weanling pigs. *Journal of Animal Science* **67:** 2996-3002.

Cromwell, G. L., Lindemann, M. D., Monegue, H. J., Hall, D. D., and Orr Jr., D. E. (1998) Tribasic copper chloride and copper sulfate as copper sources for weanling pigs. *Journal of Animal Science* **82:** 581-587.

Davis, M. E., Brown, D. C., Maxwell, C. V., Johnson, Z. B., Kegley, E. B., and Dvorak, R. A. (2004) Effect of phosphorylated mannans and pharmacological additions of zinc oxide on growth performance and immunocompetence of weanling pigs. *Journal of Animal Science* **80:** 2887-2894.

Davis, M. E., Maxwell, C. V., Brown, D. C., de Rodas, B. Z., Johnson, Z. B., Kegley, E. B., Hellwig, D. H., and Dvorak, R. A. (2002) Effect of dietary mannan oligosaccharides and (or) pharmacological additions of copper sulfate on growth performance and immunocompetence of weanling and growing/finishing pigs. *Journal of Animal Science* **80:** 2887-2894.

de Rodas, B. Z., Maxwell, C. V., Brown, D. C., Davis, M. E., Johnson, Z. B., and Fakler, T. M. (1999) Effect of diet complexity and supplemental zinc amino acid complexes on performance of nursery pigs. *Journal of Animal Science* **77** (Suppl. 1): 177 (Abstr.).

Dove C. R. (1995) The effect of copper level on nutrient utilization of weanling pigs. *Journal of Animal Science* **73:** 166-171.

Dove C. R. (1993) The effect of adding copper and various fat sources to the diets of weanling swine on growth performance and serum fatty acid profiles. *Journal of Animal Science* **71:** 2187-2192.

Dove, C. R., and Haydon, K. D. (1992) The effect of copper and fat addition to the diets of weanling swine on growth performance and serum fatty acids. *Journal of Animal Science* **70:** 805-810.

Fuller, R. L., Newland, G. M., Briggs, C. A. E., Braude, R., and Mitchell, K. G. (1960) The normal intestinal flora of the pig. IV. The effect of dietary supplement, of penicillin, chlortetracycline or copper sulfate on fecal flora. *Journal of Applied Bacteriology* **23:** 195-202.

Hahn, J. D., and Baker, D. H. (1993) Growth and plasma zinc responses of young pigs fed pharmacological levels of zinc. *Journal of Animal Science* **71:** 3020-3024.

Hill, G. M., Mahan, D.C., Carter, S. D., Cromwell, G. L., Ewan, R. C., Harrold, R. L., Lewis, A. J., Miller, P. S., Shurson, G. C., and Veum, T. L. (2001) Effect of pharmacological concentrations of zinc oxide with or without the inclusion of an antibacterial agent on nursery pig performance. *Journal of Animal Science* **79:** 934-941.

Hill, G. M., Cromwell, G. L., Crenshaw, T. D., Dove, C. R., Ewan, R. C., Knabe, D. A., Lewis, A. J., Libal, G. W., Mahan, D. C., Shurson, G. C., Southern, L. L., and Veum, T. L. (2000) Growth promotion effects and plasma changes from feeding high dietary concentrations of zinc and copper to weanling pigs (regional study). *Journal of Animal Science* **78:** 1010-1016.

Martinez, M. M., Hill, G. M., Link, J. E., Raney, N. E., Tempelman, R. J., and Ernst, C. W. (2004) Pharmacological zinc and phytase supplementation enhance metallothionein mRNA abundance and protein concentration in newly weaned pigs. *Journal of Nutrition* **134:** 538-544.

Mavromichalis, I., Peter, C. M., Parr, T. M., Ganessunker, D., and Baker, D. H. (2000) Growth-promoting efficacy in young pigs of two sources of zinc oxide having either a high or a low bioavailability of zinc. *Journal of Animal Science* **78:** 2896-2902.

McCalla, J. M., Gallaher, D. D., Johnston, L. J., Whitney, M. H., and Shurson, G. C. (1999) Evaluation of the optimal growth promoting level of dietary Zn from a Zn amino acid complex for weanling pigs. *Journal of Animal Science* **77** (Suppl. 1)**:** 64 (Abstr.)

Mullan, B. P., Wilson, R. H., Harris, D., Allen, J. G., and Naylor, A. (2002) Supplementation of weaner pig diets with zinc oxide or Bioplex™ Zinc. In: *Nutritional Biotechnology in the Feed and Food Industries: Proceedings of Alltech's 18th Annual Symposium* (T.P. Lyons and K.A. Jacques, eds.). Nottingham University Press, Nottingham, UK.

NRC. (1998) Nutrient Requirements of Swine (10th Ed.). National Academy Press, Washington DC.

O'Dell, B. L. (1989) Mineral interactions relevant to nutrient requirements. *Journal of Nutrition* **119:** 1832-1838.

Owusu-Asiedu, A., Nyachoti, C. M., and Marquardt, R. R. (2003) Response of early-weaned pigs to an enterotoxigenic *Escherichia coli* (K88) challenge when fed diets containing spray-dried porcine plasma or pea protein isolate plus egg yolk antibody, zinc oxide, fumaric acid or antibiotic. *Journal of Animal Science* **81:** 1790-1798.

Poulsen, H. D. (1995) Zinc oxide for weanling piglets. *Acta Agriculturae Scandinavica Section A, Animal Science* **45:** 159-167.

Poulsen, H. D., and Larsen, T. (1995) Zinc excretion and retention in growing pigs fed increasing levels of zinc oxide. *Livestock Production Science* **43:** 235-241.

Roof, M.D., and Mahan, D.C. (1982) Effect of carbadox and various dietary copper levels for weanling swine. *Journal of Animal Science* **55:** 1109-117.

Roselli, M., Finamore, A., Garaguso, I., Britti, M. S., and Mangheri, E. (2003) Zinc oxide protects cultured enterocytes from the damage induced by *Escherichia coli. Journal of Nutrition* **133:** 4077-4082.

Schell, T. C., and Kornegay, E. T. (1996) Zinc concentration in tissues and performance of weanling pigs fed pharmacological levels of zinc from ZnO, Zn-Methionine, Zn-Lysine, or $ZnSO_4$. *Journal of Animal Science* **74:** 1584-1593.

Smith, J. W. II, Tokach, M. D., Goodband, R. D., Nelssen, J. L., and Richert, B. T. (1997) Effects of the interrelationships between zinc oxide and copper sulfate on growth performance of early-weaned pigs. *Journal of Animal Science* **75:** 1861-1866.

Spears, J. W. (1993) Organic trace minerals in ruminant nutrition. In: *Proceedings of the 14th Canadian Western Nutrition Conference.* Calgary, Alberta. pp. 269.

Stahly, T. S., Cromwell, G. L., and Monegue, H. J. (1980) Effects of the dietary inclusion of copper and (or) antibiotics on the performance of weanling pigs. *Journal of Animal Science* **51:** 1347-1351.

Stansbury, W. F., Tribble, L. F., and Orr Jr, D. E. (1990) Effect of chelated copper sources on performance of nursery and growing pigs. *Journal of Animal Science* **68:** 1318-1322.

Van Heugten, E., Spears, J. W., Kegley, E. B., Ward, J. D., and Qureshi, M. A. (2003) Effects of organic forms of zinc on growth performance, tissue zinc distribution, and immune response of weanling pigs. *Journal of Animal Science* **81:** 2063-2071.

Veum, T. L., Carlson, M. S., Wu, C., Bollinger, D. W., and Ellersieck,

M. R. (2004) Copper proteinate in weanling pig diets for enhancing growth performance and reducing fecal copper excretion compared with copper sulfate. *Journal of Animal Science* **82:** 1062-1070.

Ward, T. L., Asche, G. A., Louis, G. F., and Pollmann, D. S. (1996) Zinc-methionine improves growth performance of starter pigs. *Journal of Animal Science* **74**(Suppl. 1)**:** 303 (Abstr.).

Wedekind, K. J., Lewis, A. J., Giesemann, M. A., and Miller, P. S. (1994) Bioavailability of zinc from inorganic and organic sources for pigs fed corn-soybean meal diets. *Journal of Animal Science* **72:** 2681-2689.

Woodworth, J. C., Tokach, M. D., Nelssen, J. L., Goodband, R. D., Quinn, P. R. O., and Fakler, T. M. (1999) The effects of added zinc from an organic zinc complex or inorganic zinc sources on weanling pig growth performance. *Journal of Animal Science* 77 (Suppl. 1)**:** 61 (Abstr.).

Zhou, W., Kornegay, E. T., Laarvan, H., Swinkels, J. W. G. M., Wong, E. A., and Lindeman, M. D. (1994a) The role of feed consumption and feed efficiency in copper-stimulated growth. *Journal of Animal Science* **72:** 2385-2394.

Zhou, W., Kornegay, E. T., Lindeman, M. D., Swinkels, J. W. G. M., Welten, M. K., and Wong, E. A. (1994b) Stimulation of growth by intravenous injection of copper in weanling pigs. *Journal of Animal Science* **72:** 2395-2403.

The role of organic minerals in modern pig production

Bruce Mullan and Darryl D'Souza
Animal Research and Development, Western Australian Department of Agriculture

Introduction

The pork industry in most countries continues to face many challenges, including often large fluctuations in profitability and hence security. This is despite there being more pork consumed in the world than any other meat. While the world demand for pork is expected to increase, especially with the improved standard of living in many developing countries, competition for these markets will be high. The industry is hence driven by a need to improve efficiency, lower the cost of production and to produce a product that meets the expectations of the consumer. Those producers and/ or countries that will continue to be involved in pig production will be those that are prepared to evaluate and adopt new technologies to remain competitive on an increasingly global market. This paper reviews how the industry has changed in recent years, some of the major challenges that face the industry and the particular role that organic minerals have in pig production.

Modern pig production

Structure of the industry

One of the biggest changes that has occurred in many countries has been the move away from the traditional farrow-to-finish family-owned unit, to multi-site contract operations. The major reason for the change to multi-site production systems is to reduce the challenge from disease. In most countries there has also been an increase in vertical integration, with the same company being involved in feed manufacturing, pig production, processing and, in some instances, the retail industry. The drive to reduce the cost of production has also seen an increase in the size of pig units, since it gives the opportunity to spread the overhead costs over a larger number of animals. For example, in Australia 87% of breeding sows are kept by approximately 24% of producers (Australian Pork Limited, 2004). In the US between 1980 and 2000, the number of piggeries declined by almost 90%, while there has been an almost seven-fold increase in the average number of pigs per operation (Stalder *et al.*, 2004). An increasing proportion of pigs are also now produced under contract with decisions on genetics, feed, building design and health programs no longer the direct responsibility of the person who is providing the day-to-day care.

Productivity

The major reason for being involved in pig production is to make a profitable return on investment. Unfortunately there is usually little that producers can do to influence the price received for their product, so most attention is focused on the cost of production and volume of product produced per unit of capital invested. Despite a relatively large amount of funds having been spent on pig research and development in many countries, the improvements in productivity over time have been modest. For example, while some producers are able to wean above 25 piglets per sow per year, the average for many is less than 20 (Close, 2004). There are many reasons why we have not seen the improvements in productivity that we might have expected. In some instances there has been sufficient profit without having to strive for improved efficiency. In other cases it is the lack of resources, such as capital for improved facilities or the lack of skilled labour that has hampered progress. Nevertheless there is growing interest in the role that nutrient supply, especially that of minerals, has on sow productivity and hence profitability.

Making certain that pigs receive the optimal balance of nutrients to meet their requirements is important if pigs are to grow or produce to their genetic potential. By far the largest cost in pork production is feed, comprising between 60 and 70% of total production costs. As a consequence, feed additives are often closely scrutinised, especially at times when the cost of the main ingredients is relatively high. There can be a temptation to remove some additives from diets as one way of reducing the cost per tonne of the complete ration. This means that those involved with the feed industry need to have a basic understanding of the mode of action of additives, what improvements in productivity have been achieved in well-controlled commercial studies, and to have an idea of the cost benefit. This is particularly important with the use of organic minerals in the breeding herd, since the benefits to using these products on, for example, the number of piglets born alive per litter, or on culling rate of sows, may take several months to show.

Close and Turnley (2004) describe how the Premier Pig Program™ has been developed to provide independent technical information and support to the pig industry worldwide. An important aspect of this program is to encourage producers to set target objectives for performance, and to then identify actions and solutions that can be taken on-farm to enhance performance. In this way productivity and economic efficiency can be improved. The program has been launched in a number of countries and has been well received by producers, an indication that part of the cause for lack of improvement in technology is a lack of technical information in a format that is easy to adopt.

Current and future challenges to the pork industry

There are a host of factors that will determine how the pig industry will be structured and operate in the future. Three factors that are of particular importance are the impact of the industry on the environment, the increased concern for the welfare of pigs, and product quality. While the requirements differ between countries, the increase in international pork trading will mean that ultimately all producers will be affected in some way.

Environment

Stalder *et al.* (2004) have documented the differences in the density of pigs between a range of countries. For example, in the Netherlands there are on average 14 pigs per hectare, whereas in Saskatchewan, Canada, the figure is 0.07 pigs per hectare. On this basis alone, it is not surprising that the pressure to reduce pig production in the Netherlands on environmental grounds is greater than it might be in Canada. However, even in countries where there are seemingly huge areas available for pig production there is still increasing concern about the impact of this intensive industry on the environment. Public concerns are mainly related to soil (accumulation and runoff of minerals from land where manure is applied), water (surface and ground water), and air quality environmental issues (Stalder *et al.*, 2004). While it is possible to reduce the environmental impact of minerals by the treatment of effluent, a more sustainable approach is to reduce the concentration in effluent by either feeding the animal closer to its requirement, and/or feeding minerals in a form that are more bioavailable to the animal.

Welfare

Animal welfare activists have had an enormous impact on the pig industry in some countries, particularly in Europe. From a nutritional perspective, it is important to satisfy the animal's requirements for essential nutrients so as to give it the best possible chance to cope with the environment in which it is housed.

Consumers

There is a growing awareness in the meat industry that the needs of customers are changing, and that we need to do more to provide what is required. Consumers require a product that they enjoy eating, is nutritious, and has been produced with high standards of food safety. Price is also a major factor that drives consumer choice, and so the cost of production has to be kept under control. Whether it is the person buying pig feed, or the person buying the end product from the supermarket, customers are going to become more demanding.

Mineral supplementation

Mineral requirements

Requirements for minerals are difficult to establish and most estimates are based on the minimum level required to overcome a deficiency symptom, and not necessarily to promote productivity or indeed, to enhance immunity (Close, 2003). Much of the research to determine mineral requirements was conducted more than 40 years ago, with genotypes and rearing systems much different to that in today's modern commercial piggeries. As a consequence, recommended mineral allowances have evolved over time and it is not surprising that when Whittemore *et al.* (2002) conducted a survey of dietary mineral additions in several European Union countries, there was a wide variation with some 3 to 4 times higher than those recommended by the ARC or NRC (Table 1). Van Lunen and Cole (1998) have suggested that the mineral needs for growth in the modern fast-growing pig are about twice the level required by the slower growing pigs of some 20-30 years ago, but the nature of research conducted in the 1960s and 1970s has not been conducted to the same extent in recent times. This is possibly because it is difficult and expensive research to undertake, and in most cases there are other areas of research considered to be of higher priority on which to spend limited funds. One research area that has increased in importance is that related to animal health, and there is increasing evidence of strong relationships between an animal's immune status and its mineral status.

Most pigs in commercial facilities are challenged by one or more diseases at some time during their production cycle. Williams (1998) has demonstrated that when there is minimal activation of the immune system, feed intake is increased and the rate and efficiency of growth is greater compared to animals subject to a disease challenge. It was therefore suggested that disease status has a direct bearing on the nutrient requirements of the animal, and Williams (1998) demonstrated this by showing how the requirement for lysine is affected by immune system activation. In regards to mineral requirements, most experiments are conducted on high health status research facilities, and we know little about the requirement for animals challenged by disease in commercial facilities. Nevertheless, we can speculate that the mineral requirement would increase, especially for those minerals with a direct role in the function of the immune system, and that organic minerals would be of greater benefit than similar minerals in the inorganic form because of their higher bioavailability.

Table 1.
Range of dietary mineral additions in several EU countries (per kg feed) (Whittemore et al., 2002)

	Piglet	Growing pig	Finishing pig	Breeding sow
Body weight (kg)	- 20	20 – 50	50 – 120	
Zinc (mg)	100 – 200	100 –200	70 – 150	80 – 125
Manganese (mg)	40 – 50	30 – 50	25 – 45	40 – 60
Iron (mg)	80 – 175	80 – 150	65 – 110	80 – 150
Copper (mg)	6 – 18	6 – 12	6 – 8	6 – 20
Iodine (mg)	0.2 –1	0.2 – 1.5	0.2 – 1.5	0.2 – 2.0
Selenium (mg)	0.2 – 0.3	0.15 – 0.3	0.2 – 0.3	0.2 – 0.4

Sources of minerals

Inorganic salts, such as sulphates, carbonates, chlorides and oxides are traditionally added to the diet to provide the correct levels to meet the animals' needs (Henman, 2001; Close, 2003). These salts are broken down in the digestive tract to form free ions that can form complexes with other dietary molecules, making them difficult to absorb. The free ions are also very reactive and interactions between various minerals have to be taken into account when developing a nutritional program. For example, when Mullan et al. (2002) fed diets containing either 0, 1.5, 3.0 or 4.5 kg/tonne of zinc oxide, the concentration of zinc in plasma increased. However, there was a negative correlation between plasma zinc and plasma copper; a 3-fold increase in plasma zinc corresponded to a 4-fold decline in plasma copper, sufficient enough for individual pigs to be deemed copper deficient. Interactions such as these may explain why at times animals do not respond to an increased supply of an inorganic mineral in the way that we might otherwise expect.

Close (2003) reviewed results from a number of studies where the bioavailability of inorganic minerals was measured. Bioavailability was defined as the degree to which an ingested nutrient in a particular source is absorbed in a form that can be utilised or metabolised by the animal. With zinc, for example, it was suggested that 75 to 80% of the ingested zinc from inorganic sources is excreted by animals. It is therefore little wonder that there is interest in using forms of minerals that are better absorbed and utilised by animals.

When trace minerals are chemically bound to a chelating agent or ligand, usually a mixture of amino acids or small peptides, much lower concentrations can be used in the diet because of the higher bioavailability. They are also less reactive with other minerals, making the design of a mineral supplementation program much more reliable. Minerals in this organic form provide the animal with a metabolic advantage that often results in improved performance.

Impact of organic minerals on the pig industry

Performance

Weaner nutrition

Zinc oxide has traditionally been added to piglet weaner diets to supply 100g of added zinc per tonne of feed (approximately 125 g zinc oxide per tonne) for the prevention of zinc deficiency. More recently the beneficial effects of adding high levels of zinc oxide to weaner diets to reduce the incidence of post-weaning diarrhoea and scours has been reported (refer also to Carlson's chapter in this publication). For example, Holm (1990) reported that in commercial trials mortality rate was reduced from 2.2 to 0.7%, and growth rate increased from 281 to 327 g/day when pigs received a diet containing 3200g of added zinc for the 2 weeks after weaning. The use of zinc oxide has been considered an inexpensive alternative to the use of antibiotics for the control of post-weaning scours, and one that has previously not required veterinary approval within the EU. As a consequence, the supplementation of diets with zinc oxide for 2 to 3 weeks after weaning has been widely practised.

However, the high concentrations of zinc in faecal matter are of concern, and the use of high levels of zinc oxide is now banned in some countries. A number of studies have thus been undertaken to evaluate the use of Bioplex™ (Alltech Inc. Nicholasville) organic zinc as a possible alternative to zinc oxide, because of its higher bioavailability. In one study, Mullan *et al.* (2002) fed pigs weaned at 21 days either a) Control diet containing no added zinc besides that included in mineral premix, b) 1500-2250 ppm zinc from zinc oxide, or c) 100 or 250 ppm zinc from Bioplex™ zinc. Piglets receiving the diet containing Bioplex™ 250 had a significantly (P < 0.05) higher growth rate, and at the end of the experiment (60 days of age) were 11 % heavier than those on the Control diet (Figure 1). These results suggested that adding 250ppm of Bioplex™ zinc to the diet of weaner pigs has advantages over the current recommendation of adding high levels of zinc oxide. However, since post-weaning diarrhoea or scours were not observed, this study was unable to directly answer the question of how well Bioplex™ zinc would control post-weaning diarrhoea or scours.

High levels of zinc have been added to weaner diets because of its known pharmacological effects. However, zinc also has a positive effect on both the immune response to pathogens and the prevention of disease by maintaining healthy epithelial tissue (Close, 2003). Carlson et al. (1998) have reported that high levels of zinc oxide alters duodenal morphology (deeper crypts and greater total thickness), and increased intestinal metallothionein concentration, which suggests that high amounts of zinc may have an enteric effect on the pig. With the move to restrict or ban the use of antibiotics in pig diets, it is important that we know more about the way minerals such as zinc might influence the impact of pathogens so that we can develop feeding strategies that are beneficial to the animal, are cost effective and friendly to the environment.

Figure 1. Average daily gain (ADG) of weaner pigs (21d) fed diets containing either zinc oxide (Control 190 ppm, ZnO at 2300 ppm) or Bioplex™ zinc (100 or 250 ppm) for the initial 39 days post-weaning. (Mullan et al, 2002)

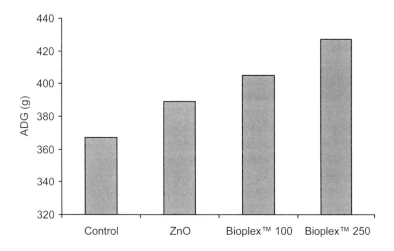

Growers and finishers

Grower and finisher pigs use by far the largest proportion of feed, and thus there is interest in any nutritional modification that will improve growth rate, feed conversion and carcass quality. Henman (2001) evaluated the impact on performance of grower-finisher pigs fed diets containing copper sulphate or Bioplex™ copper. Compared to the base diet that contained 20 ppm of copper sulphate, additional copper improved growth rate by 5% and feed conversion by 3% (Table 2). Importantly, there was no difference in performance between the pigs given 100 ppm Bioplex™ copper and those fed 200 ppm copper sulphate. It is data such as this, conducted in a commercial piggery, that provide the opportunity to evaluate the cost effectiveness of the alternative to inorganic copper.

Table 2.
The growth performance and carcass characteristics of male pigs fed diets containing two levels of copper sulphate and Bioplex™ copper.
(Henman, 2001)

Copper level	$CuSO_4$ 20 ppm	$CuSO_4$ 200 ppm	Bioplex™ Cu 100 ppm
Start weight (kg)	28.0	27.5	27.9
Final weight (kg)	88.7	90.7	91.7
Average daily gain (g)	726	731	766
Feed:gain	2.51	2.44	2.43
Average daily intake (kg)	1.82	1.78	1.86
Carcass weight (kg)	64.3	67.7	68.8
P2 fat thickness (mm)	9.6	9.6	9.7
Dressing %	74.5	74.8	75.1

In a more recent experiment, Mullan *et al.* (2004) compared copper and zinc provided in either the inorganic or organic (Bioplex™) form fed to pigs from 45 days of age (16 kg LW) until slaughter at 134 days of age. Pigs fed copper and zinc in the organic form were significantly leaner than those fed diets containing inorganic copper and zinc (11.8 vs. 13.8 mm P2, respectively; P=0.016). The authors were unable to explain the reason for this response, and the improved carcass quality of pigs fed these minerals in the organic form is the subject of current research. Due to the high proportion of costs attributable to feeding grower and finisher pigs, and also the possible impact on value of the end product, it is important that we improve our understanding of how pigs respond to organic minerals in relation to form and level of supplementation.

Breeding pigs

Perhaps the best demonstration that pigs in modern production systems are not being fed diets containing adequate amounts of minerals is that reported by Mahan and Newton (1995) for the high-producing lactating sow. They have shown that the body mineral content of sows at the end of their third parity was considerably lower when mean litter weaning weight at 21 days was above 60 kg than below 55 kg, and for both groups it was significantly less, by as much as 20%, than for unbred control animals of similar age. Thus, the higher the level of production, the greater the mineral needs of the animal. Interestingly, the levels of minerals in the diet were those proposed by NRC (1988).

Mahan and colleagues have undertaken an extensive series of experiments to determine the influence of organic minerals on performance of breeding pigs, and demonstrated very clearly the importance of supplying adequate minerals in a bioavailable form. For example, in one large study, gilts were fed diets that contained either a basal non-selenium-fortified diet, or two selenium sources (organic (Sel-plex™, Alltech Inc. Nicholasville) or inorganic (Sodium selenite)) each providing 0.15 and 0.30 ppm selenium or their combination (each providing 0.15 ppm selenium). The experiment commenced when the gilts were 28 kg and continued through until the end of their fourth parity. None of the treatments had any impact on performance during the grower period, but at 115 kg body weight, selenium levels were higher when gilts had been fed inorganic selenium compared to the basal diet, and higher still when fed organic selenium. Selenium levels in the neonate, colostrum, milk and sow tissues were higher when organic selenium was fed compared to inorganic selenium.

Since selenium is important at farrowing, indicated by the incidence of stillbirths, and during lactation because of the importance of selenium in milk to piglet vigour and health, improving the selenium status of sows will be beneficial to sow productivity. In fact, Fehse and Close (2000) demonstrated a reduction in culling rate of older parity sows, suggesting that these animals were better able to maintain productivity, when supplemented with a number of organic minerals known to have a role in reproduction.

Relatively few studies have been conducted with the breeding boar, but for a herd to achieve its potential then it is important that semen quality is also optimised. Marin-Guzman *et al.* (1997) evaluated the effects of dietary selenium and vitamin E on semen quality and its subsequent fertilisation rate in mature gilts. Boars fed low selenium diets produced a higher percentage of abnormal sperm, and while vitamin E is also important for boars, the authors considered that it might function in a different manner to that of selenium. A more recent study conducted by Jacyno *et al.* (2002) reported significant improvements in sperm concentration and sperm number ($P < 0.05$), and over a 40% reduction in defective sperm ($P < 0.01$) when 0.2ppm of Se was added to the diets of young boars in the organic form (Sel-plex™), compared with inorganic sodium selenite.

Pork quality

Food safety, price, nutritive value, meal convenience and appearance play an important role in determining whether consumers purchase meat, in addition to the type and cut of meat

(D'Souza and Mullan, 2001). However, it is the eating experience or the quality of the product that influences the consumer to re-purchase. There is intense competition in the food industry to attract and retain consumers, and it is this that has driven the agricultural industries to produce what the consumer requires, rather than what we think might be required.

A complex interaction of animal, pre-slaughter and post-slaughter factors can have a significant influence on meat quality (D'Souza and Mullan, 2001). Meat quality defects such as pale, soft, exudative (PSE) meat in pigs and poultry, and dark, firm, dry (DFD) meat in pigs, cattle and sheep still remain a major problem. While considerable research has been directed at identifying best practice to optimise meat quality, these are sometimes difficult and expensive to adopt. An alternative strategy to improve meat quality has focussed on pre-slaughter dietary nutrient supplementation, in particular the use of organic magnesium and selenium.

Magnesium

Magnesium is abundant in intracellular fluid and is an important cofactor of numerous enzyme systems (Stryer, 1988). Magnesium has a relaxant effect on skeletal muscle (Hubbard, 1973), and dietary supplementation has been shown to help alleviate the effects of stress by reducing plasma cortisol, norepinephrine, epinephrine and dopamine concentrations (Niemack et al., 1979; Kietzman and Jablonski, 1985). Consequently, studies have been conducted to investigate the influence of dietary magnesium-supplementation on reducing the effects of stress and improving meat quality.

D'Souza et al. (1988) have shown that dietary magnesium aspartate (3.2 g elemental Mg fed for 5 days pre-slaughter) supplementation significantly improved pork quality in pigs by reducing drip loss and improving pork colour and muscle pH (Table 3). The use of Bioplex™ magnesium at 1.6 g elemental magnesium for two days pre-slaughter (Table 4) similarly resulted in reduced drip loss and a lower incidence of PSE (D'Souza and Mullan, 1999). In a study that compared the influence of organic and inorganic magnesium compounds on meat quality, D'Souza et al., (2000) reported that the improvements in muscle colour, drip loss, and the reductions in the incidence of PSE were greater with organic magnesium compounds. This difference was attributed to the increased bioavailability of elemental magnesium when fed in the organic form.

Table 3.
The effect of dietary magnesium aspartate (MgAsp) supplementation and pre-slaughter handling on meat quality indicators of the *Longissimus thoracis* muscle 24hrs post-slaughter. (D'Souza *et al.* (1998).

Diet (D)	Control		MgAsp		
Handling (H)	Minimal	Negative	Minimal	Negative	Significance
Ultimate pH	5.48	5.51	5.61	5.57	D**
Surface lightness L*	48.7	49.1	45.2	47.4	D**
Drip loss, %	4.0	6.4	3.5	3.5	D**; H*
PSE, %	8	33	0	0	D*

*$P<0.05$; **$P<0.01$; ***$P<0.001$

Table 4.
The effect of dietary Bioplex™ magnesium supplementation on meat quality indicators in the *Longissimus thoracis* muscle 24hrs post-slaughter. (D'Souza and Mullan, 1999).

	Diet		Significance
	Control	Bioplex™ Magnesium	
Ultimate pH	5.39	5.40	NS
Surface lightness L*	54.10	52.30	NS
Drip loss, %	6.50	3.60	***
PSE, %	50.00	15.00	*

*$P<0.05$; ***$P<0.001$

In an Australian study conducted under commercial conditions, Hofmeyr *et al.*, (1999) have demonstrated that dietary organic magnesium supplementation is a viable method to improve meat quality in pigs. The incidence of soft, exudative (SE) pork in all three replicates was significantly reduced when pigs received a diet containing organic magnesium for two days pre-slaughter (Figure 2). The unusually high incidence of SE pork in Replicate 1 was due to a high number of halothane gene carrier pigs used in this replicate.

Figure 2.
Effect of organic magnesium supplementation on the incidence of soft and exudative (SE) pork in the *longissimus thoracis* muscle (Hofmeyr *et al.*, 1999).

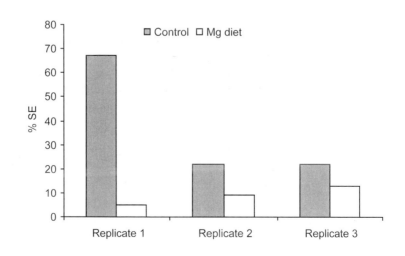

Selenium

Although inorganic selenium (sodium selenite) is regularly used as a source of selenium in diets for pigs of all ages, extensive research by Mahan and colleagues has shown that the use of organic selenium (Sel-Plex™) has additional benefits that surpass that of selenite. When organic selenium was fed to growing pigs, a linear and significant increase in the selenium content of muscle tissue was observed (Mahan *et al.*, 1999). In the same study, supplementation with inorganic selenium gave only a minimal increase in muscle selenium concentrations. Additionally, there were indications that when inorganic Se was fed it was bound to muscle tissue in a form that may be detrimental to muscle tissue, whereas that in the organic form was incorporated into the muscle proteins and did not seem to affect quality of pork loins. In a recent study, D'Souza (unpublished), investigated the use of magnesium and selenium in feed to enhance pork quality. Pork from pigs fed diets supplemented with magnesium (16g Mg Bioplex™ and 0.4g Sel-Plex™/kg of feed) had significantly improved meat colour at 24h post-slaughter and lower drip loss at 24h, 7 and 21days post-slaughter compared to pigs fed the control diet.

Apart from possible effects on pork quality, perhaps the greatest interest in feeding grower pigs organic selenium is to increase selenium concentrations in the meat, with subsequent health benefits to consumers. Schrauzer (2002) presented evidence that a daily extra-dietary supplement of 200 μg of selenium reduces cancer risk and increases resistance to viral infections in humans. In Korea this has been taken a step further where the pig industry has capitalised on selenium-enriched pork as a functional food and are currently incorporating Sel-Plex™ in pig diets. The product is marketed as selenium-enriched pork (SelenPork), as a functional food benefiting human health and nutrition. Consumer feedback also indicates that Koreans regard SelenPork as being juicier and having better appearance (D'Souza and Mullan, 2001).

Use of organic minerals for meat quality by industry

Supplementing pig feeds with organic magnesium and selenium has been shown to have positive effects on pork quality, which is of direct benefit to the processing sector through a reduction in drip loss, and to consumers through an improvement in eating quality and nutrient content. Despite this, the adoption rate of both practices has been slow in most countries. It is common in many countries for producers to be paid on the basis of carcass quality (e.g. % lean or depth of backfat) rather than on aspects of meat quality. This is partly due to it being more difficult to measure meat quality on-line, but also due to many processors failing to recognise the value in improvements. Unless producers are rewarded financially for improving meat quality, then the adoption of these nutritional strategies will remain low. However, in many countries the link between retailers, processors and producers is becoming stronger, and as such it is only a matter of time before the use of organic minerals are considered part of best practice.

Environmental impact

The expansion and concentration of the pig industry in many areas of the world has caused increased concern about the disposal of effluent. Most attention is given to the levels of nitrogen and phosphorus, but trace minerals such as copper and zinc are also important since they too can cause problems to aquatic organisms or to grazing livestock if the effluent is not contained and/or treated. Inorganic copper and zinc have for some time been fed at pharmacological levels, well above the animal's requirements, to promote growth and prevent scouring and diarrhoea, respectively. However, the high concentrations in piggery effluent, and the subsequent damage that can result, has led the Animal Feed Committee of the European Union to propose maximum inclusion levels that are well below current authorized levels (Close, 2003). Hence there is interest in evaluating the use of organic trace minerals, such as Bioplex™ copper and Bioplex™ zinc, because of their higher bioavailability compared to inorganic forms.

Zinc

Mullan et al., (2002) evaluated the use of Bioplex™ zinc included at either 100 or 250 ppm as an alternative to using high concentrations of zinc oxide (1500-2250 ppm) in the diet of pigs weaned at 21 days of age (see weaner nutrition earlier in this chapter). These diets were compared to a control diet that only contained the base level of zinc from the standard weaner premix being used at that time. The diets were fed for 19 days post-weaning and faecal samples were then taken and analysed for zinc. The concentration of zinc in faecal material was almost four times higher when inorganic zinc was fed at therapeutic levels compared to the base level contained in the control diet (Table 5). However, when zinc was fed in the organic form (Bioplex™ zinc), the concentration in faecal material was similar to that in the control animals.

Wu et al. (2001) has also reported similar differences in the zinc concentration in faecal matter when pigs were fed either 2000 ppm zinc from zinc oxide, as compared to those fed 200 or 400 ppm organic zinc. Provided pig performance is not compromised when organic zinc is used, then the above two studies demonstrate that the use of organic forms of zinc is one way to reduce the zinc concentration in piggery effluent.

Table 5.
Concentration of zinc (ppm) in feed and faecal samples on a dry matter basis (Mullan *et al.*, 2002)

Treatment	Control	Zinc oxide	Bioplex™ 100	Bioplex™ 250	P =	l.s.d.
Feed	190	2300	260	370		
Faeces	2290	8910	1960	1830	0.001	931

Copper

Smits and Henman (2000) evaluated the performance of grower and finisher pigs fed diets supplemented with either copper sulphate (150 ppm Cu) or organic copper (40 ppm Cu). Those pigs fed the diets containing organic Cu at 40 ppm achieved similar levels of performance to those fed 150 ppm Cu from copper sulphate (Table 6). However, the quantity of copper excreted in the faeces was 3 to 4 times lower in the pigs fed the organic copper. Pierce *et al.*, (2001) have also measured the faecal copper content of growing pigs when fed either a control diet, or diets containing copper sulphate or Bioplex™ copper. Those pigs fed the organic copper had similar performance to those fed an inorganic source of copper, but had a 46% decrease in faecal copper concentrations.

Table 6.
The growth performance and faecal Cu excretion of pigs fed different Cu sources (Smits and Henman 2000)

Diet	Control (no added Cu)	CuSO$_4$ (150 ppm Cu)	Bioplex™ Cu (40 ppm Cu)
Growers (30-60 kg)			
Feed intake (kg/d)	1.94	2.05	2.08
Growth rate (kg/d)	0.90	0.95	0.96
Feed : Gain (kg/kg)	2.15	2.16	2.21
Faecal Cu (mg/kg DM)	130	853	275
Finishers (60-90 kg)			
Feed intake (kg/d)	2.35	2.59	2.65
Growth rate (kg/d)	0.85	0.87	0.84
Feed : Gain (kg/kg)	2.84	2.98	3.02
Faecal Cu (mg/kg DM)	108	776	198

In a similar study, this time with weaner pigs, Carlson (2001) measured the faecal output of copper when diets contained either 50 or 100 ppm of organic (Bioplex™) copper, or 250 ppm copper sulphate. Faecal output of copper was substantially higher when fed as copper sulphate (Figure 3) and there was no significant impact on growth performance. Wu *et al.*, (2001) have also results that demonstrate the beneficial impact on copper excretion when Bioplex™ copper was fed instead of copper sulphate in nursery pig diets. Thus it seems that the benefits to growth of using copper supplementation can be maintained through the use of organic forms of copper, rather than copper sulphate, greatly reducing the level of copper in effluent and hence reducing the impact on the environment.

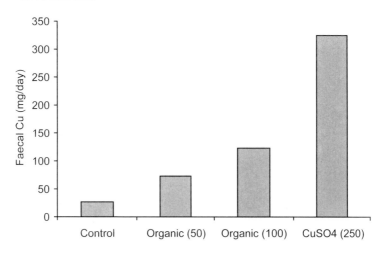

Figure 3. Faecal output of copper for weaner pigs fed either a control diet, or diets containing either 50 or 100 ppm organic copper, or 250 ppm of copper sulphate (Carlson, 2001).

Conclusion

There is increasing pressure on the pig industry world-wide to become more efficient, to reduce the cost of producing meat that consumers desire while taking into account the environmental impact of pig production. Organic minerals have an important role to play in the modern pig industry because of their higher bioavailability. As we continue to improve our knowledge of how minerals impact on pig performance then commercial producers and feed manufacturers will be able to evaluate the use of these minerals as a partial or full replacement for the inorganic forms currently being used.

References

Australian Pork Limited (2004). *Australian Pig Annual 2003*, Australian Pork Limited, Deakin West, Australia.

Carlson, M.S. (2001). Dietary trace elements for the growing pig. In: *Concepts in Pig Science* (eds. T.P. Lyons and K.A. Jacques). Nottingham University Press, Nottingham, UK. pp. 147-156.

Carlson, M.S., Hoover, S.L., Hill, G.M., Link, J.E., and Turk, R.J. (1998). Effect of pharmacological zinc on intestinal metallothionein concentration and morphology in nursery pigs. *Journal of Animal Science* **76** (Suppl. 1.): 57.

Close, W.H. (2004). Achieving production and economic targets: The Premier Pig Program™. In: *Proceedings from Alltech's 18ᵗʰ Asia-Pacific Lecture Tour*, pp 85-102

Close, W.H., and Turnley, K. (2004). Creating technical and educational forums that help pig producers meet performance and economic goals: the Premier Pig Program™. In: *Biotechnology in the Feed Industry, Proceedings of the 20ᵗʰ Annual Symposium* (eds. T.P. Lyons and K.A. Jacques) Nottingham University Press, Nottingham, UK. pp 113-119.

Close, W.H. (2003). Trace mineral nutrition of pigs revisited: meeting production and environmental objectives. *Recent Advances in Animal Nutrition in Australia*, University of New England, NSW **14:**133-142.

D'Souza, D.N., and Mullan, B.P. (2001). Dietary nutrient supplements improve meat quality. In: *Biotechnology in the Feed Industry, Proceedings of the 17ᵗʰ Annual Symposium* (eds. T.P. Lyons and K.A. Jacques) Nottingham University Press, Nottingham, UK. pp 305-317.

D'Souza, D.N., Warner, R.D., Leury, B.J., and Dunshea, F.R. (2000). The influence of dietary magnesium supplement type, and supplementation dose and duration, on pork quality and the incidence of PSE pork. *Australian Journal of Agricultural Research* **51:**185.

D'Souza, D.N., and Mullan, B.P. (1999). The influence of dietary magnesium Bioplex™ supplementation on pork quality. *Alltech Biotechnology Pig Research Report*.

D'Souza, D.N., Warner, R.D., Leury, B.J., and Dunshea, F.R. (1998). The effect of dietary magnesium aspartate supplementation on pork quality. *Journal of Animal Science* **76:** 104.

Fehse, R., and Close, W.H. (2000). The effect of the addition of organic trace elements on the performance of a hyper-prolific sow herd. In: *Biotechnology in the Feed Industry, Proceedings of the 16ᵗʰ Annual Symposium* (eds. T.P. Lyons and K.A. Jacques) Nottingham University Press, Nottingham, UK. pp 309-325.

Henman, D. (2001). Organic mineral supplements in pig nutrition: performance and meat quality, reproduction and environmental responses. In: *Biotechnology in the Feed Industry, Proceedings of the 17ᵗʰ Annual Symposium* (eds. T.P. Lyons and K.A. Jacques) Nottingham University Press, Nottingham, UK. pp 297-304.

Hofmeyr, C.D., Dunshea, F.R., Walker, P.J., and D'Souza, D.N. (1999). Magnesium supplementation to reduce the incidence of soft exudative pork under commercial conditions. In: *Manipulating Pig production VII* (ed. P.D. Cranwell). Australasian Pig Science Association: Werribee, Australia. pp 179.

Holm, A. (1990). E. *coli* associated diarrhea in weaner pigs: zinc oxide added to the feed as a preventative measure? *Proceedings International Pig Veterinary Society Congress,* pp154.

Hubbard, J.I. (1973). Microphysiology of vertebrate neuromuscular transmission. *Physiology Reviews* **53:** 674.

Kietzmann, M., and Jablonski, H. (1985). Blocking of stress in swine with magnesium aspartate hydrochloride. *Praktischer Tierarzt* **661:**311.

Jacyno, E., Kawecka, M., Kamyczek, M., Koiodziej, A., Owsianny, J., and Delikator, B. (2002) Influence of inorganic Se and vitamin E and organic Se and vitamin E on reprodutive performance of young boars. *Agricultural and Food Science in Finland* **11:** 175-184

Mahan, D.C., Cline, T.R., and Richert, B. (1999). Effects of dietary levels of selenium-enriched yeast and sodium selenite as selenium sources fed to growing-finishing pigs on performance, tissue selenium, serum glutathione peroxidase activity, carcass characteristics, and loin quality. *Journal of Animal Science* **77:** 2172-2179

Mahan, D.C., and Newton, E.A. (1995). Effect of organic and inorganic selenium sources and levels on sow colostrums and milk selenium content. *Journal of Animal Science* **73:** 151-158.

Marin-Guzman, J., Mahan, D.C., Chung, Y.K., Pate, J.L., and Pope, W.F. (1997). Effects of dietary selenium and vitamin E on boar performance and tissue responses, semen quality, and subsequent fertilization rates in mature gilts. *Journal of Animal Science* **75:** 2994-3003.

Mullan, B.P., Hernandez, A., and Pluske, J.R. (2004) Influence of the form and rate of Cu and Zn supplementation on the performance of growing pigs. In: *Biotechnology in the Feed Industry, Proceedings of the 20th Annual Symposium* (eds. T.P. Lyons and K.A. Jacques) Nottingham University Press, Nottingham, UK. abs.

Mullan, B.P., Wilson, R.H., Harris, D., Allen, J.G., and Naylor, A. (2002). Supplementation of weaner pig diets with zinc oxide or Bioplex™ zinc. In: *Biotechnology in the Feed Industry, Proceedings of the 18th Annual Symposium* (eds. T.P. Lyons and K.A. Jacques) Nottingham University Press, Nottingham, UK. pp 419-424.

Niemack, E.A., Stockli, F., Husmann, E., Sanderegger, J., Classen, H.G., and Helbig, J. (1979). Einfluss von Magnesium-Aspartat-Hydrochorid auf Kannibalismus, Transportstress und den Electrolytegehalt im Herzen von Schweinen. *Magnesium Bulletin* **3:** 195.

National Research Council (NRC). (1988). *Nutrient Requirements of Swine*. 9th edition, National Academy Press, Washington, D.C.

Pierce, J., Driver, J., Herter-Dennis, J., and Henman, D. (2001). Reducing phosphorus and copper excretion from poultry and swine using phytase and organic minerals. In: Addressing Animal Production and Environmental Issues. *Proceedings of the International Symposium* (eds. G.B. Havenstein). College of Agriculture and Life Sciences, North Carolina State University, Raleigh, NC.

Schrauzer, G.N. (2002). Selenium and human health: The relationship of selenium status to cancer and viral disease. In: *Biotechnology in the Feed Industry, Proceedings of the 18th Annual Symposium* (eds. T.P. Lyons and K.A. Jacques) Nottingham University Press, Nottingham, UK. pp 263-272.

Smits, R.J., and Henman, D.J. (2000). Practical experiences with Bioplexes in intensive pig production. In: *Biotechnology in the Feed Industry, Proceedings of the 16th Annual Symposium* (eds. T.P. Lyons and K.A. Jacques) Nottingham University Press, Nottingham, UK. pp 293-300.

Stalder, K.J., Powers, W.J., Burkett, J.L., and Pierce, J.L. (2004). Reducing the environmental impact of swine production through nutritional means. In: *Biotechnology in the Feed Industry, Proceedings of the 20th Annual Symposium* (eds. T.P. Lyons and K.A. Jacques) Nottingham University Press, Nottingham, UK. pp 149-157.

Stryer, L. (1988). Glycolysis. In: *Biochemistry,* 3rd Edition. W.H. Freeman and Company, NY. pp 352.

Van Lunen, T.A., and Cole, D.J.A. (1998). Growth and body composition of highly selected boars and gilts. *Animal Science* **67:** 107-116.

Whittemore, C.T., Close, W.H., and Hazzledine, M.J. (2002). The need for nutrient requirement standards for pigs. *Pig News and Information* **23:** 67N-74N.

Williams, N.H. (1998). Impact of immune system activation on pig growth and amino acid needs. In: *Progress in Pig Science* (eds. J. Wiseman, M.A. Varley and J.P. Chadwick), Nottingham University Press, Nottingham, UK. pp 583-588.

Wu, C., Tsunoda, A., Bollinger, D.W., Carlson, M.S., Veum, T.L., and Tibbetts, G.W. (2001). Reducing pharmacological levels of copper and zinc in nursery pig diets: response to zinc and copper proteinates. In: *Biotechnology in the Feed Industry, Proceedings of the 17th Annual Symposium* (eds. T.P. Lyons and K.A. Jacques) Nottingham University Press, Nottingham, UK. pp 285-295.

Trace mineral requirements of poultry - validity of the NRC recommendations

S Leeson

Department of Animal & Poultry Science, University of Guelph, Guelph, Ontario, N1G 2W1

Introduction

Trace mineral needs of poultry are usually met by premixes that represent no more than 0.25% the cost of a diet. Consequently there has been little incentive to redefine trace minerals for broilers, layers or turkeys. A review of published information in scientific journals over the last 15 years indicates that less than 1.5% of research effort has been expended on trace minerals. When there are no overt deficiencies or excess of trace minerals in a diet, trace minerals have little impact on general bird performance. The resurgence of interest in certain aspects of nutrition has been brought about by concerns for the environment and particularly the level of all nutrients in manure. It seems inevitable that regulatory concerns will be raised about the level of other components in manure, one group of which will be trace minerals and associated contaminants. Today in Ontario some rural well water contains 0.2 ppm zinc. These relatively high levels are likely to be a consequence of various agricultural practices, and zinc content of poultry manure will be a contributor to this situation. As trace mineral levels in poultry diets come under closer scrutiny, providing excess to requirements will have to be curtailed.

Trace mineral requirements - the NRC specifications

The National Research Council operates under the mandate of the National Academy of Sciences based in Washington, D.C. Over the last 50 years or so, the NRC has itself formed sub-committees in order to define the nutrient requirements of various animal species including most of the important farmed animals together with needs for laboratory animals, cats and dogs. Over the last 20 years, the Poultry sub-committee has published recommendations on nutrient requirements each 7-10 years (1977, 1984, 1994). In Europe, the now defunct Agricultural Research Council likewise published nutrient recommendations for farm animals, again every 10 years or so.

The mandate of the NRC species subcommittees is to provide unbiased reviews and recommendations regarding nutrient requirements of various animal species. The last NRC Poultry Subcommittee was established in 1992, the outcome of which was the 9th Revised Edition of Nutrient Requirements of Poultry published in 1994. Within this publication are listed the requirements for trace minerals of egg-layers, breeders, broilers, turkeys, pheasant and waterfowl. In establishing any nutrient requirement value, the committee members are given one simple, albeit very restrictive directive, and must base their recommendations only on data published in refereed journals. The idea behind this mandate is to prevent the use of potentially biased commercial data. This directive is particularly restrictive to estimating trace mineral needs, since there has been a lack of scientific research and publication on this topic since the 1960's, and relies on on very dated literature for estimates of trace mineral needs. The improved growth rate of broilers and turkeys and the increased egg output of modern layer strains that has occurred over the last 40 years is well recognised. For this reason, the NRC estimates are often criticized as not representing the needs of modern strains of commercial poultry.

Table 1 shows the year of publication upon which the trace mineral requirements (NRC 1994) are based. There is obviously a dearth of research in trace mineral nutrition over the last 30-40 years.

Table 1.
Year of research used in estimate of trace mineral requirements (NRC, 1994)

Trace mineral	Pullets	Layers	Broilers
Mg	1949, 1960, 1963	1967, 1968, 1969	1947, 1960, 1960, 1961, 1963, 1975
Mn	1939, 1971	1939, 1969, 1971	1939, 1983
Zn	1958, 1959, 1961, 1972, 1972	1986	1958, 1958, 1958, 1960, 1961, 1983, 1984, 1990
Fe	1961, 1961, 1964, 1968	1981	1964, 1968 1979, 1982
Cu	1961	1978	1979

Another point of interest is the type of diets used in these studies. Most often semi-purified or purified research diets are used, since the researcher is often unsure as to the content and/or bioavailability of trace minerals in conventional feedstuffs. Also, the trace mineral used in these experimental diets is invariably of the highest purity possible obtained at great cost from chemical supply companies. One could therefore question the relevance of NRC (1994) trace mineral requirements for modern commercial poultry. The situation is further confounded by the fact that many of the NRC (1994) requirement values are in fact "estimates" rather than actual requirements. These estimates are highlighted in bold font within the NRC (1994) publication and indicate that there is insufficient data available for a definite requirement value. Rather the "estimates" are approximations based on extrapolation from work conducted with other ages of bird and/or from other species. Table 2 outlines the proportion of estimated values for trace mineral specifications.

Table 2.
NRC (1994)
trace mineral
specifications

	Species	% Estimated data
Brown egg:	Pullets	100%
	Layers	100%
Broiler:	After 3 weeks	100%
Broiler Breeder:	No data available	
Turkey:	After 4 weeks	100%

The most comprehensive trace mineral requirement values are given for white-egg layers. Although there is no estimate for copper, the other values are defined, since there has been considerable work carried out with this strain of bird. However these estimates are much different to values currently used commercially, and such differences highlight another concern with the NRC (1994) values, in that they carry no measure of "insurance" and are absolute requirement values for birds under minimal stress. Table 3 outlines NRC (1994) trace mineral needs of layers compared to commercial values. No doubt the commercial values reflect a measure of insurance, yet many other nutrients rarely carry such 200-500% excess as seen with trace minerals. The NRC (1994) trace mineral values are absolute requirements, often estimated from studies using purified ingredients, such as casein and starch. In commercial diets, the major feed raw materials will provide significant quantities of trace minerals, although it is unlikely that these minerals are 100% available.

Table 3.
Trace mineral
(ppm) requirements
of a Brown egg
layer at 115g feed/d
intake

Mineral	NRC (1994)	Commercial	Factor
Cu	?	10	-
Fe	45	80	x2
Mn	20	80	x4
Zn	35	80	x2
Se	0.06	0.30	x5

Table 4 shows the total level of trace minerals provided by corn and soybean meal in a typical broiler starter diet, compared to NRC (1994) requirements and commercial values.

109

Table 4.
Contribution of
corn and soybean
meal to trace
mineral totals
in a broiler starter
(ppm)

Mineral	Corn + Soy	NRC (1994)	Commercial	Corn-Soy % Commercial
Mn	12	60	80	15
Cu	11	8	8	140
Fe	120	80	80	150
Zn	20	40	80	25
Se	0.06	0.15	0.3	20

Theoretically, corn and soybean meal provide the needs of the young broiler for copper and zinc. Unfortunately, we know very little about the bioavailability of trace minerals in ingredients such as corn and soybean. O'Dell *et al.* (1972) and Nwokolo and Bragg (1980) show 40-70% availability of Mg, Mn, Cu and Zn in canola meal and 50-78% availability in soybean meal. There is virtually no information available to account for such variability, and so predicting the bioavailability of trace minerals in common ingredients becomes a tenuous exercise. Some other ingredients can contain very high levels of trace minerals, where for example defluorinated phosphates have been reported to contain up to 10,000 ppm Fe, and that this is up to 50% bioavailable (Henry *et al.*, 1992). At this level, 1% dietary phosphate will supply 50 ppm bioavailable iron, which is close to the requirement for most classes of poultry. Obviously suppliers of phosphates are not likely to guarantee minimum levels of iron, and so the source is likely to be disregarded or discounted when establishing an ingredient matrix.

More recent mineral analyses have been conducted in spring 2002 on feed ingredients used in various trace mineral studies (table 5). It is interesting to note that values are quite different to other published values (e.g. NRC, 1994; Leeson and Summers, 1997) and reflects the variable uptake of trace minerals by plants.

Table 5.
Trace mineral
content (ppm) of
selected feed
ingredients

Raw material	Zinc	Manganese	Iron	Copper
Corn	12	10	107	11
Soybean meal	37	19	184	15
Meat Meal	97	7	285	12
Wheat shorts	76	104	203	16

Another important variable factor in the study of trace mineral needs, and one that is not fully documented within NRC (1994), is the bioavailability of specific minerals from different salts. Traditionally trace minerals are provided as inorganic oxides, sulphates and, occasionally, carbonates. There is limited information describing the mineral bioavailability from various salts (Ledoux *et al*, 1991; Smith *et al.*, 1994; Roberson and Edwards, 1994; Peshi and Bakalli,

1996). In general, sulphates are thought to have higher bioavailability than do oxides. Another area of discrepancy in such studies is the choice of response criteria. While growth rate and feed efficiency may be the most important from a commercial viewpoint, bone accretion of trace minerals may well be a more sensitive indicator for minerals such as zinc and manganese.

It is important to realize that factors such as disease or high environmental temperatures influence the animal's requirement for trace minerals at the dietary level. Belay *et al.*, (1992) reported that levels of both faecal and urinary magnesium increased under hot environments, and that needs for this mineral can be increased by up to 50% under certain conditions.

Too much mineral?

Because inorganic trace minerals are inexpensive, there is a tendency to over-formulate to ensure a generous safety factor. The interactions between charged inorganic trace minerals are well known, and so excess of one individual mineral can negatively impact metabolism of one or more other minerals. Such antagonism is more likely to occur when high inclusion levels are used and when unknowingly, other major ingredients are rich in certain minerals.

In a preliminary trial to just 17d, we have seen improved growth rate with birds fed diets devoid of supplemental manganese. In this study, the unsupplemented control diet contained 12 mg Mn/kg diet, which appeared to be adequate for broilers of this age under trial conditions. However it is not suggested that this reflects commercial requirements, rather the mode of action may well be through antagonism of other minerals when 70 mg Mn/kg is added to the control diet.

Table 6.
Performance of male broilers fed corn soy diets with or without supplemental manganese

	0-17d weight gain (g)	0-17d FCR
Control + Mn (70 ppm)	360[b]	1.87[a]
Control - Mn	439[a]	1.55[b]

Appleby and Leeson, unpublished

Confounding effect of enzymes

Enzymes are now routinely used in many poultry diets, and these may have an effect on liberating trace minerals from within complexes that are normally indigestible. Such activity may occur with oligosaccharidases such as xylanases, ß-glucanases and

111

especially phytase enzymes. Phytase undoubtedly increases the bioavailability of trace minerals from phytic acid found in feed grain including corn, wheat and soybean meal. Theoretically for each 6 moles phosphorus liberated, there will be 1 mole each of Fe, Mg and Zn released. Roberson and Edwards (1994) concluded that if phytase is used, then it may not be necessary to use supplemental zinc while levels of other cationic minerals such as Mn and Fe can also be reduced. Yi *et al.* (1996) showed improved retention of zinc from "natural" ingredients when phytase was added to the diet (Table 7). Using regression analyses, Yi *et al.* (1996) suggested that 100 U of phytase released approximately 1 mg of zinc. Therefore 600 U phytase will provide around 10% of the zinc needs for a young broiler.

Table 7.
Effect of phytase on zinc utilization

Zinc (ppm)	Phytase (U/kg)	Zinc retention	
		%	mg/bird
0	0	37.9	0.77
5	0	35.8	1.06
10	0	35.4	1.25
20	0	34.2	1.49
0	150	39.2	0.82
0	300	44.0	1.02
0	450	43.0	1.00
0	600	44.8	1.03

Organic trace minerals

The potential negative impact from oversupply of dietary trace minerals, coupled with the likelihood of legislation regarding manure loading has lead to a resurgence in research involving organic trace minerals. Organic minerals are usually chelates of protein/amino acids containing minerals, whose consistent bioavailability equates more closely to that of amino acids i.e. 90-95%. Mineral proteinates typically contain amino acids, dipeptides, tripeptides or proteins *per se*, and are thought to enhance digestibility and availability of the mineral sequestered by the ligand. Improved digestibility may be due to better solubilization, greater stability in the lumen and/or the ligand serving as an efficient carrier for the mineral across the brush border. Once absorbed, there is also the potential for greater retention, since there is less likelihood of secretion or excretion prior to incorporation in end-product molecules. Proteinates seem ideal choices in formulating diets containing lower levels of trace minerals, where knowledge of bioavailability is much more critical.

As an initial step in investigating the use of Bioplex® minerals for reducing trace mineral levels in manure, a study was conducted with caged broiler chickens. Broiler diets were formulated with mineral sulphates supplying 100 ppm Zn, 90 ppm Mn, 30 ppm Fe and 5 ppm Cu. These sulphates were assumed to be 70% bioavailable. The same level of bioavailable minerals were contributed by Bioplex® minerals, and further reduced to 80%, 60%, 40% or 20% of these levels (Table 8).

Table 8.
Trace mineral inclusion levels (ppm)

	Inorganic	Available*	Bioplex Level 100%	80%	60%	40%	20%
Zinc	100	70	70	56	42	28	14
Manganese	90	63	63	50	38	25	13
Iron	30	18	18	14	11	7	3.6
Copper	5	3	3	2.4	1.8	1.2	0.6

*assumes 70% availability

All other trace minerals and vitamin levels were constant across the 6 treatments. Each treatment was tested with 6 replicate groups of 8 caged birds to 17d and thereafter 5 replicate groups of 5 caged birds to 42d. Table 9 shows the body weight and feed efficiency of broilers fed the various levels of trace minerals.

There were surprising few effects of mineral supplementation, where birds fed just 20% of a normal level of Bioplex® trace minerals grew quite well considering the cage environment. There were no overt problems with bird health, and no differences seen in mortality. During the 15-17d period and the 39-42d period, a balance study was conducted, and feed and excreta analysed for trace minerals.

Table 9.
Broiler response to diet trace minerals

		Body weight (g) 17d	42d	Feed:Gain 0-17d	0-42d
Inorganic		489	2217	1.45	1.75
Bioplex®	100%	470	2351	1.51	1.70
	80%	472	2239	1.47	1.73
	60%	467	2285	1.53	1.72
	40%	444	2185	1.48	1.74
	20%	459	2291	1.50	1.69
	± SD	36	97	.08	.05
		NS	NS	NS	NS

Based on this balance data, trace mineral excretion for a farm housing 100,000 male broilers was calculated for each of the trace minerals under study (Table 10).

Table 10.
Calculated
mineral output in
manure from a
farm growing 5
crops of 100,000
male broilers/yr

		kg mineral/year			
		Zinc	Manganese	Iron	Copper
Inorganic		470[a]	273[a]	535	19[a]
Bioplex®	100%	318[b]	217[b]	523	17[ab]
	80%	294[b]	185[b]	491	18[ab]
	60%	309[b]	172[cd]	494	16[ab]
	40%	299[b]	156[d]	487	16[ab]
	20%	292[b]	130[e]	446	15[b]
	± SD	37	13	50	1.7
		**	**	NS	*

The use of Bioplex® minerals (calculated to contribute the same level as inorganic salts in the diet), resulted in reduced mineral output. This reflects the 70% bioavailability assigned to the inorganic salts, and that diets with Bioplex® may have contained 30% less mineral per se. Alternatively the Bioplex® minerals may be even more bioavailable relative to the inorganic salts, although the trial was not designed to answer this question.

In a subsequent trial, broilers were grown on litter to 42d. Trace minerals were provided either as inorganic salts or Bioplex® minerals, reduced to 14% or 7% of the total inorganic minerals in the diet. Results are shown in Table 11.

Table 11.
Broiler
performance in
response to trace
mineral source

	Body wt. gain		Feed:Gain	
	0-20d	20-41d	0-20d	20-41d
Inorganic control	747[a]	1888	1.35	1.73
Bioplex®≡14% control	725[b]	1880	1.39	1.68
Bioplex®≡7% control	706[c]	1892	1.38	1.70

There was an indication of poorer growth with the Bioplex® minerals to 20d although after this time, growth rate and feed efficiency were acceptable. Bioplex® at 14% of control levels was comparable in cost to the inorganic premix used in the control feed.

Reduced levels of trace minerals as Bioplex® have also been investigated for laying hens. Caged SCWL hens were fed corn-soy diets with regular levels of trace minerals (Cu, Zn, Mn, Fe) as inorganic salts, or 20% of these total levels as Bioplex® minerals. A third treatment involved no supplemental trace minerals. Diets were fed for eight 28d periods starting when birds were 28 weeks of age. There was no effect of diet on egg production, although there was a consistent trend for layers fed no trace minerals to produce fewer eggs (Table 12). Eggshell equality was unaffected.

Table 12. Effect of trace mineral source on egg production (28-60 weeks age)

Trace Mineral Treatment	Egg Production (%)								Total Egg Mass (Kg)	Total Eggs
	1[1]	2	3	4	5	6	7	8		
Inorganic	96.0	95.8	90.9	93.4	91.5	89.1	87.5	86.4	12.5	203.7
Bioplex[2]	94.1	95.2	91.4	93.2	91.9	88.0	86.8	85.5	12.4	202.0
None	93.4	94.4	90.1	91.9	89.8	87.6	86.9	85.9	12.0	200.3
SD	4.8	3.7	3.6	4.0	4.8	8.2	7.5	8.4	0.8	10.6
Sig.	NS	NS	NS	NS	NS	NS	NS	NS	NS	NS

NS, no significant difference [1]28d period [2]20% of inorganic mineral level

There was a noticeable loss in egg weight when no minerals were fed (Table 13).

Table 13.
Effect of trace mineral source on egg weight

Trace mineral treatment	Egg Weight (g)							
	1[1]	2	3	4	5	6	7	8
Inorganic	59.4 ab	59.4	60.2	61.1 ab	61.2	62.6	62.7	63.6
Bioplex®	59.6a	59.6	60.6	61.7a	62.0	63.0	63.4	63.9
None	58.2b	58.8	59.4	60.0b	60.2	61.3	61.6	62.3
SD	1.9	1.9	2.4	2.0	2.3	2.4	2.5	2.6
Sig.	*	NS	NS	*	NS	NS	NS	NS

*$P<.05$; ** $P<.01$; NS, no significant difference [1]28d period

Within the first 28d of the study, there was a 1g loss in egg size ($P<0.05$) and this effect was consistent for the remainder of the study. Excreta were assayed for minerals when birds were 45 weeks of age (Table 14). Using Bioplex® minerals, there was 60-70% reduction in manure content of Zn and Mn, and an 11% reduction for Cu. Interestingly, the mineral content of excreta for birds fed Bioplex® minerals or no supplemental minerals, was quite similar.

Table 14.
Layer manure minerals (ppm DM)

Trace mineral treatment	Zn	Mn	Cu
Inorganic	665.8a	770.5a	53.8
Bioplex®	222.9b	167.8b	47.5
None	218.8b	149.6b	38.3
SD	41.2	29.3	12.3
Sig.	**	**	NS

**, $P<.01$; NS, no significant difference Note: Birds were Shaver White age 38 weeks in Period 1.

Conclusions

The NRC (1994) nutrient requirement values are often criticized for being unrealistically low for modern strains of birds housed under commercial conditions. Certainly the levels for trace minerals are very low compared to commercial practice. However our apparent oversupply of trace minerals (relative to NRC 1994) is now being questioned relative to nutrient loading of manure. Mineral proteinates, such as Bioplex®, give us greater confidence of bioavailability, and so lower inclusion levels are feasible. In the preliminary studies detailed here it seems as though we can feed broilers and layers Bioplex® in corn-soy based diets at just 20% of the regular level of trace minerals, without any loss in performance. At this level, Bioplex® minerals are comparable in cost to inorganic trace mineral premixes, but with the associated advantage of dramatically reduced manure mineral accumulation.

116

If these data are confirmed in subsequent studies, then it would seem that the NRC (1994) estimated for trace minerals are in fact valid, or at least more valid compared to our thoughts some 5-10 years ago.

References

Albert, A., (1962). Stability constraints of trace minerals. *Federal Proceeding* **20**: 137.

Belay, T., Wiernusz C.J. and Teeter R.G. (1992). Mineral balance and urinary fecal mineral excretion profile of broilers housed in thermoneutral and heat distressed environments. *Poultry Science* **71**: 1043-1047.

Henry, P.R., Ammerman C.B., Miles R.D. and Littell R.C. (1992). Relative bioavailability of iron in feed grade phosphates for chicks. *Journal of Animal. Science* **70**: 228.

Ledoux, D.R., Henry P.R., Ammerman C.B., Rao P.V., Miles R.D. (1991). Estimation of the relative bioavailability of inorganic copper sources for chicks using tissue uptake of copper. *Journal of Animal. Science* **69**: 215.

Leeson, S. and Summers J.D. (1997). Commercial Poultry Nutrition 7th Rev. Ed.

National Research Council, (1994). Nutrient Requirements of Poultry. 9th Rev. Ed. NAS-NRC, Washington, D.C.

Nwokolo, E. and Bragy D.B. (1980). Biological availability of minerals in rapeseed meal. *Poultry Science* **59**: 155-158.

O'Dell, B.L., Burpo C.E. and Savage J.E. (1972). Evaluation of zinc availability in foodstuffs of plant and animal origin. *Journal of Nutrition* **102**: 653-660.

Pesti, G.M. and Bakalli R.I. (1996). Studies on the feeding of cupric sulfate pentahydrate and cupric citrate to broiler chickens. *Poultry Science* **75**:1086.

Roberson, K.D. and Edwards H.M. (1994). Effects of $1,25(OH)_2 D_3$ and phytase on Zn utilization in broiler chicks. *Poultry Science* **73**: 1312-11326.

Smith, M.O., Sherman I.L., Miller L.C. and Robbins K.R. (1994) Bioavailability of manganese from different sources in heat-distressed broilers. *Poultry Science* **73**: 163.

Yi, Z., Karnegay E.T. and Dembow D.M. (1996). Supplemental microbial phytase improves zinc utilization in broilers. *Poultry Science* **75**: 540-546.

Minerals, disease, and immune function

M. T. Kidd
Mississippi State University, Department of Poultry Science, Mississippi State, MS 39762-9665

Introduction

It is of utmost importance for poultry producers to execute necessary precautions to prevent disease-induced morbidity and mortality. The precautions typically include vaccination programs, coccidiostats, biosecurity programs, and good management. It has not been until recently that nutritional regimes have been implemented to heighten immunity with the aim to prevent and/or control diseases. Nutritional regimes to improve health are sometimes scrutinized as any diet cost increase is calculated, but improvements in health typically are not. Research in the 1980's and 1990's gave rise to numerous reports delineating the essentiality of trace minerals and immune responsiveness. This paper deals with our current knowledge of trace mineral needs and immunocompetence, as well as recent research dealing with heightened immunity/disease prevention by optimizing trace mineral needs.

Recommended trace mineral needs

Estimated trace mineral recommendations per kg of diet (NRC, 1994) for broilers throughout life (1-56 d) are: Cu, 8 mg; I, 0.35 mg; Fe, 80 mg; Mn, 60 mg; Se, 0.15 mg; and Zn, 40 mg. These recommendations, of which over half are predicted rather than based from empirical research, are primarily based on growth rate of chickens, not immunity of broilers. It must be pointed out that it is very difficult to predict trace mineral needs when sufficient data, i.e., element titrations or predictive models based on research, is lacking. Moreover, research published on trace minerals since the 1994 NRC publication primarily deals with deficiencies or adequate and supplemented levels, rather than dose responsiveness. Hence, published reports assessing trace mineral needs for immunity are needed to make accurate predictions in practical settings.

Several minerals are involved in preventing or tackling disease via immune function. The key elements concerned for poultry are zinc (Zn), copper (Cu), selenium (Se), manganese (Mn) and iron (Fe).

Mineral status during infection

Variation in circulating levels of trace minerals occurs during an innate immune response in the bird. During an innate immune response, especially that originating from bacteria, there is an increase in circulating levels of Cu, but a decrease in circulating levels of Zn and Fe (Klasing et al., 1987). Organs, especially the liver, sequester circulating pools of Fe and Zn for host protection. Hence, many bacteria require available Fe for growth. Conversely, circulating Cu is increased during an innate immune response. As Cu is increased in plasma, ceruloplasmin (a Cu-containing protein) is also increased as mediated via IL-1ß (Klasing et al., 1987). Thus, Cu research is warranted in avian disease models as bacteria and protozoa (Laurent et al., 2001) have been shown to increase IL-1ß. Furthermore, optimization of immune cell function with Zn and the bird's ability to sequester Zn during infection are topics that require more research.

Zinc

Zn is present in numerous metalloenzymes functioning both structurally and catalytically. It is the only trace mineral to be required for functionality of enzymes in all six classes: oxidoreductase (e.g., superoxide dismutase), transferease (e.g., DNA polymerase), hydrolase (e.g., alkaline phosphatase), lyase (e.g., carbonic anhydrase), isomerase (e.g., phosphomannose isomerase), and ligase (e.g., tRNA synthetase). Mononuclear phagocytes (heterophils, monocytes, and macrophages) produce superoxide ion used to destroy pathogens, deeming Zn-superoxide dismutase vital for the integrity of these immune cells. The role of Zn in cellular biology is diverse and it has been shown to offer host protection in many species against bacteria, fungi, parasites, and viruses. Its role in poultry immunology/disease resistance is of key importance.

Infection (especially when caused by bacteria) results in low circulating zinc levels (hypozincaemia), but its systemic decline is more poorly understood than that of Fe. Cellulitis occurs in broilers when skin lacerations from e.g. scratches become infected with bacteria and is of major significance to the poultry industry due to economic loss through carcass condemnations. The combination of vitamin E (48 IU/kg of diet) and complexed Zn (40 mg/kg of diet) has been reported to give a significant decrease in cellulitis in broilers (Downs et al., 2000). Rostan et al. (2002) published a review on Zn needs for skin and concluded that although Zn's role in cellular metabolism has received much attention, its critical role as a skin anti-oxidant has been overlooked. In a similar role, Zn has been shown to act as a protective agent in hearts with deficient blood supply (Powell et al., 1990). Progeny from broiler breeders fed 150 mg Zn and 163 mg Mn/kg of diet had increased left ventricle plus septum and total ventricular weights, but not improved ascites resistance, in comparison to birds fed 75 mg Zn and 80 mg Mn/kg of diet (Virden et al., 2004). A review by Rivera et al. (2003) highlighted the protective role of trace minerals on the immune response during parasitic infections, and Zn modulation on immune responsiveness was discussed. Future research should evaluate the role of Zn on innate immune responses following an enteric challenge in broilers.

Concerning general immunity, numerous advantages to adequate or excessive Zn levels have been described in poultry and possible mechanisms of action discussed (Kidd et al., 1996). The improvements in immunity (primarily cellular and innate immune response) via increased Zn status have been demonstrated in broiler breeders (Dozier, 2004), progeny from broiler breeders (Kidd et al., 1992, 1993), broilers (Bartlett and Smith, 2003), and turkeys (Kidd et al., 1994a). These improvements in immunity also improve disease resistance. For example, young female turkeys fed increased Zn (in form of Zn-methionine) had improved blood clearance of E. coli in vivo (Kidd et al., 1994b). The former effect indicates the heightened phagocytic ability of macrophages of spleen origin as mediated by increased dietary Zn. In summary, the improvements to Zn in immunity may prevent mortality. Virden et al. (2003) demonstrated reduced early mortality in progeny chicks from hens fed diets supplemented with increased Zn and Mn in the form of amino acid complexes. Future research should address Zn needs in practical settings for improvements in livability and immunity in commercial poultry fed antibiotic free diets with and without common challenges.

Selenium

The beneficial properties of Se in poultry have been comprehensively reviewed by Surai (2002). Similar to that of Zn, Se has received considerable attention in poultry research concerned with immunity and disease resistance. Hegazy and Adachi (2000) fed chicks diets enriched with Se and noted improved antibody production to Salmonella. Improvements in antibody production in chickens as mediated by increased dietary Se were also noted with sheep red blood cells (a T-dependent antigen) in the presence of E. coli induced stress (Larsen et al., 1997). In addition, birds fed diets fortified with Se have improved T-cell function (Marsh et al., 1987) and monocyte phagocytosis (Dietert et al., 1983). Benefits in disease conditions have also been observed in birds fed Se fortified diets. For example, Colnago et al. (1984) fed 0.25 or 0.50 mg Se/kg of diet and noted improved immunity against Eimeria tenella. Much of the research discussed addresses Se needs in the presence of vitamin E. Dietary level and source of Se should be considered in modern poultry production to optimize anti-oxidant properties and disease resistance.

Manganese

The role of Mn in immune function is less understood than that of other trace minerals. Reports in the 1970's and 1980's indicated that Mn supplementation in a number of experiments, including hens, elevated antibody titers and maintained this elevation over time. Similar to Zn and Cu, Mn is also important for cellular superoxide dismutase, which is primarily found in the mitochondria. The enzymes role in disease has been assessed by Macmillan-Crow and Cruthirds (2001) who demonstrated that mice expressing only 50% of normal Mn superoxide dismutase levels had increased susceptibility to oxidative stress and impaired mitochondrial function due to high levels of reactive oxygen intermediates.

The absorption of Mn in poultry is poorer than other trace minerals in comparison to other species, indicating that it should be supplied in the diet at levels in excess of standard requirements (Underwood, 1977). In addition, coccidiosis infections have been shown to decrease intestinal absorption of Mn (Turk et al., 1982). Smialowicz et al. (1985) demonstrated that intramuscular injections of $MnCl_2$ enhanced macrophage function, subsequent research in turkeys is in agreement with that of mice (Ferket and Kidd, 1997). Hence immune responsiveness and disease resistance of chickens fed diets varying in Mn warrants attention.

In ovo trace mineral effects: Future possibilities?

Providing poultry (especially broilers and turkeys) access to feed and water as soon as possible post hatch is critical to assure adequate flock performance. The functionality of the immune system is also important as the bird leaves the environment of the egg and is immediately exposed to oxygen, pathogens, and vaccines. Hence, *in ovo* feeding of various minerals may serve as a means to heighten early chick growth and livability. Tako et al. (2004) administered Zn-methionine *in ovo* (amnion injection at 17 d of incubation) and found that hatched chicks had improved absorptive and digestive functions. Gore and Qureshi (1997) administered vitamin E *in ovo* at 18 d of incubation and noted improved macrophage and antibody responses in hatched chicks. These improvements to *in ovo* administered vitamin E were observed in the 4th and 5th week post hatch. It may be that *in ovo* Se, coupled with vitamin E, could prove beneficial for immunity and growth of poultry post hatch. Future *in ovo* research with Se and Zn warrants attention-especially due to the high degree of polyunsaturated fatty acids in the embryo lipid fraction.

Acknowledgement

Journal Article Number PS10571 from the Mississippi Agricultural and Forestry Experiment Station supported by MIS-322140. Use of trade names in this publication does not imply endorsement by the Mississippi Agricultural and Forestry Experiment Station of the products, nor similar ones not mentioned.

References

Bartlett, J. R. and Smith M. O. (2003) Effects of different levels of zinc on the performance and immunocompetence of broilers under heat stress. *Poultry Science.* **82**:1580-1588.

Colnago, G. L., Jensen L. S., and Long P. L. (1984). Effect of selenium and vitamin E on the development of immunity to coccidiosis in chickens. *Poultry Science.* **63**:1136-1143.

Dietert, R. R., Marsh J. A. and Combs G. F. Jr. (1983) Influence of dietary selenium and vitamin E on the activity of chicken blood phagocytes. *Poultry Science* **62**:1412 (abstract).

Downs, K. M., Hess J. B., Macklin K. S., and Norton R. A. (2000) Dietary zinc complexes and vitamin E for reducing cellulitis incidence in broilers. *Journal of. Applied. Poultry Research.* **9**:319-323.

Dozier, W. A. (2004). Mineral needs of broiler breeders. *Proceedings of Arkansas. Nutrition Conference* CD-ROM.

Ferket, P. R. and Kidd M. T. (1997). Organic zinc sources and performance and health in poultry. p 37-43 In: *Proceedings of the Maryland Nutrition Conference.* Baltimore, Maryland, USA.

Gore, A. B. and Qureshi M. A. (1997). Enhancement of humoral and cellular immunity by vitamin E after embryonic exposure. *Poultry Science* **76**:984-991.

Hegazy, S. M. and Adachi Y. (2000.) Comparison of the effects of dietary selenium, zinc, and selenium and zinc supplementation on growth and immune response between chick groups that were inoculated with Salmonella and aflatoxin or Salmonella. *Poultry Science* **79**:331-335.

Kidd, M. T., N. B. Anthony, and S. R. Lee, 1992. Progeny performance when dams and chicks are fed supplemental zinc. *Poultry Science* **71**:1201-1206.

Kidd, M. T., Anthony N. B., Newberry L. A., and Lee S. R. (1993). Effect of supplemental zinc in either a corn-soybean or a milo corn-soybean meal diet on the performance of young broiler breeders and their progeny. *Poultry Science* **72**:1492-1499.

Kidd, M. T., Qureshi M. A., Ferket P. R., and Thomas L. N. (1994a). Dietary zinc-methionine enhances mononuclear-phagocytic function in young turkeys. *Biological Trace Element Research* **42**:217-229.

Kidd, M. T., Qureshi M. A., Ferket P. R., and Thomas L. N. (1994b). Blood clearance of *Escherichia coli* and evaluation of mononuclear-phagocytic system as influenced by supplemental zinc-methionine in young turkeys. *Poultry Science* **73**:1381-1389.

Kidd, M. T., Ferket P. R., and Qureshi M. A. (1996). Zinc metabolism with special reference to its role in immunity. *World's Poultry Science Journal* **52**:309-324.

Klasing, K. C., Laurin D. E., Peng R. K., and Fry M. (1987). Immunologically mediated growth depression in chicks: Influence of feed intake, corticosterone and interleukin-1. *Journal of Nutrition* **117**:1629-1637.

Larsen, C. T., Pierson F. W., and Gross W. B. (1997). Effect of dietary selenium on the response of stressed and unstressed chickens to Escherichia coli challenge and antigen. *Biological Trace Element Research* **58**:169-176.

Laurent, F., Mancassola R., Lacroix S., Menezes R., and Naciri M. (2001). Analysis of chicken mucosal immune response to Eimeria tenella and Eimeria maxima infection by quantitative reverse transcription-PCR. *Infection Immunity* **69**:2527-2534.

Macmillan-Crow, L. A. and Cruthirds D. L. (2001). Invited review: Manganese superoxide dismutase in disease. *Free Radical Research* **34**:325-336.

Marsh, J. A., Dietert R. R., and Combs G. F. Jr. (1987). Effect of dietary selenium and vitamin E in the chicken on con A induced splenocyte proliferation. *Progressive Clinical Biology Research* **238**:333-345.

National Research Council. 1994. Nutrient Requirements of Poultry. 9th Rev. ed. National Academic Press, Washington, DC, USA.

Powell, S. R., Saltman P., Uretzky G., Chevion M. (1990). The effect of zinc on reperfusion arrhythmias in the isolated perfused rat heart. *Free Radical Biology and Medicine* **8**:33-46.

Rivera, M. T., De Souza A. P., Araujo-Jorge T. C., Castro S. L., and Vanderpas J. (2003). Trace elements, innate immune response and parasites. *Clinical Chemistry Laboratory Medicine* **41**:1020-1025.

Rostan, E. F., DeBuys H. V., Madey D. L. and Pinnell S. R. (2002). Evidence supporting zinc as an important anti-oxidant for skin. *International Journal of Dermatology* **41**:606-611.

Smialowicz, R. J., Luebke R. W., Rogers R. R., Riddle M. M. and Rowe D. G. (1985). Manganese chloride enhances natural cell-mediated immune effector cell function: Effects on macrophages. *Immunopharmacy* **9**:1-11.

Surai, P. F., (2002). Selenium in poultry nutrition 2. Reproduction, egg and meat quality and practical applications. *World's Poultry Science Journal* **58**:431-450.

Tako, E., Ferket P. R., and Uni Z. (2004). Zinc-methionine enhances the intestine development and functionality in the late term embryos and chicks. *Poultry Science* **83**(Suppl. 1): 267.

Turk, D. E., Gunji D. S., and Molitoris P. (1982). Coccidial infections and manganese absorption. *Poultry Science* **61**:2430-2434.

Virden, W. S., Yeatman J. B., Barber S. J., Zumwalt C. D., Ward T. L., Johnson A. B., and Kidd M. T. (2003). Hen mineral nutrition impacts progeny livability. *Journal of Applied Poultry Research* **12**:411-416.

Virden, W. S., Yeatman J. B., Barber, S. J. Willeford K. O., Ward T. L., Fakler T. M., Wideman R. F.Jr., and Kidd M. T. (2004). Immune system and cardiac functions of progeny chicks from dams fed diets differing in zinc and manganese level and source. *Poultry Science* **83**:344-351.

Lessons in human mineral nutrition: what can we learn?

Liadhan McAnena
Northern Ireland Centre for Diet and Health, University of Ulster

Introduction

Approximately fifteen minerals are considered to be essential in humans. Among the macrominerals, calcium, magnesium and phosphorus have a structural role in bone; potassium, sodium and chlorine are important as electrolytes. Primary deficiency of any of these six nutrients is very rare in humans – indeed, the interest surrounding dietary sodium results from the probability of too much rather than too little. However, among the trace elements (those constituting less than 0.01% of human body weight (Solomons and Rutz, 1998), deficiencies of iron, zinc, selenium and iodine frequently present substantial problems in human populations. Deficiencies of copper, molybdenum and manganese are only seen in some, highly specialised circumstances. From a veterinary point of view, copper is probably the trace mineral most often associated with deficiency disease, whereas in humans, iron deficiency is the most widespread, and iodine deficiency is arguably the cause of most suffering. Chromium and fluoride are not normally associated with deficiency diseases, but they may be considered essential nutrients because they can confer beneficial health effects.

This review will concentrate mainly on the four trace elements that cause primary deficiencies in human populations, together with copper which assumes such importance in animal nutrition, and it will consider their functions, the homeostatic mechanisms that regulate their status in the body, the means used to assess their status, and the genetic variations, and interactions among nutrients, which influence the body's trace mineral requirements.

Iron

Practically all of the iron in the human body (4 - 5g) is tightly bound to proteins: haemoglobin and myoglobin (the oxygen-carrying pigments of erythrocytes and muscle cells) the storage proteins of the reticuloendothelial system (which refers to the bone marrow, the liver, spleen and macrophages); and transport proteins in the plasma. In healthy conditions, virtually no iron is free in ionic form in the plasma and tissues (Strain and Cashman, 2002). Iron can switch between divalent and trivalent forms, and this key property provides both the basis of most of its physiological functions and the reason for its characteristic protein binding. The potential oxidative damage which iron might otherwise cause to biomolecules, such as proteins, fatty acids and nucleic acids, is limited by protein sequestering. Besides its roles in oxygen transport and transport, iron is also a component of very many tissue enzymes, for example, the cytochromes which are involved in electron transport and energy metabolism.

Iron is widely distributed in food; meat, eggs, vegetables and cereals are all good sources. Typical Western diets contain 10-15 mg of iron/day. In the British diet, although meat products are a rich source of iron, cereal products provide about one-third of dietary intake (British Nutrition Foundation website). Dietary iron in animal protein is supplied in the form of haem iron i.e. bound to a porphyrin group. Haem iron makes up about 10% of dietary iron (FSAI, 1999) but contributes over 40% of total iron absorbed in the intestine (Strain and Cashman, 2002). Non-haem iron, mostly found in plant and dairy foods, consists of ferric salts as well as enzymes in which iron is bound to the sulphur atoms of cysteine residues. These enzymes are often called iron-sulphur proteins.

Iron absorption

Iron absorption occurs mainly in the duodenum and healthy adults absorb about 15% of the total iron contained in a mixed diet (FSA, 2003). Intestinal mucosal cells carry a specific receptor, which recognises haem molecules, which are endocytosed into the cells, where iron is released from the haem molecule by the enzyme haem oxygenase. Non-haem iron absorption by mucosal cells follows a different mechanism, also involving receptors on the cell surface. The rate of absorption is inversely related to mucosal cells' non-haem iron content. This iron uptake is apparently regulated by one, or several, cell surface proteins but their identity is not yet certain.

Haem iron absorption is little affected by diet, but non-haem absorption is strongly influenced by dietary components. Dietary components may form complexes with iron which are insoluble, or in which the iron is so tightly bound that it cannot be absorbed. Generally, dietary constituents that solubilise iron enhance absorption, and compounds that either precipitate or polymerise iron decrease absorption. Ascorbate maintains iron in solution in the intestine by reducing it to the divalent state. Citrate, fructose and amino acids act as ligands promoting absorption. Vitamin A, ß-carotene, alcohol and haem iron are also enhancers of absorption. The presence of meat, fish or poultry within a meal increases non-haem iron absorption approximately four-fold. Inhibitors include: calcium salts, for example, phosphate; phytate and polyphenols such as those found in tea (Strain and Cashman, 2002).

It should be noted that the terms haem and non-haem iron refer only to the dietary source; their mechanisms of absorption differ, but once in the bloodstream, both forms enter the same iron pool. Absorbed iron is moved out of the intestinal cell into the plasma by mechanisms which are not yet clear. In the plasma it is bound to transferrin for transport. The total iron-binding capacity of plasma is about one-third saturated when iron status is replete. All nucleated cells have transferrin receptors on their surface, and tissue cells take up the transferrin molecule, endocytose it, then release the iron. Bone marrow cells manufacturing erythrocytes take up 80% of the transferrin-bound iron in plasma (FSA, 2003). When erythrocytes die, the iron present in haemoglobin is returned to iron stores; so very little iron is lost from the body but rather it is "recycled". Iron is stored in the reticuloendothelial system, bound to proteins such as ferritin and haemosiderin.

Iron requirements

Daily iron dietary requirements are estimated from the amount necessary to cover basal iron losses, menstrual losses and growth needs. Basal iron losses are small. Sweat and epithelial cells shed continuously from the surface skin and lining of the gastrointestinal tract result in the loss of less than 1 mg iron/day. Iron circulating in plasma is protein-bound, so it cannot pass through the glomerulus; loss of iron in urine is negligible (< 0.1 mg/day). Owing to menstrual losses, women of reproductive age lose another 12-15 mg of iron every month. To replace iron lost from the body, therefore, males and non-menstruating females need to absorb 1 mg/day, and women of reproductive age require about 1.4 mg/day (FAO/WHO, 2001). Daily dietary iron requirements throughout life, as defined by the UK Department of Health, are shown below (DoH, 1991). The Lower Reference Nutrient Intake (LRNI) is the amount of iron which is enough for only the 2.5% of the population who have particularly low requirements. The RNI is enough to meet the needs of 97.5% of the population.

Age	LRNI iron (mg/day)	RNI iron (mg/day)
0-3 months	0.9	1.7
4-6 months	2.3	4.3
7-12 months	4.2	7.8
1-3 years	3.7	6.9
4-6 years	3.3	6.1
7-10 years	4.7	8.7
11-18 years male	6.1	11.3
female	8.0	14.8
19-50 years male	4.7	8.7
female	8.0	14.8
50+ yrs	4.7	8.7

Table 1.
Recommended
daily intakes of
iron for humans

Iron homeostasis, to prevent iron deficiency or overload, is carried out by up- or down-regulating intestinal iron absorption, according to body stores and to physiological requirement, which is very closely related to the rate of erythrocyte production.

Iron deficiency

When iron deficiency occurs, it can be seen to develop in a series of stages (Yip and Dallman, 1996). First, the depletion of stored tissue iron, as tissue ferritin in liver, bone marrow and spleen, is mirrored by decreasing concentrations of ferritin protein in the plasma. Second, depletion of plasma iron (which is transported as transferrin) results in decreased transferrin saturation. As the cells' requirement for iron increases, more transferrin receptors are expressed on cell surfaces. A portion of the receptor molecule is secreted into the plasma where it can be measured as "soluble" transferrin receptor. In late stages of iron deficiency, there is insufficient haemoglobin for red blood cell formation, and other physiological functions. By the time iron-deficiency anaemia can be detected, with characteristic decreased erythrocyte volume and haemoglobin content (microcytic hypochromic anaemia) there is also decreased activity of intracellular iron-containing enzymes such as the cytochromes, catalase and peroxidases.

Iron deficiency affects two billion people, in virtually all countries. In infants and children it is associated with low birthweight, prematurity, increased perinatal morbidity, reduced resistance to infections, impaired psychomotor development and retarded growth. In adults, it causes fatigue and reduced work performance, and may cause reproductive impairment. The population groups most at risk of iron deficiency are those with high physiological requirements for tissue growth, such as young children, adolescents and women of childbearing age, and those with diseases or lifestyles that cause decreased iron absorption or increased iron loss. Poor iron absorption can result from diseases producing intestinal malabsorption, for example, coeliac disease. Many gastrointestinal diseases, including peptic ulcer, inflammatory bowel disease, stomach and colorectal cancer, can cause chronic blood loss in faeces, often imperceptible to the patient. Non-steroidal anti-inflammatory drugs, such as aspirin or ibuprofen, are gastric irritants, and long-term use can cause chronic gastrointestinal bleeding. High iron losses are associated with chronic blood loss, for example, menorrhagia (excessive menstrual blood loss). Iron deficiency is also seen in individuals with inadequate iron intake associated with poor income. Cow's milk iron deficiency anaemia is sometimes seen in infants aged 9-24 months whose diet consists primarily of cow's milk. Absorption of iron from cow's milk is very low compared to human milk, which contains a protein called lactoferrin. The presence of lactoferrin results in iron absorption of about 50% (FSA, 2003).

Iron toxicity

The human body has no means of iron excretion; instead, intestinal iron absorption is down-regulated to prevent iron toxicity, when dietary intakes are high (FSAI, 1999). No safe upper level for total iron intake has been established either in the UK or by the EU, as the available data from human or animal studies were considered insufficient. However, the US Food and Nutrition Board have defined a Tolerable Upper Intake Level of 45 mg iron/day as the highest level which could safely be consumed on a daily basis by most individuals.

Iron toxicity may occur in individuals with genetic diseases. Hereditary haemochromatosis (HH) is the most common genetic disease in Ireland, estimated to affect up to 1 in 200 people of Irish descent (Edwards and Kushner, 1993). It is an autosomal recessive condition caused by mutations in the HFE gene, resulting in uncontrolled iron uptake in intestinal and liver cells. Iron is deposited in the liver, pancreas, heart, joints, and pituitary gland. Treatment, by phlebotomy, can prevent the progress of tissue damage, which can otherwise produce cirrhosis, primary liver cancer, diabetes and cardiomyopathy. HH is very often undiagnosed until late in life but the diagnosis rate has risen in recent years. Another condition, African or Bantu siderosis is also probably genetic but it may also be associated with a high-iron diet. Unfortunately, the gene responsible has not yet been identified.

The toxicity of iron stems from its redox activity, which may promote the formation of free radicals. These atoms or molecules with an extra or unpaired electron are very unstable and extremely reactive. Under normal circumstances, however, the protein binding of iron ensures that free radical generation is minimised.

Assessing iron status

Several methods should be used in combination to obtain an accurate diagnosis of iron status. Normal plasma ferritin values are in the range 15-300 μg/l. Values below 12 μg/l suggest that tissue iron stores have become depleted. Transferrin saturation is normally about one-third (FSA, 2003). Changes in haemoglobin content or packed cell volume are insensitive measures of iron status, as anaemia is a late sign of iron depletion. Unfortunately, earlier changes are less often measured, so it is difficult to estimate how widespread sub-clinical iron deficiency might be. However, given the prevalence of overt iron-deficiency anaemia, with its serious costs in health and productivity, the consequences of sub-optimal iron status are likely to be considerable.

Iodine

The physiological function of iodine is as an essential constituent of the hormones thyroxine (T4) and tri-iodothyronine (T3), produced by the thyroid gland. Thyroid hormones regulate basal metabolic rate, cellular oxygen consumption, cellular integrity and enzyme synthesis (Hetzel and Clugson, 1999). The average adult human body contains about 10-20 mg of iodine, of which 70-80% is stored in the thyroid gland, the only significant store of iodine (SCF, 2002). Iodine status can be assessed by thyroid function.

Rich dietary sources of iodine include marine fish, shellfish, seaweeds, sea salt and fortified salt. Cereals and grain contain variable amounts, determined by the soil iodine level. In the UK, cow's milk is a good source of iodine, probably mainly because of supplemented cattle feed (FSA, 2003). Milk makes a greater contribution in children's diet because of their higher milk consumption. Inorganic iodine in foods, generally in the form of iodide, is readily absorbed, largely from the small intestine. The thyroid gland traps about 60 μg iodine/day from the plasma, and the amount is regulated according to the body's requirements (FAO/ WHO, 1989). The process is largely mediated by thyroid-stimulating hormone (TSH) secreted by the pituitary gland. TSH stimulates the thyroid to take up more iodine, enabling it to produce more thyroid hormones. Iodine-containing T4 is taken up by most tissues. Excess iodine is excreted largely in the urine.

Iodine requirements

The UK LRNI for iodine in adults is 70 μg/day and the RNI 140 μg/day (DoH, 1991). Thyroid function is subject to influence by other factors; for example, deficiencies of vitamin A, zinc, iron and copper can result in hypothyroidism. Thyroid hormone synthesis can also be impaired by substances present in certain foods. Termed goitrogens, they occur naturally in cabbage, broccoli, sprouts, turnips, soybeans, peanuts and walnuts. Another goitrogen, thiocyanate, can be produced by degradation of the cyanogenic glycosides present in corn, maize, cassava, potato, cauliflower. The effect of goitrogens in food can be overcome by adequate intakes of dietary iodine.

Iodine deficiency

Iodine deficiency results in an increase in stillbirths, perinatal and infant mortality, neurological and intellectual impairment, and enlargement of the thyroid gland known as goitre. In response to low levels of circulating T4, TSH activity increases, stimulating the cells of the thyroid gland to become larger and more efficient at trapping iodine from plasma. The gland becomes enlarged as a compensatory mechanism. Goitre is estimated to affect some seven million people (SCF, 2002). It is treatable by iodine supplementation. It cannot be eliminated by changing dietary habits because food grown in iodine-deficient regions can never provide enough iodine for the people and livestock living there. The deficiency results from geologic rather than social or economic conditions, and so it must be corrected by supplying iodine from external sources.

Thyroid hormones are necessary for the development of the nervous system in the foetus and infant. Iodine deficiency in a foetus can result in cretinism. Symptoms include deafness, squint, motor spasticity and severe mental retardation. Iodine deficiency is the most common cause of preventable mental retardation. Goitre and cretinism are frequently endemic in areas where the soils are iodine deficient, and 1.6 billion people worldwide are estimated to live in such areas. WHO estimates that nearly 50 million people have mental impairments caused by iodine deficiency.

Iodine toxicity

There are insufficient data from experimental studies to establish a UK safe upper level for iodine intake, but the European Commission's Scientific Committee on Food (SCF) has defined a tolerable upper intake level of 600μg as the maximum level of chronic daily iodine intake unlikely to pose a risk of adverse health effects. Toxicity causes hyperthyroidism, producing symptoms such as rapid heart rate, trembling, excessive sweating and loss of weight. Iodine toxicity is sometimes seen after the implementation of salt iodisation programmes. During long-term iodine deficiency, the goitrous thyroid gland may develop hyperfunctioning autonomous nodules, which then respond strongly to supplemental iodine, resulting in hyperthyroidism (FSA, 2003). Iodine toxicity has also occurred after widespread salt iodisation was implemented in countries which contain some iodine-sufficient areas, so the supplementation has resulted in areas of excess dietary iodine.

Selenium

Selenium plays an important role in immune function. Deficiency has been linked to the occurrence, virulence or disease progression of some viral infections, for example the progression of HIV to AIDS (Schrauser and Sacher, 1994). Adequate selenium intake is also required for human fertility, in men and women; normal sperm development requires sperm capsule selenoprotein, which probably has a structural role in the sperm tail; and there is evidence to suggest that selenium deficiency increases the risk of miscarriage (Barrington et al, 1996). Some evidence suggests that at intakes higher than those traditionally regarded as nutritionally adequate, selenium may have beneficial effects in protecting against cancer (FAO/WHO, 2001). Selenium is an essential component of the enzyme iodothyronine deiodinase, a selenoprotein which regulates the inter-conversion of active and inactive forms of iodothyronines. Other known selenoenzymes include the antioxidants glutathione peroxidase (GPx) and selenoprotein W, and selenoprotein P which accounts for 60 to 80% of the selenium in human plasma but whose function is unknown.

Selenium is found widely in the environment. Good food sources include fish, meat, nuts, eggs and cereal. There is considerable variation in selenium levels in food, depending on the soil selenium content. Some areas are deficient, others rich (FSA, 2003); for example European soils are poorer in selenium than USA. Total Diet Studies, a national dietary survey the UK Department for Environment, Food and Rural Affairs, indicates that selenium status in the UK has fallen in the past 20 or 30 years. This is thought to be partly because of increased consumption of bread made from European, rather than imported Canadian, wheat, in accordance with EU policies.

Most of the selenium in food is thought to be present as the amino acid derivatives selenomethionine or selenocysteine (DoH, 1991).

Organic forms of selenium, on particular the amino acid derivatives selenomethionine and selenocysteine, are more readily absorbed than inorganic sulphides and selenides. Plant foods generally contain more a greater proportion of organic selenium compounds than animal foods.

After absorption, some selenium is transported in the plasma bound to albumin while the rest is bound to very low density lipoproteins. Selenium is lost in urine, faeces, expelled air, hair, nails and breast milk. The UK RNI is 75 μg selenium/day for men and 60 μg/day for women. During lactation, a further 15 μg/day, approximately, is required. Selenium status is affected by several factors, such as the antioxidant vitamins A, E and C. Selenium is an antioxidant nutrient; vitamin E can ameliorate some of the symptoms of selenium deficiency and vice versa (Strain and Cashman, 2002).

Selenium deficiency

Two main diseases are associated with selenium deficiency: Kashin-Bek disease (an osteoarthropathy identified in Siberia) and Keshan disease. Keshan disease is a selenium-responsive cardiomyopathy affecting children and women of child-bearing age. In China in the late 1970s, the link between Keshan disease and low selenium status was discovered during an outbreak of epidemic proportions. The onset of Keshan disease is thought to be precipitated by the normally harmless Coxsackie virus, in selenium-deficient individuals (18, 19). Large-scale selenium supplementation trials involving more than 1.5 million children have virtually eradicated new cases of Keshan disease.

Iodine and selenium interactions

Autopsies of Keshan disease casualties revealed that up to 80% had goitre complications. Selenium is involved in normal thyroid metabolism, as already noted; it is required for the synthesis of active thyroid hormone (T3). Patients with sub-acute or latent Keshan disease had thyroid hormones in the normal range but higher serum concentration of the precursor hormone, T4, than control subjects. It appears that low selenium status may block optimum thyroid metabolism and decrease T4 deiodisation (Strain and Cashman, 2002).

Selenium toxicity

Selenium toxicity is well documented in animals but less known in humans. In seleniferous areas of China, chronic toxicity, or selenosis, has occurred after long-term consumption of foods with very high selenium content (Yang and Zhou, 1994). Acute selenium poisoning causes intense irritation of eyes, nose, mouth and lungs. Chronic exposure also produces nausea, anorexia and "garlic breath" caused by exhaled dimethyl selenide. The UK safe upper level of intake is 450 μg/day. The EU Scientific Committee on Food has determined a tolerable upper intake level of 300 μg selenium/ day.

Assessing selenium status

Currently, there is considerable debate as to the best index of selenium status. In clinical practice, hair, toenail or plasma selenium are often used as an index of recent intake. However, plasma selenium has recently been shown to be altered in the acute-phase immune response. Measurement of selenium in urine can detect excess but not deficiency. Activity of GPx in erythrocytes and plasma may provide an accurate measure (FSA, 2003). GPx activity plateaus before normal plasma concentrations of selenium are exceeded, however, so it is not useful to detect toxicity.

Zinc

Zinc has long been believed to be associated with wound healing and healthy tissue. It is required for DNA synthesis and for the activity of many enzymes, including alcohol dehydrogenase. It is also a crucial component of a family of proteins called the zinc "finger proteins". Over 100 zinc finger proteins are known and their functions are extraordinarily diverse. They include transcription activation, protein folding and assembly, and lipid binding. Zinc ions are essential for the structure and function of zinc finger proteins. The zinc finger regions are repeated cysteine- and histidine-containing domains that bind zinc in a tetrahedral configuration.

Zinc is known to have important roles in human reproduction. The effects of androgens and oestrogens are mediated by zinc finger proteins. Zinc is required for synthesis of luteinising hormone and follicle-stimulating hormone, gonadal differentiation, testicular growth, formation of sperm, testicular steroidogenesis and fertilization. Zinc also has a critical role in the structure and function of biomembranes, probably because it stabilises thiol groups and phospholipids and occupies sites that might otherwise contain transition metals with redox potential such as iron. Zinc is also involved in the quenching of free radical reactions. Loss of zinc from a membrane may be associated with increased susceptibility to oxidative damage, structural strains and alterations in specific receptor sites and transport systems (O'Dell, 2000).

Because zinc is essential in plants and animals, it is widely distributed in human diets. Good sources include oysters, fish, sea-foods, meats, whole grains and legumes. The UK RNI of zinc for adult men and women is 9.5 mg/day and 7.0 mg/day, respectively, and the LRNI is 5.5 mg/day and 4.0 mg/day (SCF, 2002).

Zinc absorption

About 20-40% of dietary zinc is absorbed from the intestine, by both passive diffusion and an active transport pump (FSA, 2003). Absorption is regulated by metallothionein, a protein synthesised in the intestinal mucosal cells in response to high levels of divalent metals, which binds metal ions and limits their absorption. A number of dietary factors also affect absorption. For example, competitive interactions exist between zinc and other cations, such as iron and copper. High iron content in the diet decreases zinc absorption. Ligands, such as phytate, form insoluble complexes with zinc and prevent absorption, and calcium increases binding of zinc by phytate (Oberleas et al. 1966). Amino acids such as histidine, methionine and cysteine, however, are thought to facilitate zinc absorption by removing zinc from the zinc-calcium-phytate complexes (Mills, 1985). Other modifiers include dietary fibre, ascorbic acid, fructose, sucrose, and polyphenols (tannins) found in soya, leafy vegetables, coffee and tea (Sanstrom and Lonnerdal, 1989).

In the plasma, 40% of circulating zinc is tightly bound, incorporated into a-macroglobulin. The rest is more loosely bound to albumin, transferrin and caeruloplasmin (FAO/WHO, 2001). This is thought to be the nutritionally relevant fraction. Zinc is excreted in the faeces via pancreatic and intestinal secretions, and is also excreted in the urine. It is also lost in lactation and during turnover of skin, hair and nails, and in semen and menstrual blood. No 'storage pool' or 'nutritional reserves' of zinc have been identified, so humans are relatively dependent upon a constant renewed supply of the metal (Strain and Cashman, 2002).

Zinc deficiency

Clinical zinc deficiency is rare, but is found with increased loss of zinc from body, for example, with widespread burns. It has also been reported in alcoholics. Zinc deficiency was first recognised as a condition that could affect humans, in the Middle East in the 1970s when studies of young men who had been rejected for army service because of their dwarf-like stature revealed a clinical syndrome involving anaemia plus other symptoms: skin changes, growth retardation and hypogonadism. This syndrome was found to be related to zinc deficiency (Prasad et al., 1961). Adequate zinc intake is essential to maintain immunocompetence, and zinc deficient individuals show increased susceptibility to a variety of infectious agents (Shankar and Prasad, 1998). Other clinical manifestations of severe zinc deficiency include impaired taste, delayed sexual maturation, impotence and hypospermia, alopecia, night blindness, eye and skin lesions, delayed wound healing, immune deficiencies and behavioral disturbances.

Inherited acrodermatitis enteropathica (AE) is a rare genetic (autosomal recessive) error of zinc metabolism. The mutated gene has been localized to chromosome 8 and is thought to produce a defective anionic exchange mechanism on the mucosal cell surfaces. Both the binding of zinc to the mucosal cells, and the translocation of zinc across the plasma membrane into the cell are impaired, resulting in decreased zinc absorption (Hambidge, 2000). AE is lethal, usually within the first few years of life if left untreated. With life-long high-dose oral zinc treatment the prognosis is good, probably owing to increased uptake and transfer of zinc by a less specific mechanism.

Experimental evidence suggests that zinc status may be involved in the pathogenesis of anorexia nervosa (Varela et al., 1992). In rats, zinc deficiency reduces food intake to about 50% of the diet of zinc-adequate rats, and these signs disappear upon zinc repletion. There is also some evidence that anorexic patients may stop losing weight, and increase weight when zinc is given.

Zinc toxicity

Because zinc is not stored in the human body, and because excess intakes usually result in reduced absorption and increased excretion, acute zinc toxicity is rare. However, prolonged intakes of zinc supplements have been associated with a range of biochemical and physiological changes. Most of these are probably symptoms of copper depletion, as copper and zinc compete directly for absorption in the intestine. Sufferers from haemochromatosis may absorb larger amounts of zinc, which suggests a possible increased risk of zinc-induced copper deficiency (FSA, 2003). The EU Scientific Committee on Food recommends a tolerable upper intake level of 25 mg zinc/day (SCF, 2002), and the same intake is recommended in the UK as a safe upper level (FSA, 2003).

Assessing zinc status

Zinc status is difficult to assess accurately in humans. It is often measured by urinary zinc, as excretion decreases during deficiency.

Zinc concentration in plasma may also be measured but is prone to changes related to inflammatory status. A plasma copper:zinc ratio greater than 2.0 is suggested to be related to zinc deficiency. Zinc in erythrocytes and hair may indicate longer-term status. Neutrophil alkaline phosphatase activity may also be a possible zinc status index.

Copper

Copper is present in all tissues and is an essential component of a number of enzymes and proteins. Copper-containing proteins include cytochrome C oxidase, which is involved in energy production; caeruloplasmin, an acute phase protein involved in inflammation, superoxide dismutase (SOD) (an antioxidant enzyme), amine oxidases (involved in brain chemistry), collagen formation, growth control and the chromatin scaffold proteins which maintain chromosome structure. Copper is widespread in foods and particularly good sources include green vegetables, fish, oysters, liver, nuts and mushrooms.

Absorption

Copper is absorbed primarily in the duodenum, through an active transport mechanism and passive diffusion (McAnena and O'Connor, 2002). Absorption is regulated by metallothionein, which is secreted by mucosal cells in response to high concentrations of metal ions such as copper and zinc. Metallothionein, however, has a higher affinity for copper than for zinc, and so high concentrations of zinc can impair copper absorption both indirectly, and directly, as already noted (Cousins, 1985). High dietary iron probably affects copper absorption only when copper status is already low or marginal. Copper excretion, which is mainly via the bile, can be up-regulated or down-regulated according to the body's needs. Very little copper is excreted by the kidneys.

Copper deficiency

The RNI for adults aged 19-50yrs is 1.2mg copper/day. The symptoms of copper deficiency are seen in many organ systems, with anaemia, neutropenia, osteoporosis and cardiac disorders; but because copper is widespread in food, and absorption and excretion are tightly regulated, clinical copper deficiency is rare. It is usually seen only in malnourished infants, and in patients with Menkes syndrome, an X-linked recessive disorder of copper absorption and transport. In Menkes syndrome, copper is absorbed but retained in the intestinal cells. Clinical manifestations are progressive mental deterioration, hypothermia, hypopigmentation, connective tissue abnormalities and death in early childhood (Mercer, 2001).

Although overt copper deficiency is rare, some evidence suggests that copper intakes from typical Western diets may be barely adequate. Dietary copper intakes of 1.1 mg /day for men and 0.9 mg/day for women were reported in the FoodCue Study, a multi-centre European survey (Kehoe et al., 2000). Marginal copper deficiency has been shown experimentally to have adverse effects including decreased glucose tolerance, abnormal electrocardiograms, hyperlipidaemia and increased clotting factors. It is probable that a lifelong marginal deficiency can contribute to ill health.

Copper toxicity

Haemodialysis patients and subjects with chronic liver disease are potentially sensitive to copper excess (Lyle et al.,1976). Another condition called Wilson's disease is an autosomal recessive inherited disorder of copper metabolism. Where there is a failure of normal copper excretion into the bile. As a result, copper accumulates and causes toxicity in the liver and brain. Clinical manifestations may include liver disease, and neurological and psychiatric disturbances (Loudiano and Gitlin, 2000).

Indian Childhood Cirrhosis is a fatal disorder associated with accumulation of massive levels of copper in the liver (O'Neill and Tanner, 1989). It has been attributed to boiling and storing milk in copper and brass vessels, but there also seems to be an element of genetic predisposition. Similar cases have also been reported non-Indian children in the US and Europe. In the UK a safe upper level of 10mg copper/day is recommended (FSA, 2003). The EU Scientific Committee on Food, however, recommends a tolerable upper intake level of 5 mg copper/day.

Assessing copper status

Currently there is no adequate index of copper status. A robust index of nutritional status should be specific, predictable, sensitive and accessible for measurement. Currently used (but unsatisfactory) indices include serum and hair copper concentrations, and activity of copper-containing enzymes such as caeruloplasmin, diamine oxidase and SOD (Milne, 1998).

Manganese

The human body contains 10 – 20 mg of manganese, distributed throughout the tissues, and at higher concentrations in tissues rich in mitochondria. A few manganese metalloenzymes are known to exist and include mitochondrial manganese SOD, arginase, pyruvate carboxylase, and glutamine synthetase. Manganese activates numerous other enzymes such as glycosyl transferases, hydrolyases and kinases. Sources of manganese include cereals, legumes, ginger and leafy vegetables and especially tea, a single cup of which may provide 0.4 to 1.3 mg (WHO, 1996).

Absorption, which occurs along the whole intestine, is very low and is inversely related to the level of iron and calcium in the diet (SCF, 2002). The question of how to assess manganese status in human is currently under investigation; the activity of manganese-dependent enzymes appear sensitive to low intake, but may not be specific. Manganese deficiency in humans has only ever been reported once: in a volunteer who received for two weeks a purified vitamin K-free diet, which also, accidentally, contained only 0.1 mg manganese/day (Strain and Cashman, 2002). This diet resulted in weight loss, dermatitis, a decline in blood lipids and reddening of black hair. Osteoporosis has been associated with low blood levels of manganese (Raloff, 1986). In UK there is no specific recommendation for minimum or maximum manganese intake, but the EU Scientific Committee for Food considered a "safe and adequate intake" to be 1-10 mg/day, and the US Food and Nutrition Board has set an "estimated safe and adequate daily dietary intake" of 2-5 mg/day. Manganese toxicity has been reported in mine workers breathing manganese-laden dust (FSA, 2003).

Molybdenum

Molybdenum is essential for certain enzymes in the metabolism of DNA and sulphites. Xanthine oxidase and dehydrogenase convert hypoxanthine to xanthine, and then to uric acid. Aldehyde oxidase oxidises and detoxifies various pyrimidines, purine pteridines and related compounds. Sulphite oxidase converts sulphite to sulphate (FNB, 2001).

Sources of molybdenum include wheat flour and germ, legumes and meat. Absorption of molybdenum varies over a wide range: 25 – 93% (FSA, 2003) and a carrier-dependent active process exists in the stomach and proximal intestine. As with ruminants, there appears to be an antagonistic copper-molybdenum interaction in humans, and molybdenum is sometimes used to treat the toxic accumulation of copper seen in Wilson's disease.

No RNI has been set for molybdenum, but the US Food and Nutrition Board has chosen 2.3 mg/day for men and 1.8 mg/day for women as a recommended adequate intake. This value is based on an estimate of molybdenum intake by the general population, which is assumed to be adequate. Molybdenum deficiency in humans has only ever been reported in one patient receiving prolonged total parenteral nutrition, and in a rare, fatal, autosomal recessive disorder involving defective hepatic synthesis of a molybdenum-containing cofactor (SCF, 2002). Excess intake may be associated with altered metabolism of nucleotides and with impaired copper bioavailability. High intakes of molybdenum have been associated with increased risk of gout. (FSA, 2003). Gout is characterized by deposition, in the joints, of sodium urate crystals, which may be caused by stimulation of xanthine oxidase by high molybdenum intake. The EU Scientific Committee for Food has set a safe upper level of 0.6 mg molybdenum/day.

Chromium

Chromium can exist in a variety of oxidation states, but the trivalent and hexavalent forms are the most important biologically. Hexavalent chromium compound do not exist in nature; chromium in foods is in the trivalent form. The role of chromium is uncertain, but it may act in an organic complex which influences and extends the action of insulin (SCF, 2002). It also has a possible role in lipoprotein metabolism, in stabilizing the structure of nucleic acids and in gene expression, but no chromium-containing protein has been identified to date.

Chromium is widespread in foods; particularly rich sources include meat, whole grains, lentils and spices and molasses, but intestinal absorption of chromium is low (Strain and Cashman, 2002). In humans, chromium deficiency has only been observed in patients on long-term parenteral nutrition (Jeejeebhoy et al., 1977). No Dietary Reference Values have been set for chromium, but the US Food and Nutrition Board have determined an adequate daily intake as 30 mg/day for men and 20 mg/day for women.

There has recently been some concern about chromium picolinate supplements, which are widely utilized to enhance "fat burning". Some evidence, albeit from *in vitro* studies, has linked chromium intake to DNA damage. Dietary chromium intake can be measured by plasma or serum levels, but body chromium status cannot be accurately assessed by fasting plasma or serum concentrations, because chromium tissue stores do not rapidly equilibrate with blood chromium. Elevated serum chromium, however, may be a good indicator of excessive exposure (FSA, 2003).

Fluoride

Although fluoride has no known metabolic role in the body, it is known to activate certain enzymes and inhibit others. Its function in human health is in the crystalline structure of teeth and bones where it forms calcium fluorapatite (Cerlewski, 1997). It also inhibits bacterial acid production and, by its interactions with calcium and phosphate, enhances the remineralisation of enamel when it is partially demineralised by organic acids (52, 53). It has been demonstrated epidemiologically that exposure to inadequate amounts of fluorine places the individual at increased risk of dental caries (54).

Fluorine is present at low levels in practically all plant and animal foodstuffs, and at higher concentrations in fluoridated water, in some marine fish and in tea. Tea leaves concentrate fluoride to the extent where a single cup, even made with un-fluoridated water, may provide at least 0.25 mg of fluoride. This makes a substantial contribution to the Average Intake of 3 mg/day, as determined by the US Food and Nutrition Board in 1997.

Fluoride is well absorbed in the intestine and transported in the circulation bound to albumin. It is excreted by the kidneys, and urinary fluoride can be used to assess fluoride intake. Chronic fluoride toxicity produces enamel and skeletal fluorosis. Dental fluorosis can result in tooth discoloration and surface irregularities. Skeletal fluorosis produces symptoms including calcification of ligaments, osteosclerosis and hypercalcification of vertebrae, which can cause neurological deficits (Strain and Cashman, 2002).

References

Barrington, J.W, Lindsay, P, James, D, Smith, S and Roberts, A (1996) Selenium deficiency and miscarriage: A possibly link? *British Journal of Obstetrics and Gynaecology.* **103**(2):130-132

Beck, M.A, Esworthy, R.S, Ho, Y.S and Chu, F.F. (1998) Glutathione peroxidase protects mice from viral-induced myocarditis. *Faseb Journal.***12**(12):1143-1149

British Nutrition Foundation http://www.nutrition.org.uk/

Cerklewski, F.L. (1997) Fluorine. In: *Handbook of nutritionally essential minerals*, Editors O'Dell BL, Sunde RA. New York: Marcel Dekker, Inc. 583-602

Cousins, R.J (1985) Absorption, transport and hepatic metabolism of copper and zinc: Special reference to metallothionein and ceruloplasmin. *Physiological Reviews*; **65**:238-30

DoH (Department of Health) (1991) Dietary Reference Values for Food Energy and Nutrients for the United Kingdom In: *Report on Health and Social Subjects* No. **41**. London: HMSO 01 132 1397 2

Edwards C.Q and Kushner, J.P. (1993) Screening for hemochromatosis. *New England Journal of Medicine* **328**:1616-20

FAO/WHO (1989) Expert Committee on Food Additives. Monograph 661. Iodine. WHO International Programme on Chemical Safety Food Additives Series **24**

FAO/WHO (2001) Human vitamin and mineral requirements. Report of a joint FAO/WHO expert consultation. Bangkok, Thailand

FNB (2001) Food and Nutrition Board. Institute of Medicine: Molybdenum. In: Dietary Reference Intakes: Vitamin A, Vitamin K, Arsenic, Boron, Chromium, Copper, Iodine, Iron, Manganese, Molybdenum, Nickel, Silicon, Vanadium and Zinc. National Academies Press: Washington, D.C. p. 420-441

FSAI (Food Safety Authority of Ireland) (1999) Recommended Dietary Allowances for Ireland.

FSA (2003) Expert Group on Vitamins and Mineral: Review of Zinc. Food Standards Agency, UK

FSA (2003) Expert Group on Vitamins and Minerals Review of Iodine. Food Standards Agency, UK

FSA (2003) Expert Group on Vitamins and Minerals: Review of Chromium. Food Standards Agency, UK

FSA (2003) Expert Group on Vitamins and Minerals: Review of Copper. Food Standards Agency, UK

FSA (2003) Expert Group on Vitamins and Minerals: Review of Iron. Food Standards Agency, UK

FSA (2003) Expert Group on Vitamins and Minerals: Review of Manganese. Food Standards Agency, UK

FSA (2003) Expert Group on Vitamins and Minerals: Review of Selenium. Food Standards Agency, UK

FSA, (2003) Expert Group on Vitamins and Minerals: Review of Molybdenum. Food Standards Agency, UK

Hambidge, M. (2000) Human zinc deficiency. *Journal of Nutrition.***130** (5S Suppl):1344S-1349S

Hetzel, B.S and Clugston, G.A. (1999) Iodine. In: *Nutrition in Health and Disease*. 9th vol. Editors, Shils, M, Olson, J.A, Shike, M and Ross A.C. Baltimore: Williams & Wilkins;253-264

Jeejeebhoy, K.N, Chu, R.C, Marliss, E.B, Greenberg, G.R and Bruce-Robertson, A (1977) Chromium deficiency, glucose intolerance and neuropathy reversed by chromium supplementation in a patient receiving long-term parenteral nutrition. *American Journal of Clinical Nutrition* **30**: 531-538

Kehoe, C.A, Turley, E, Bonham, M.P, O'Connor, J.M, McKeown, A, Faughnan, M.S, Coulter, J.S, Gilmore, W.S, Howard, A.N,

Strain, J.J. (2000) Response of putative indices of copper status to copper supplementation in human subjects. *British Journal of Nutrition* **84** (2)**:**151-156

Levander, O.A. (2000) Coxsackievirus as a model of viral evolution driven by dietary oxidative stress. *Nutrition Review* **58** (2 Pt 2):S17-24

Loudiano, G and Gitlin, J.D. (2000) *Seminars in Wilson's Disease;* **20** (3)**:**353-364

Lyle, W.H, Payton, J.E and Hui, M. (1976) Haemodialysis and copper fever. *Lancet* **1:**1324-1325

McAnena, L.B and O'Connor, J.M. (2002) Measuring Intake of Nutrients and their Effects: the Case of Copper. In: *The Nutrition Handbook for Food Processors*, Editors: CJK Henry and C Chapman. CRC & Woodland Publishing Ltd. pp117-141

Mercer, J.B. (2001) The molecular basis of copper-transport diseases. *Trends in Molecular Medicine* **7** (2)**:**64-69

Mills, C (1985). Dietary interactions involving trace elements. In: *Annual Review of Nutrition*. Editors, Olson R, Beutler E and Broquist H. Annual Reviews Inc., Palo Alto, CA, vol **5**, pp 173-193

Milne, D.B. (1998) Copper intake and assessment of copper status. *American Journal of Clinical Nutrition* **67**:1041s-1045S

Oberleas, D., Muhrer, M.E, O'Dell, B.L (1966) Dietary metal complexing agents and zinc bioavailability in the rat. *Journal of Nutrition* **90**: 56-62

O'Dell, B.L. (2000) Role of zinc in plasma membrane function *Journal of Nutrition* **130**(5S Suppl):1432S-1436S

O'Neill, N.C and Tanner, M.S. (1989) Uptake of copper from brass vessel by bovine milk and its relevance to Indian childhood cirrhosis. *Journal of Pediatric Gastroenterology and Nutrition* **9** (2)**:**167-172

Prasad, A.S, Halsted, J.A and Nadimi, M. (1961) Syndrome of iron deficiency anemia, hepatosplenomegaly, hypogonadism, dwarfism, and geophagia. *American Journal of Medicine* **31**:532-546

Raloff, J. (1986) Reasons for boning up on manganese. *Science;***130**:199

Sandström, B. and Lönnerdal, B. (1989). Promoters and antagonists of zinc absorption. In: *Zinc in Human Biology*. Editor, Mills C.F. p.57-78. Devon, U.K., Springer-Verlag

SCF (Scientific Committee on Foods) (2002) Opinion on the Tolerable Upper Intake Levels of Iodine. European Commission, Brussels.

SCF (Scientific Committee on Foods) (2002) Opinion on the Tolerable Upper Intake Levels of Zinc. European Commission

SCF (Scientific Committee on Foods) (2002) Opinion on the

Tolerable Upper Intake Levels of Manganese. European Commission, Brussels

SCF (Scientific Committee on Foods) (2002) Opinion on the Tolerable Upper Intake Levels of Molybdenum. European Commission

SCF (Scientific Committee on Foods) (2002) Opinion on the Tolerable Upper Intake Levels of Chromium. European Commission, Brussels

Schrauzer, G.N. and Sacher, J. (1994). Selenium in the maintenance and therapy of HIV infected patients *Chemical and Biological Interactions* **91**(2-3), 199-205

Shankar, A.H. and Prasad, A.S. (1998) Zinc and immune function: the biological basis of altered resistance to infection. *American Journal of Clinical Nutrition.* **68**:447S-463S

Solomons, N.W, Ruz, M. (1998) Trace element requirements in humans: An update. *Trace Element Experimental Medicine* **11**:177-195

Strain, J.J and Cashman, K.D. (2002) Minerals and Trace Elements. In: *Introduction to Human Nutrition.* Editors, Gibney, MJ, Vorster, HH and Kok, FJ

Varela, P, Marcos, A, Navarro, M.P. (1992) Zinc status in anorexia nervosa. *Annals of Nutrition and Metabolism* **36**:197–202

WHO (1996) Guidelines for drinking-water quality, 2nd edition Vol 2: *Health criteria and other supporting information.* World Health Organization, Geneva

Yang, G. and Zhou, R (1994) Further observations on the human maximum safe dietary selenium intake in a seleniferous area in China. *Journal of Trace Elements, Electrolytes, Health and Disease.* **8**: 159-165

Yip, R and Dallman, P.R. (1996) Iron. In: *Present Knowledge in Nutrition.* 7th ed. Editors, Ziegler EE, Filer LJ. ILSI Press, Washington D.C., USA p. 277-292

Minerals and anti-oxidants

Peter F. Surai
Head of Anti-oxidant Research, Alltech (UK) Ltd., Stamford, Lincs

Introduction

Animal health depends on many factors and it is increasingly appreciated that diet plays a pivotal role in maintaining health and preventing disease. Among many dietary factors, minerals have special importance in the maintenance of fast growth, reproduction and immuno-competence in poultry production. This concept is based on understanding the contribution of minerals in reducing the detrimental effects of free radicals and toxic metabolites on immune processes in the animal's body.

Natural mineral anti-oxidants in feed ingredients

The anti-oxidant/pro-oxidant balance can be modulated by sub-optimal diets and poor nutrient intakes, or positively affected by dietary supplementation. Therefore, feed components can change this balance and may influence such effects as the rate of ageing and disease resistance in human and animals. The most important step in balancing oxidative damage and anti-oxidant defence in the animal's body is enhancing anti-oxidant capacity by optimising the dietary intake of anti-oxidant compounds.

Animal feeds contain a range of different compounds that possess anti-oxidant activities, many of them being minerals or mineral–dependent. The key minerals in animal feed are listed below, and many of these are involved in anti-oxidation (Surai, 2002; Surai and Dvorska, 2002).

Selenium

- trace element
- essential part of a range of selenoproteins, including glutathione peroxidase (GSH-Px), thioredoxin reductase (TrxR), iodothironine

deiodinase (ID) and some others. In the animal and human body 25 selenoproteins have been identified to date

- food ingredients contain variable concentrations of Se, but most of them are deficient in this element
- physiological requirement is low, but if not met, anti-oxidant system is compromised with detrimental consequences for animal health
- toxic in high doses
- there are two major sources of Se for animals: a natural source in the form of various selenoamino acids including selenomethionine and selenocysteine or inorganic selenium in the form of selenite or selenate
- organic selenium supplementation has physiological and biochemical benefits for animals, including poultry.

Zinc

This is the second most abundant trace element in mammals and birds and is a component of over 300 enzymes participating in their structure or in their catalytic and regulatory actions in most species. It takes part in:

- anti-oxidant defence as an integral part of SOD
- hormone secretion and function (somatomedin-c, osteocalcin, testosterone, thyroid hormones, insulin, growth hormone)
- keratin generation and epithelial tissue integrity
- bone metabolism being an essential component of the calcified matrix
- nucleic acid synthesis and cell division
- protein synthesis
- catalytic, structural and regulatory ion for enzymes and transcription factors and participates in the metabolism of carbohydrates, lipids and proteins
- sexual development and spermatogenesis
- immune function
- appetite control via acting on the central nervous system

Organic Zn has higher availability in comparison to inorganic sources and is considered to be more beneficial for animal health.

Copper

Copper is an essential component of a range of physiologically important metalloenzymes and takes part in:

- anti-oxidant defence as an integral part of SOD
- cellular respiration
- cardiac function
- bone formation
- carbohydrate and lipid metabolism
- immune function
- connective tissue development
- tissue keratinization
- myelination of the spinal cord

The main Cu-containing enzymes are shown in Table 1. Inorganic copper has a strong pro-oxidant effect and (if not bound to proteins) can stimulate lipid peroxidation in feed or the intestinal tract (Surai et al., 2003a). Organic copper does not possess pro-oxidant properties and can improve the copper status of animals.

Table 1. Copper-containing enzymes in animals and humans (Adapted from Nath, 1997).

Common name	EC number	Functional role	Known or possible consequence of deficiency
Cytochrome c oxidase	1.9.3.1	Electron-transport chain	Muscle weakness; cardiomyopathy, brain degeneration
Superoxide dismutase	1.15.1.1	Free radical detoxification	Membrane damage; other free radical damage
Thyrosinase (monophenol monooxygenase)	1.14.18.1	Melanin production	Failure of pigmentation
Dopamine -ß-hydroxylase	1.14.17.1	Catecholamine production	Neurological effects
Lysyl oxidase	1.4.3.13	Cross-linking of collagen and elastin	Vascular rapture; loose skin and joints; osteoporosis
Ceruloplasmin	1.16.3.1	Ferroxidase, anime oxidase; Cu transport	Anaemia; deficient supply of Cu to other tissues
Clotting factor V		Blood clotting	Bleeding tendency

Iron

Iron has a vital role in many biochemical reactions taking part in:

- anti-oxidant defence as an essential component of catalase
- energy and protein metabolism
- heme respiratory carrier
- oxidation/reduction reactions
- electron transport system

Iron is a very strong pro-oxidant and if not bound to proteins can stimulate lipid peroxidation. This is especially relevant to the digestive tract where lipid peroxidation can be stimulated, causing enterocyte damages and decreased absorption of nutrients (Surai et al., 2003a). If iron is included in the premix in inorganic form, it can stimulate vitamin oxidation during storage. Therefore organic iron is a solution to avoid these problems and improve the iron status of animals.

Manganese

Manganese plays an important role in body metabolism as an essential part of a range of enzymes taking part in:

- anti-oxidant protection as an integral part of SOD
- bone growth and egg shell formation
- carbohydrate and lipid metabolism
- immune and nervous function
- reproduction

As with other organic minerals, manganese seems to be better assimilated from the diet

From this brief list of mineral functions, it can be clearly seen that most are relevant to immune function, via involvement in the anti-oxidation processes.

The need for anti-oxidant defence

Free radicals are atoms or molecules containing one or more unpaired electrons. Most biologically relevant free radicals are derived from oxygen and nitrogen, the so-called reactive oxygen species (ROS) and reactive nitrogen species (RNS). Both these elements are essential, but in certain circumstances are converted into free radicals. These are highly unstable, and their reactive capacity makes them capable of damaging biologically relevant molecules such as DNA, proteins, lipids or carbohydrates (Surai, 2002).

The animal's body is under constant attack from free radicals, formed as a natural consequence of the body's metabolic activity and the immune system's strategy for destroying invading micro-organisms (Table 2). For example, under normal physiological conditions about 3-5% of the oxygen taken up by the cell undergoes univalent reduction leading to the formation of free radicals (Singal et al., 1998). About 10^{12} O_2 molecules are processed by each rat cell daily with 2% leakage from cells, yielding a total of 2 $\times 10^{10}$ molecules of ROS per cell per day (Chance et al., 1979). Furthermore Helbock et al. (1998) have calculated that the DNA in each cell in a rat is hit by about 100,000 free radicals a day and each cell sustains as many as 10,000 potentially mutagenic (if unrepaired) lesions per day arising from endogenous sources of DNA damage (Ames and Gold, 1997). If oxidative lesions are not repaired and exposure increases with age, then an old rat can accumulate approximately 66,000 oxidative DNA lesions per cell (Ames, 2003). An interesting calculation has been made by Halliwell (1994) where it was assumed that in mitochondria about 1-3% of oxygen consumed might leak from the electron transport chain forming superoxide radicals. They calculated that an adult at rest utilises approximately 3.5 ml O_2 per kg body weight per minute or 352.8 litres per day (assuming 70 kg body mass) or 14.7 moles per day. Therefore if 1% of the oxygen becomes superoxide this equate to 0.147 moles per day or 53.66 moles per year or about 1.72 kg per year of superoxide radicals. This represents a substantial increase in physiological stress levels.

Internally generated	External sources
Mitochondria	Cigarette smoke
Phagocytes	Radiation
Xanthine oxidase	UV light
Reactions with Fe and with other	Pollution
transition metals	Certain drugs
Arachidonate pathways	Chemical reagents
Peroxisomes	Industrial solvents
Exercise	
Inflammation	
Ischemia and reperfusion	

Table 2. Selected sources of free radicals (Adapted from Surai, 2002)

Such calculations demonstrate the substantial free radical production in the body and the great potential for damage to tissues and cells. The internal and external sources of free radicals are shown in Table 2. It is interesting that free radicals also work as physiological mediators and signalling molecules; therefore complete removal of free radicals from the cell could have detrimental consequences.

In the case of the immune system, the problem is exacerbated as immune cells produce free radicals and use them to destroy pathogens (Surai, 2002). High oxygen concentration is potentially toxic for living organisms, as first described in laboratory animals in 1878 (Knight, 1998).

Living organisms have evolved specific anti-oxidant protective mechanisms to deal with the free radicals constantly produced by cells. These mechanisms helped organisms to survive in an atmosphere when oxygen concentration was increasing millennia ago, and are described by the general term "anti-oxidant system" (Halliwell and Gutteridge, 1999; Surai, 2002). In nature there are thousands of compounds possessing anti-oxidant properties that are able to neutralise free radicals. They can be fat-soluble (vitamin E and carotenoids, coenzyme Q, etc.) and water-soluble (ascorbic acid, glutathione, bilirubin, taurine, etc.), or synthesised in the body (ascorbic acid, glutathione or taurine) or have to be delivered via feed (minerals, vitamin E, carotenoids).

There is a range of mineral-dependent anti-oxidant enzymes, which can be synthesised in the body and are able to effectively deal with free radicals, but require feed-derived mineral co-factors to do so. For example, Se in the form of selenocysteine is an essential part of a family of enzymes called glutathione peroxidases (GSH-Px) and thioredoxin reductases (TR) Zn, Cu and Mn are integral parts of another anti-oxidant enzyme family called superoxide dismutases (SOD) and iron is an essential part of the anti-oxidant enzyme called catalase. When these metals are delivered in feed in sufficient amounts the body can synthesise anti-oxidant enzymes. In contrast deficiency of these elements causes oxidative stress and damages to biological molecules and membranes.

How anti-oxidants work

Biological anti-oxidants react with free radicals or precursor metabolites converting them into less reactive molecules and preventing or delaying oxidation of biological molecules. The most important and well-characterised natural anti-oxidants in the animal's body are vitamins E and C. Plant pigments such as carotenoids have anti-oxidant capacity. Protective anti-oxidant compounds are located in organelles, subcellular compartments or the extracellular space enabling maximum cellular protection to occur.

In fact all anti-oxidants in the body are working together to achieve physiological defence. The anti-oxidant 'team' acts to control levels of free radical formation, as a coordinated system where deficiencies in one component impacts the efficiency of others. For example, ascorbate can help vitamin E to recover from oxidation to become active again. If relationships in this team are effective, where the individual has a balanced diet and sufficient intake of anti-oxidants, then even low doses of such anti-oxidants as vitamin E or Selenium can be effective. When the anti-oxidant system finds itself in high stress conditions, if free radical production is increased dramatically, without external help it will be difficult to prevent damage to organs and cells. Such external help can be provided by dietary supplementation with increased doses of natural anti-oxidants, especially minerals such as selenium. For nutritionists or feed formulators the challenge is to understand when the anti-oxidant team requires help and how much of this help can justify extra feed expense, because anti-oxidants are typically expensive components of the diet. A list of possible stresses in poultry production includes the following (Surai, 2002):

- *Time* between an egg being laid and it's cooling down for storage. Eggs should be collected frequently in hotter climates. In such conditions free radical damages to lipids and proteins can occur and anti-oxidant protection is beneficial.

- *Egg storage before incubation* often associated with lipid peroxidation within egg membranes, particularly those containing high levels of PUFAs. Increased Se concentration in combination with other anti-oxidants (vitamin E and carotenoids) can be an effective means to prevent damaging effects of free radicals produced within the egg.

- *Temperature, humidity and carbon dioxide concentration* fluctuations during incubation can affect embryonic development, oxidation and phosphorylation in tissues leading to free radical production. For example, high carbon dioxide concentrations during the incubation period has been shown to jeopardise the liveability of the embryo.

- *Day 19 of embryonic development* is an important point when risk of lipid peroxidation is very high. At this stage chick tissues are characterised by comparatively high levels of polyunsaturated fatty acids (PUFA). At the same time natural anti-oxidant reserves have not reached a sufficient level for innate protection. At this stage of development 'piping' occurs; and oxygen availability for tissues increases. Low anti-oxidant status in combination with high temperature, humidity, and PUFAs can increase susceptibility to lipid peroxidation.

- *Hatching time* is considered as an environmental stress for the chick. At this point natural anti-oxidant concentrations have reached a maximum, but high levels of lipid unsaturation in tissues and decreasing concentration of ascorbic acid can limit vitamin E recycling and high temperature and humidity increase risk of lipid peroxidation.

- *Delay in collecting chicks from incubator.* Since not all chicks are hatched at the same time (eggs from older breeders hatch earlier than those from young flocks and chicks from smaller eggs hatch earlier than those from large eggs), some may be in the incubator for 2-12 hours longer than others. This puts pressure on anti-oxidant defence capacity. Furthermore, any delay in food and/or water intake after hatching usually negatively affect a number of performance parameters, and delays the maturation of the enzymatic systems that control metabolism, free radical production and anti-oxidant protection systems.

- *Transportation from hatchery to farm* is another source of stress. For breeding companies where chicken transportation can involve several thousand miles, a very high degree of stress should be associated with temperature fluctuation and dehydration.

- *Sub-optimal temperatures in the poultry house.* Cold tolerance as well as feather cover is influenced by thyroid hormone activity, which is Se-dependent.

- *High levels of ammonia and CO_2 in poultry house as a result of inadequate ventilation* can substantially decrease anti-oxidant system efficiency.

- *Disease challenge.* Phagocytic immune cells produce free radicals in the process of killing internalised pathogens. Without adequate anti-oxidant nutrient reserves, cellular membranes and important organelles, can be damaged by the free radicals thereby reducing the effectiveness of the immune cell. In addition, Se is considered to have a specific role in immune system regulation, which is independent of its anti-oxidant functions.

- *Vaccination* is a substantial stress; and in some cases using vitamin E as a vaccine adjuvant can help improve vaccination efficiency.

- *Induced moulting with feed withdrawal* is an important stress condition where decreased efficiency of heterophil function increases bird susceptibility to various infections.

- *Mycotoxins in the feed* can decrease anti-oxidant assimilation from the feed and increase their requirement to prevent damaging effects of free radicals and toxic products of mycotoxin metabolites. It is now recognised that at least 25% of world's grains are contaminated with mycotoxins.

- *Heavy metals and other toxins (dioxin, pesticides, fungicides, herbicides, etc.) in the feed* can also cause an oxidative stress, decreasing immunocompetence, productive and reproductive performances and increasing a requirement for anti-oxidants.

- *Oxidized fat in the diet* increases the exposure to free radicals, inducing stress in the intestine and increasing anti-oxidant requirement to prevent damage to tissues. When a chicken diet includes fat which has undergone high temperature treatment, resulting peroxides can contribute substantially to oxidative stress.

- *Extensive preventive medication (coccidiostats or other veterinary drugs in the diet)* can limit dietary anti-oxidant uptake or increase stress conditions, e.g. monensin can stimulate lipid peroxidation in the chicken liver. Similarly, oral furazolidone treatment of chickens has been associated with a decreased vitamin E concentration and increased lipid peroxidation in their liver.

- *Vitamin A excess* in the diet has been shown to cause oxidative stress, decreasing vitamin E and carotenoid concentrations in tissues and increasing tissue susceptibility to lipid peroxidation.

The list of potential stresses can vary from one poultry farm to another, but overproduction of free radicals and the critical need for anti-oxidant protection are common factors.

Three levels of anti-oxidant defence

There are certain anti-oxidant considerations for adequate defence that the nutritionist must take into account when deciding the level of exposure the animal faces. Protective anti-oxidant compounds are located in organelles, subcellular compartments or in extra-cellular space, enabling maximum protection. The anti-oxidant system of the living cell includes three major levels of defence (Niki, 1996; Surai, 1999; Surai, 2002):

- The first level of defence is responsible for prevention of free radical formation by removing precursors of free radicals or by inactivating catalysts and consists of three anti-oxidant enzymes namely SOD, GSH-Px and CAT plus metal-binding proteins (Figure 1).

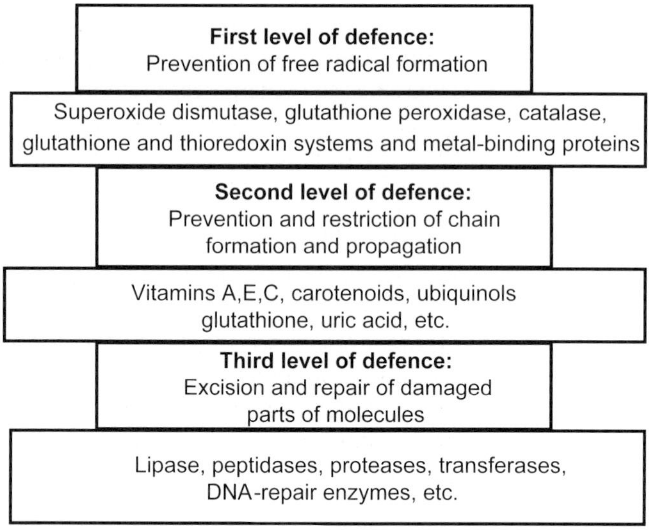

Figure 1.
Three levels of
antioxidant
defence in animal
cells (Adapted
from Surai, 2002)

The figure content:

First level of defence: Prevention of free radical formation
Superoxide dismutase, glutathione peroxidase, catalase, glutathione and thioredoxin systems and metal-binding proteins
Second level of defence: Prevention and restriction of chain formation and propagation
Vitamins A,E,C, carotenoids, ubiquinols glutathione, uric acid, etc.
Third level of defence: Excision and repair of damaged parts of molecules
Lipase, peptidases, proteases, transferases, DNA-repair enzymes, etc.

- Since the superoxide radical is the main free radical produced under physiological conditions in the cell (Halliwell, 1994) the enzyme superoxide dismutase (EC 1.15.1.1) is considered to be the main element of the first level of anti-oxidant defense in the cell (Surai, 1999). This enzyme transforms the superoxide radical in the following reaction:

$$2O_2^{\cdot} + 2H^+ \xrightarrow{\hspace{0.5cm} SOD \hspace{0.5cm}} H_2O_2 + O_2$$

Superoxide dismutase was discovered by McCord and Fridovich in 1969 who discovered the enzymatic activity in preparations of carbonic anhydrase or myoglobin that inhibited the aerobic reduction of cytochrome C by xanthine oxidase. This discovery opened up a new era in free radical research. At present, three distinct isoforms of SOD have been identified in mammals, and their structure and protein content have been described (Zelko *et al.*, 2002). SOD1, or Cu-Zn-SOD (previously called haemocuprein, Bannister, 1988), was the first enzyme of this family to be characterised and is a copper and zinc-containing compound that is found almost exclusively in intracellular cytoplasmic spaces. It exists as a 32 kDa homodimer and is present in the cytoplasm and nucleus of every cell type examined (Zelko *et al.*, 2002).

The second member of the family has manganese (Mn) as a cofactor and is called Mn-SOD. It was shown to be a 96 kDa homotetramer, located exclusively in the mitochondrial matrix, a prime site of superoxide radical production (Halliwell and Gutteridge, 1999).

Therefore the expression of Mn-SOD is considered to be essential for the survival of aerobic life and the development of cellular resistance to oxygen radical-mediated toxicity (Fridovich, 1995). Mn-SOD is an inducible enzyme and its activity is affected by cytokines and oxidative stress. In fact, Mn-SOD has been shown to play a major role in promoting cellular differentiation and in protecting against hyperoxia-induced pulmonary toxicity (Fridovich, 1995). In 1982 a third SOD isozyme was discovered by Marklund and co-workers and called extracellular superoxide dismutase (EC-SOD), due to its exclusive extracellular location. EC-SOD is a glycoprotein with a molecular weight of 135,000 kDa with high affinity for heparin. However, there are some species-specific variations in molecular weight. EC-SOD is present in various organisms as a tetramer or, less commonly, as a dimer and contains one copper and one zinc atom per subunit, which are required for enzymatic activity (Fattman et al., 2003). The expression pattern of EC-SOD is highly restricted to the specific cell type and tissues where its activity can exceed that of Cu-Zn-SOD or Mn- SOD. The fourth form of the enzyme Fe-SOD was isolated from various bacteria but is not found in animal tissues (Michalski, 1992). Furthermore, a novel type of nickel-containing SOD was purified from the cytosolic fractions of Streptomyces species (Youn et al., 1996). The biosynthesis of SODs, in most biological systems, is well controlled. In fact, exposure to increased oxygen levels, increased intracellular fluxes of O_2^- and metal ions perturbation, and exposure to environmental oxidants appear to influence the rate of SOD synthesis in both prokaryotic and eukaryotic organisms (Hassan, 1988).

The hydrogen peroxide formed by SOD action can be detoxified by GSH-Px or CAT which reduce it to water as follows:

$$H_2O_2 + 2GSH \xrightarrow{\text{GSH-Px}} GSSG + 2H_2O$$

$$2H_2O_2 \xrightarrow{\text{Catalase}} 2H_2O + O_2$$

Catalase (CAT) (EC 1.11.1.6) is a tetrameric iron dependent enzyme consisting of four identical subunits of 60 kDa containing a single ferriprotoporphyrin group per subunit. It plays an important role in the acquisition of tolerance to oxidative stress in the adaptive response of cells (Mates et al., 1999). In mammalian cells, NADPH is bound to catalase protecting it from inactivation by H_2O_2 (Chaudiere and Ferrari-Illiou, 1999). Since GSH-Px has a much higher affinity for peroxide than CAT (Jones et al., 1981) and wider distribution in the cell (catalase is located mainly in peroxisomes), peroxide removal from the cell is very much dependent on GSH-Px. Recently it has been shown that thioredoxin peroxidases are also capable of directly reducing hydrogen peroxide (Nordberg and Arner, 2001). It is interesting that the levels of anti-oxidant enzymes are regulated by gene expression as well as by post-translational modifications (Fujii and Taniguchi, 1999).

Transition metal ions accelerate the decomposition of lipid hydroperoxides into cell-toxic products such as aldehydes, alkoxyl radicals and peroxyl radicals:

$$LOOH + Fe^{2+} \longrightarrow LO^* + Fe^{3+} + OH^-$$
$$LOOH + Fe^{3+} \longrightarrow LOO^* + Fe^{2+} + H^+$$

Therefore, metal-binding proteins (transferrin, lactoferrin, haptoglobin, hemopexin, metallothionenin, ceruloplasmin, ferritin, albumin, myoglobin, etc.) also belong to the first level of defence. It is necessary to take into account that inorganic and charged iron and copper compounds are powerful promoters of free radical reactions and their availability in "catalytic" forms must be carefully regulated *in vivo* (Halliwell, 1999). To ensure this, organisms have evolved to keep transition metal ions safely sequestered in storage or transport proteins. In this way the metal-binding proteins prevent formation of hydroxyl ions by preventing them from participation in radical reactions. For example, transferrin binds iron (about 0.1% of the total body reserves), transports it within the plasma pool and attaches it to the transferrin receptor, where it will not be able to catalyse free radical reactions. Ferritin is considered to be involved in iron storage (about 30% of total body reserves) within the cytosol in various tissues including liver and spleen.

The majority of iron in the body (55-60%) is associated with hemoglobin within red cells and about 10% with myoglobin in muscles (Galey, 1997). A range of other iron-containing proteins (mainly enzymes) can be found in the body including NADH dehydrogenase, cytochrome P450, ribonucleotide reductase, proline hydroxylase, tyrosine hydroxylase, peroxidases, catalase, cyclooxygenase, aconitase, succinate dehydrogenase, etc. (Galey, 1997). Despite the importance of iron in numerous biochemical reactions, iron can be dangerous when not carefully managed via proteins. In fact, under certain stress conditions, a release of free iron from the normal storage sites can occur, whereby the superoxide radical can release iron from ferritin and H_2O_2 degrades the heme of hemoglobin to liberate iron (Halliwell, 1987). Recently it has been suggested that pro-oxidant properties of inorganic iron could have detrimental consequences for the digestive tract (Surai et al., 2003). Therefore, organic iron should be the nutritionist's choice for dietary supplementation.

Ceruloplasmin is a copper-binding protein that mediates free radical metabolism. Under physiological conditions it binds six or seven copper ions per molecule, preventing their participation in free radical generation. About 5% of human plasma copper is bound to albumin or amino acids, the rest being bound to ceruloplasmin. Furthermore ceruloplasmin possesses anti-oxidant properties, being able to scavenge superoxide radical (Yu, 1994). It is now quite clear that metal sequestration is an important part of extracellular anti-oxidant defence. Similar to inorganic iron, inorganic copper is also a strong pro-oxidant in the digestive tract (Surai et al., 2003) and therefore organic copper is a preferential form of dietary supply.

Unfortunately this first level of anti-oxidant defence in the cell is not sufficient to completely prevent free radical formation and some radicals do escape through the preventive first level of anti-oxidant safety screen initiating lipid peroxidation and causing damage to DNA and proteins. Therefore the second level of defence consists of chain-breaking anti-oxidants - vitamin E, ubiquinol, carotenoids, vitamin A, ascorbic acid, uric acid and some other anti-oxidants. Glutathione and thioredoxin systems play a substantial role in the second level of anti-oxidant defence (Surai, 2002). Chain-breaking anti-oxidants inhibit peroxidation by reducing the propagation reaction as much as possible, limiting the potential cascade reaction and proliferation of free radicals. They prevent the propagation step of lipid peroxidation by scavenging peroxyl radical intermediates in the chain reaction:

$$LOO^* + Toc \longrightarrow Toc^* + LOOH$$

(LOO^* is lipid peroxyl radical; Toc - tocopherol, Toc^* - tocopheroxyl radical, LOOH – lipid hydroperoxide).

Vitamin E, the most effective natural free radical scavenger identified to date, is the main chain breaking anti-oxidant in the cell. However, hydroperoxides produced in the reaction of vitamin E with the peroxyl radical are toxic and if not removed they impair membrane structure and functions (Gutteridge and Halliwell, 1990). In fact, lipid hydroperoxides are not stable and in the presence of charged transition metal ions can decompose producing new free radicals and cytotoxic aldehydes (Diplock, 1994). Therefore hydroperoxides have to be removed from the cell in the same way as H_2O_2, but catalase is not able to detoxify these compounds and only Se-dependent GSH-Px can deal with them converting hydroperoxides into non-reactive products (Brigelius-Flohe, 1999) as follows:

$$ROOH + 2GSH \xrightarrow{\text{GSH-Px}} ROH \text{ (non-toxic)} + H_2O + GSSG$$

Thus, vitamin E performs only half the job in preventing lipid peroxidation by scavenging free radicals and forming hydroperoxides. The second part of this important process of anti-oxidant defence is due to Se-GSH-Px. It is necessary to underline, that vitamin E and selenium work in a tandem; and even very high doses of dietary vitamin E cannot replace Se which is needed to complete the second part of anti-oxidant defence as mentioned above. Thus, Se (as an integral part of the GSH-Px and thioredoxin reductase) belongs to the first and second levels of anti-oxidant defence. Indeed, anti-oxidant interactions and recycling is a key mechanism of the effective anti-oxidant defence (Figure 2).

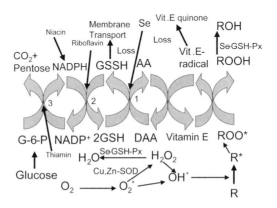

Figure 2.
Radical formation and antioxidant defence (Adapted from Surai, 2002)

As a result of anti-oxidant action of vitamin E the tocopheroxyl radical is formed. This radical can be reduced back to an active form of α-tocopherol by coupling with ascorbic acid oxidation. Ascorbic acid can be regenerated back from the oxidised form by recycling with glutathione which can receive a reducing potential from NADPH, synthesised in the pentose phosphate cycle of carbohydrate metabolism. Enzymes involved in vitamin E recycling are as follows: 1. Se-dependent thioredoxin reductase; 2.Glutathione reductase; 3.Glucose-6-phosphate dehydrogenase. Due to incomplete regeneration (the efficiency of recycling is usually less than 100%) in biological systems, the anti-oxidants have to be obtained from the diet (vitamin E and carotenoids) or synthesised in the tissues (ascorbic acid and glutathione).

It has been suggested that anti-oxidant/pro-oxidant balance in the digestive tract, in individual cells and in the whole body is responsible for regulation of many different physiological processes and ultimately responsible for maintenance of good health (Surai, 2002;Surai et al., 2003;Surai et al., 2004; Figure 3).

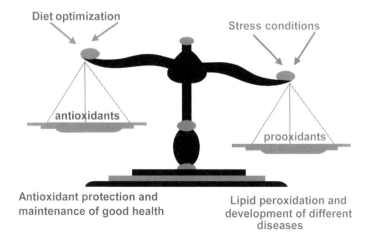

Figure 3.
Antioxidant-
prooxidant balance
in the cell (Adapted
from Surai, 2002)

Mineral anti-oxidants and their correct application, in terms of forms used and delivery systems, exert a major influence on poultry production, in particular their role in reproduction and immunocompetence.

Male fertility

The principle anti-oxidant minerals associated with male fertility are selenium and zinc. In order to be fertile, spermatozoa is characterised by high motility and acrosome integrity. To be motile, the spermatozoa needs intact mitochondria (energy-producing stations in the cell) and high membrane flexibility and fluidity, membrane properties which require a high level of polyunsaturated fatty acids (Surai et al., 2003). Spermatozoa from all animal species is characterised by extremely high proportions of such fatty acids (Figure 4) and, as a result, they become very vulnerable to oxidative stress due to overproduction of free radicals. To deal with such problems the anti-oxidant system of the spermatozoa includes fat-soluble and water-soluble chain-breaking anti-oxidants as well as enzymes.

Understanding the involvement of selenium in maintenance of semen quality has been generated from data on selenoproteins. In particular, there are several selenoproteins, which are found in spermatozoa, including the enzyme GSH-Px, which are responsible for preventing damaging effects of free radicals and toxic metabolites on spermatozoa. Specific sperm nuclear GSH-Px was identified in 2001 (Pfeifer et al., 2001). It seems likely that thioredoxin reductase (TR) is also involved in anti-oxidant defence in spermatozoa, but this has yet to be confirmed. A specific sperm capsular

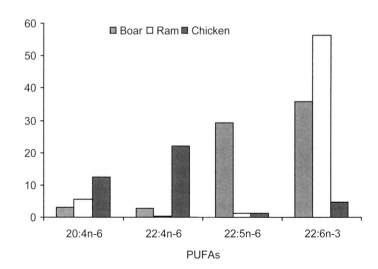

Figure 4.
Polyunsaturated
fatty acids
(PUFAs) in
semen (Adapted
from Surai, 2003)

selenoprotein, located in the midpiece of spermatozoa, has recently been identified as a form of Se-dependent GSH-Px. Mitochondria, a main source of free radicals due to energy production in the spermatozoa, are located in the midpiece, making anti-oxidant protection in this location of the cell a crucial factor for motility and effective fertility. This has been demonstrated in studies where Se-deficiency has been shown to cause sperm abnormalities in this region (Surai, 2002), resulting in decreased fertilising ability. Organic selenium dietary supplementation was seen to be more efficient in improving semen morphology than selenite in these cases (Edens, 2002). Experiments with Sel-Plex in cockerel diets has further proved that organic selenium increases duration of fertility (Agate et al., 2000).

Zinc is an important mineral for male fertility maintenance. As mentioned above, zinc is an integral part of superoxide dismutase, an enzyme of the first level of anti-oxidant defences. Zinc deficiency is associated with decreased testosterone levels, sperm count, motility and production and supplemental Zn is proven to be helpful in treating male infertility (Sinclair, 2000). The role of zinc in mammalian spermatozoa can be presented as follows (Hidiroglou and Knipfel, 1984):

- Semen and its constituents contain comparatively high zinc concentration

- Zinc deficiency results in retarded development of testicular growth with marked atrophy of tubular epithelium and reduced zinc contents of testis, epididymis, and dorsolateral prostate.

- Zinc deficiency decreases output of pituitary gonadotrophins and androgen production, and zinc turnover involves testosterone as well as pituitary hormones.

- Metabolic regulation of sperm is mediated through zinc as a regulator of enzyme activity in the semen.

- Within spermatozoa, zinc is closely associated with sulfhydryl groups and disulfide linkages and is concentrated in the tail.

- Zinc in seminal plasma influences the oxygen consumption of the spermatozoa and, nuclear protein activity (Wong et al., 2000).

- Control of motility of sperm by zinc involves control of energy utilization through ATP systems involved in contraction and through regulation of phospholipid energy reserves.

Indeed, reproductive failures in the female and in spermatogenesis are manifestations of zinc deficiency (Hidiroglou et al., 1979). Involvement of dietary minerals in male reproduction is shown in Figure 5.

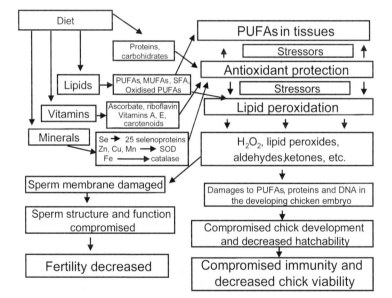

Figure 5. Nutrition, antioxidant defences and poultry reproduction

Embryonic development

Chick embryo tissues contain a high proportion of polyunsaturated fatty acids in the lipid fraction. Tissues of newly hatched chicks express a range of antioxidant defences, including natural anti-oxidants and enzymes (superoxide dismutase, glutathione peroxidase and catalase) as well as mineral cofactors (Se, Zn, Mn and Fe) (Surai, 2002). Se, Cu, Fe and manganese are delivered from the maternal diet via the egg and the others are synthesised in the tissues.

It is necessary to underline that maternal diet composition is a major determinant of anti-oxidant system development during embryogenesis and in early postnatal development. Minerals such as selenium are transferred from feed into egg and further to embryonic tissues. Research indicates that increased supplementation of the maternal diet can substantially increase Se concentrations in developing chick tissues and significantly decreases susceptibility to lipid peroxidation. A positive effect of Se supplementation of the maternal diet has been observed at day 5 and 10 post-hatch when vitamin E concentrations in the liver and plasma were significantly elevated compared to controls. Recent results indicate that increased concentration of Se in the egg was associated with increased Se concentration in the chicken liver until 3 weeks posthatch and in the breast muscle and plasma Se concentration was elevated during 4 weeks of the postnatal development of the chicken.

Postnatal development of the chick is associated with changes in the anti-oxidant defence strategy. The main protection from oxidation in newly hatched chicks is afforded through high concentrations of natural anti-oxidants, mainly vitamin E and, in wild birds, carotenoids in tissues. However, during the first 10 days post-hatch, vitamin E and carotenoid concentrations in the chicken liver decreases 20-fold; and the same is true for turkeys, ducks and geese. To compensate for this decrease, activity of GSH-Px in the liver significantly increases. As a result, this Se-dependent enzyme becomes the major anti-oxidant defence during postnatal development of the chicken. There is some evidence to show that under commercial conditions, inclusion of organic selenium into the breeder's diet is associated with improved hatchability. Furthermore organic selenium supplementation of the maternal diet decreases chick mortality for the first two weeks posthatch confirming the relationship between anti-oxidant defences and chicken viability (Surai, 2002).

Immune system

The immune system of the animal is based on natural 'innate' (inherited from the mother) and adaptive or 'acquired' (formed through experience of pathogen exposure) immunity. Innate immunity is dependent on the efficient function of phagocytic cells, namely neutrophils and macrophages (Figure 6). These cells are equipped with an array of microbicidal weapons, such as proteases, that hydrolyse protein, disrupting membranes, and are stored in granules in the cell cytoplasm. Furthermore, these cells have a powerful system for generating large amounts of ROS and they use them as an effective weapon to destroy pathogens. However, on release from the storage, phagosome organelle, the same free radicals can damage biological molecules, compromising phagocyte function and reducing acquired immunity. Phagocytes also produce communication molecules (e.g. eicosanoids, cytokines) that are used for signalling between various immune cells, so protecting their function is essential to other areas of immune function as well.

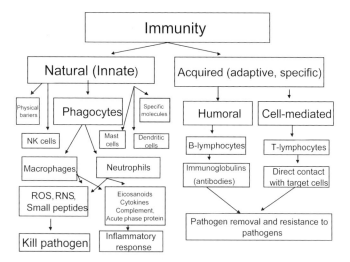

Figure 6. General scheme of immune system (Adapted from Surai, 2002)

Invading pathogens are controlled by both the innate and acquired branches of the immune system. The establishment of acquired immunity is not sufficiently fast to eradicate micro-organisms encountered by the young animal, and innate immunity is mainly responsible for recognition of invading pathogens by specific receptors. Binding of pathogens to recognition receptors induces the production of ROS and RNS, pro-inflammatory cytokines and communicating molecules which are responsible for sending regulatory signals to the acquired immune system (Werling and Jungi, 2003).

Acquired immunity is based on the activity of B- and T-lymphocytes, which produce antibodies to specific invading substances (B-lymphocytes) or bind (T-lymphocyte) and remove them from the cell. Specific acquired immune responses rely on the major histocompatibility complex's (MHC) recognition of peptide antigens taken from the pathogen to activate a variety of T cells (helper and cytotoxic cells) that interact with B cells to produce antibodies (Castle, 2000).

Acquired immunity is characterised by the ability to recognise up to 10^{11} distinct structures and is tightly regulated to turn on or off a response. The aim is to eradicate pathogens without destroying the animal's own cells. In the healthy animal resistance to infection relies on a balance between the innate and acquired immunity. Regulation of the immune system is extremely complex, and it is only recently that science has started to understand the co-ordination of the body's response to disease. It seems likely that communication between immune cells is a crucial factor of immunocompetence.

If we imagine that immune system is a fighting force against pathogens than we would expect them to have suitable communications systems to receive and send signals to each other to ensure a correct response. Key immune cells, such as macrophages, neutrophils, T- and B-lymphocytes, have receptors on their surface that perform this function. These receptors are extremely sensitive to communicating molecules, but they are also sensitive to free radicals and can be easily damaged, potentially limiting or damaging the communication system. In such a situation without proper communication the immune system becomes useless. Indeed, immune cells may begin fighting each other, eventually destroying immunocompetence and causing autoimmune reactions.

Immune cells require chemicals to destroy the pathogens they are fighting as well as protection to ensure they do not destroy themselves. Immune cells protect themselves with natural anti-oxidants such as Se-GSH-Px and thioredoxin reductase. Macrophages destroy pathogens using an overproduction of free radicals, which can cause damage to specific enzymatic systems resulting in decreasing efficiency of the immune cell with each oxidative burst and result in apoptosis.

Se- and vitamin E deficiencies are associated with reduced functions of both innate and acquired immunity. In particular phagocytic functions, lymphocyte proliferation and antibody production may be compromised (Surai, 2002). Se supplementation has been shown to improve immunocompetence and increase resistance to various diseases. This has been demonstrated in a variety of animals including poultry, cows, sheep, horses, pigs, fish, cats and dogs. A summary of the effect of a compromised anti-oxidant system on the immune system is shown in Figure 6.

The importance of a delicate balance of the immune system is reflected by observations showing that an over-reacting immune system has similar detrimental consequences to immuno-suppression. For example, in some individuals, the immune system recognises host antigens as "non-self", attacking them and producing tissue damage leading to chronic inflammatory or autoimmune diseases. The immune system can also become sensitised to usually benign antigens from the environment causing allergies (Calder, 2001). It seems likely that in these immune system impairments miscommunication between immune cells plays a crucial role, and protection afforded by mineral-dependant systems is essential.

The immune system is functionally immature at birth. Therefore postnatal development of the immune system is associated with accumulation of polyunsaturated fatty acids and a need for anti-oxidant protection. Therefore, expression of selenoproteins in immune cells in early development is a crucial factor in a regulation of the immunocompetence development. However, selenium reserves in the newly born or hatched animals are very limited when inorganic selenium is used in the maternal diet. In contrast, organic selenium, for example in the form of Sel-Plex, is shown in a number of studies to be able to significantly increase Se concentration in colostrum, milk and egg. The supply of selenium is absolutely essential for the formation of effective anti-oxidant defences, resulting in effective immune system maturation and immunocompetence.

It is proven that such anti-oxidant compounds as vitamin E, selenium and carotenoids are involved in immunomodulation (Surai, 2002). However, the levels of the dietary anti-oxidants showing those effects are usually several times higher than that necessary for chicken growth and development. Furthermore, other trace minerals, including Zn, Cu and Fe are also involved in immune system regulation as enzyme components.

Again, zinc is required as a catalytic, structural and regulatory ion for enzymes and transcription factors, and is thus a key trace element in many homeostatic mechanisms of the body, including immune responses. Low zinc bioavailability results in limited immuno-resistance to infection in aging (Ferencik and Ebringer, 2003). It is necessary to underline that a variety of in vivo and in vitro effects of zinc on immune cells depend on its concentration, e.g. major immune cells show decreased function after zinc depletion. In monocytes especially, all functions are impaired, whereas in natural killer cells, cytotoxicity is decreased, and in neutrophil granulocytes, phagocytosis is reduced (Ibs and Rink, 2003). Furthermore, the normal functions of T cells are impaired and B cells undergo apoptosis. Impaired immune functions due to zinc deficiency are reversed on supplementation. However, high dosages of zinc have negative effects on immune cells and show alterations that are similar to those observed with zinc deficiency (Ibs and Rink, 2003). Organic Zn is characterised by improved availability in comparison to inorganic sources and is considered to be beneficial for animal health.

The immune system requires copper to perform several functions, but little is known about its direct mechanism of action (Percival, 1998). For example, some of the recent data from various studies showed that interleukin 2 is reduced in copper deficiency and is likely the mechanism by which T cell proliferation is reduced. It is important to note that even in marginal deficiency, when common indexes of copper are not affected by the diet, the proliferative response and interleukin concentrations are still reduced (Percival, 1998). Copper deficiency is also associated with a decreased number of neutrophils. Their ability to generate superoxide anion and kill ingested micro-organisms is also reduced in both overt and marginal copper deficiency. In many experiments it has been proven that Cu deficiency reduces antibody production, although cell-mediated immunity is more resistant to Cu deficiency. However, Cu deficiency appears to reduce production of interferon and tumour necrosis factor by mononuclear cells (Spears, 2000). Inorganic copper has a strong pro-oxidant effect and if not bound to proteins could stimulate lipid peroxidation in feed or even more importantly in the intestinal tract. Organic copper does not possess pro-oxidant properties and can improve the copper status of animals

Iron is a vital metal for the proliferation of all cells including those of the immune system. Indeed iron plays an essential role in immuno-surveillance, because of its growth promoting and differentiation-inducing properties for immune cells as well as its interference with cell mediated immune effector pathways and cytokine activities (Weiss, 2002). Iron is also crucial in the proliferation of tumour cells and micro-organisms, as it is involved in mitochondrial respiration and DNA synthesis. Iron deficiency causes several defects in both the humoral and cellular immunity. One of the most profound changes is a reduction in peripheral T cells and atrophy of the thymus (Bowlus, 2003). Growing evidence suggests that T cells may regulate iron metabolism perhaps through interactions with the non-classical major histocompatibility complex gene HFE.

Iron is a very strong pro-oxidant and, if not bound to proteins, can stimulate lipid peroxidation. This is especially relevant to digestive tract where lipid peroxidation can cause enterocyte damage and decreased absorption of nutrients, particularly those with anti-oxidant properties. If iron is included in a premix in inorganic form it can stimulate vitamin oxidation during storage. Therefore organic iron supplementation is a solution to avoid such problems and improve iron status of animal.

Disease resistance and improvements in immune response via anti-oxidants

The main goal in improving the immune system is to increase resistance to various diseases, and this area has been extensively studied with chickens. Feeding a combination of vitamin E with Se has been known to reduce mortality and increase body weight gain in chickens infected with *Eimeria tenella* (Colnago et al., 1984).

168

The same authors showed that dietary supplementation with selenium or vitamin E reduced mortality and increased body weight gain of non-immunized chickens infected with *E. tenella* in three out of four experiments. When chicks were inoculated with virulent Marek's disease virus at 10 days of age, selenium (dosed at 0.6 mg/kg) decreased the morbidity and mortality of the flock. In particular, selenium has been demonstrated to increase the ability of cells to remove ROS and lipid peroxides, and decrease the degree of tissue damage caused by ROS (Huang and Chen, 1996). Another experiment examined the effect of anti-oxidant supplementation against Infectious Bursal Disease (IBD). One day old chicks were fed on a diet containing selenium at 0.086 mg/kg, 0.3 mg/kg or 0.6 mg/kg. The chickens were infected with IBD virus at 39 days of age. Ten days later the mortality rates for the 0.086, 0.3 and 0.6 mg/kg diets were 33.3% 12.4% and 10.6%, respectively. Infection-induced inhibition of T lymphocyte transformation was lower in the selenium supplemented birds (Bu *et al.*, 1996).

In other trials, when Se was added to the feed of White Leghorn chickens prior to challenge with either *E. coli* or sheep erythrocyte antigen, the incidence of death or lesions was reduced from 86% to 21% at the optimal dose of Se (0.4 mg/kg feed; Larsen *et al.*, 1997). Lower Se values have been measured in birds infected with *Ascaridia galli* compared with controls, and this has been related to a lower degree of Se absorption, and the regeneration of the intestinal mucosa in infected birds (Damyanova *et al.*, 1995).

Nutritional strategies to prevent oxidation damage

Animals are capable of synthesising anti-oxidant enzymes, but dietary availability of Se, Mn, Zn and Cu are among major restrictions for this synthesis. For example, recently it has been shown that availability and efficiency of selenium in animal nutrition greatly depends on the dietary sources of this element. Indeed, animal dietary formulation is based on the supplementation with selenium as a safety margin to prevent selenium deficiency and to maintain good health and high reproductive performances of animals. Recently it has been suggested that, during evolution, all animals have adapted only to use the organic form of selenium (Surai, 2002). Indeed all feed ingredients contain selenium only in organic form, mainly as various seleno-amino acids. This means that inorganic selenium (selenite or selenate) is not a suitable substitute. There is a principal difference in absorption and metabolism between these two forms of selenium. Organic selenium is actively absorbed in the intestine as amino acid employing similar selective uptake mechanisms as other amino acids. In contrast, inorganic selenium is passively absorbed as a mineral. Because of these differences in uptake only selenomethionine can build Se reserves in the body (mainly in muscles). Since selenomethionine is not synthesised in animals, only plants can synthesize SeMet, there are no Se tissue reserves formed when inorganic selenium is used. Other forms of seleno-aminoacids (for example, Se-cysteine) are not a reserve form of the element. This principal difference can explain why organic selenium is more effective than inorganic one, especially in stress conditions, when uptake efficiency is crucial.

To compare and contrast commercial situations, we can consider two different scenarios of anti-oxidant defence in poultry. The first, and most common, scenario is for animals fed inorganic selenium in the diet. Under physiological stress, the body responds by using anti-oxidant reserves and, more importantly, by synthesising additional selenoproteins (Figure 7). In this case the main limitation is the absence of tissue selenium reserves and a restricted ability to synthesise additional selenoproteins, resulting in inadequate anti-oxidant protection when overproduction of free radicals is encountered. In this scenario we would expect the immune system, general health and reproduction to be compromised.

It is necessary to realise that dramatic differences in physiological stress are not required to cause such events. Sometimes a small difference, which is difficult to notice, can trigger enough radicals to cause a major problem. Indeed several cumulating, consecutive stresses may dramatically affect animal behaviour and health. This is especially important for newly born animals including birds, since their anti-oxidant mechanisms are not mature and they are dependent on anti-oxidant maternal delivered via the egg (birds) or colostrum and milk (mammals). Since inorganic selenium is not well transferred to the egg and even less effective in transferring to the milk we could not expect an anti-oxidant system improvement through this route in this scenario.

The alternative scenario would be when organic selenium is fed (Figure 8). This leads to selenium reserves being accumulated in the form of selenomethionine in tissue. Under stress conditions, protein catabolism by proteosomes releases Se, which can be used for the synthesis of additional selenoproteins to prevent any damaging effects of free radical overproduction. This is especially important since many stresses are associated with a decrease in feed consumption. As a result of such syntheses, selenoproteins can reduce lipid peroxidation, benefiting animals by maintaining immunocompetence and reproductive performance. As selenomethionine is transferred to the egg and to the milk and colostrum, newly hatched chicks or new-born animals benefit as a result of their improved anti-oxidant system.

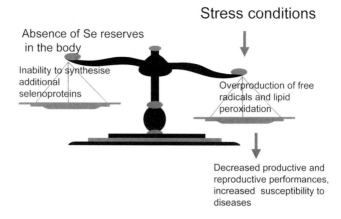

Figure 7.
Inorganic selenium scenario in poultry production (Adapted from Surai, 2002)

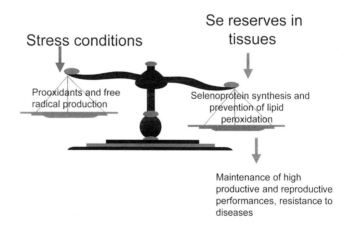

Figure 8.
Organic selenium scenario in poultry production (Adapted from Surai, 2002)

It is important to realise that this scenario has limitations in terms of level of stresses we are considering. For example, when high levels of toxins are present in the diet or environmental stresses are high, the body response may not be sufficient to prevent pathobiological changes in animal body. On the other hand, this model can be effective for a range of everyday stress conditions.

The development and commercial application of products such as Sel-Plex, which have guaranteed composition and proven efficacy shown in research and commercial trials opens a new era in animal nutrition. It provides opportunities not only for improvement of animal health and productivity but also for production of Se-enriched meat, milk, eggs and other foods that can improve human diets. A comparison between Sel-Plex and selenite, based on published data, clearly showed advantages of the natural form of Se in comparison to selenite (Table 3). Therefore, it seems appropriate that selenite be considered as a drug, and should be used accordingly. For example, when Se deficiency is diagnosed

Parameter	Organic selenium (Sel-Plex™)	Selenite
Absorption	Similar to Methionine with active transport in the gut	Similar to other mineral with passive transport in the gut
Accumulation	Building Se reserves by non-specific incorporation of SeMet into the proteins	Not accumulated in the body
Toxicity	At least 3 times less toxic than selenite	Highly toxic, can penetrate via skin causing problems
Bioavailability	Higher bioavailability in comparison to selenite to animals and human	Very low availability for ruminants due to reduction by rumen microbes
Anti-oxidant activity	SeMet possess anti-oxidant properties per se and could scavenge NO and other radicals	Possess pro-oxidant properties and could stimulate free radical production when reacting with GSH
Effect on DNA	SeMet stimulate DNA-repair enzymes	Selenite can cause DNA damage
Transfer to eggs, milk and meat	Transferred to egg, milk and meat giving a possibility to produce designer/ functional food	Poorly transferred to eggs, milk and meat
Transfer via placenta	Better transferred via placenta than selenite	Poorly transferred via placenta
Reactions with other elements	Neutral, ascorbic acid promotes SeMet assimilation from the diet	Highly reactive, reduced to metallic, unavailable selenium by ascorbic acid
Protective effect in stress conditions	Provide additional protection due to Se reserves in the body	Cannot provide additional protection due to absence Se reserves in the body
Effect on drip loss	Did not affect drip loss	Increases drip loss
Environmental issues	Better retention in tissues, less released with faeces and urine	Low retention in tissues and high release with faeces and urine
Stability during storage and feed processing	Stable	Stable
Classification based on the mode of action	Feed additive	Drug

Table 3.
Major differences between organic selenium (Sel-Plex™) and selenite

based on clinical signs, selenite would be the preparation of the choice. Using it via feed, water or injection will solve the short-term or acute Se deficiency, which has been demonstrated under various experimental conditions with chickens, pigs and cattle. The beneficial effect of organic selenium for animals can be even higher when it is used in combination with other organic minerals, namely Zn, Cu, Fe and Mn. It has been proven that these minerals are more effectively absorbed and metabolised in the body and this could be a major advantage for poultry, pig, dairy and beef industries.

Conclusions

Research has shown that we are living in the world of free radicals. Humans, chickens, pigs, cows and all other animal species are exposed to free radical attack in everyday life and that is why an integrated anti-oxidant system has evolved in every cell to prevent damage to biologically important molecules including DNA, proteins and lipids. Some anti-oxidants are synthesised in the body, however diet forms the major source of anti-oxidants. From the hundreds of dietary compounds possessing anti-oxidant activities, selenium, zinc, iron, manganese and vitamin E are considered to be the core of anti-oxidant defence. It has been appreciated that the efficiency of anti-oxidants depends on their form in the diet, and in recent years it has been proven that organic selenium (e.g. Sel-Plex) has important advantages in comparison to inorganic selenium.

Benefits of organic selenium have been proven for many species, including chicken, pigs, cows, sheeps and fish. It seems likely that an optimal combination of organic selenium and vitamin E in the diet is a key for an effective anti-oxidant defence. However, there is a need for further research in this field to establish those optimal combinations for each species depending on age, productivity and other relevant technological conditions. Inorganic copper and iron are major stimulators of lipid peroxidation in digestive tract, using organic forms of these elements can avoid their detrimental activity and help maintaining high productive and reproductive performance of poultry and farm animals reared under commercial conditions.

References

Agate, D.D., O'Dea, E.E. and Rustad, M.E. (2000). Effects of dietary selenium on laying hen fertility as assessed by the periviteline sperm hole assay. *Proc. Poultry Research and Production*

Symposium, Alberta Poultry Research Centre, pp.1-4.

Ames, B.N. (2003) An Enthusiasm for Metabolism. *J. Biol. Chem.* **278**: 4369-4380.

Ames, B.N. and Gold, L.S. (1997). The causes and prevention of cancer: gaining perspective. *Environ. Health. Perspect.* **105** Suppl 4: 865-873.

Bannister, W.H. (1988). From haemocuprein to copper-zinc superoxide dismutase: a history on the fiftieth anniversary of the discovery of haemocuprein and the twentieth anniversary of the discovery of superoxide dismutase. *Free Radical Research Communications* **5**: 35-42.

Bowlus, C.L. (2003). The role of iron in T cell development and autoimmunity. *Autoimmun Rev.* **2**: 73-78.

Brigelius-Flohe, R. (1999). Tissue-specific functions of individual glutathione peroxidases. *Free Radical Biology and Medicine* **27**: 951-965.

Bu, Z.G., Huang, K.H. and Chen, W. F. (1996). Study on the cell mediated immunity mechanism in the selenium-enhanced resistance of chicks to infectious bursal disease. *Chinese Journal of Veterinary Science* **16**: 273-276

Calder, P.C. (2001). Polyunsaturated fatty acids, inflammation, and immunity. *Lipids* **36**: 1007-1024

Castle, S.C. (2000). Clinical relevance of age-related immune dysfunction. *Clinical Infectious Diseases* **31**: 578-585

Chance, B., Sies, H. and Boveris, A. (1979). Hydroperoxide metabolism in mammalian organs. Physiol Rev. **59**: 527-605.

Chaudiere, J., Ferrari-Iliou, R. (1999). Intracellular antioxidants: from chemical to biochemical mechanisms. *Food and Chemical Toxicology* **37**: 949-962

Colnago, G.L., Jensen, L.S. and Long, P.L. (1984). Effect of natural feedstuffs added to a semi-purified diet on *Eimeria tenella* infection. *Poultry Science* **63**: 2145-2152

Damyanova, A., Teodorova, S. and Gabrashanska, M. (1995). Content of some microelements in chickens with ascaridiasis under combined drug treatment. *Parasitology Research* **81**: 549-552

Diplock, A.T. (1994). Antioxidants and disease prevention. In: *Molecular Aspects of Medicine*. Volume. 15, Edited by H. Baum, H. Pergamon Press, Oxford and New York, pp. 295-376

Edens, F. (2002). Practical applications for selenomethionine: broiler breeder production. *Proceedings of 18th Alltech's Annual Symposium*, Edited by Lyons, T.P. and. Jacques, K.A., Nottingham University Press, Nottingham, UK, pp. 29-42

Fattman, C.L., Schaefer, L.M. and Oury, T.D. (2003). Extracellular superoxide dismutase in biology and medicine. *FreeRadical Biology and Medicine* **35**: 236-256

Ferencik, M. and Ebringer, L. (2003). Modulatory effects of selenium and zinc on the immune system. *Folia Microbiol (Praha)* **48**: 417-426

Fridovich, I. (1995). Superoxide radical and superoxide dismutases. *Annual Review of Biochemistry* **64**: 97-112

Fujii, J. and Taniguchi, N. (1999). Down regulation of superoxide dismutases and glutathione peroxidase by reactive oxygen and nitrogen species. *Free Radical Research* **31**:301-308

Galey, J-B. (1997). Potential use of iron chelators against oxidative damage. In: Antioxidants in disease mechanisms and therapy. Edited by Sies, H., Academic Press, San Diego, pp. 167-203

Gutteridge, J.M.C. and Halliwell, B. (1990). The measurement and metabolism of lipid peroxidation in biological systems. *Trends in Biochemical Sciences* 129-135

Halliwell, B. (1994). Free radicals and antioxidants: A personal view. *Nutrition Reviews* **52**: 253-265

Halliwell, B. (1999). Antioxidant defence mechanisms: from the beginning to the end (of the beginning). *Free Radical Research* **31**: 261-272

Halliwell, B. (1987). Oxidants and human disease: some new concepts. *FASEB Journal* **1**: 358-364

Halliwell, B. and Gutteridge, J.M.C. (1999). Free Radicals in Biology and Medicine. Third Edition. Oxford University Press, Oxford.

Hassan, H.M. (1988). Biosynthesis and regulation of superoxide dismutases. *Free Radical Biology and Medicine* **5**: 377-385

Helbock, H.J., Beckman, K.B., Shigenaga, M.K., Walter, P.B., Woodall, A.A., Yeo, H.C. and Ames, B.N. (1998). DNA oxidation matters: the HPLC-electrochemical detection assay of 8-oxo-deoxyguanosine and 8-oxo-guanine. *Proc. Natl. Acad. Sci.* **95**: 288-293.

Hidiroglou, M. (1979). Trace element deficiencies and fertility in ruminants: a review. *J. Dairy Sci.* **62**: 1195-1206.

Hidiroglou, M. and Knipfel, J.E. (1984). Zinc in mammalian sperm: a review. *J Dairy Sci.* **67**: 1147-1156.

Huang, K.H. and Chen, W. F. (1996). Effect of selenium on the resistance of chickens to Marek's disease and its mode of action. *Acta Veterinaria et Zootechnica Sinica* **27**: 448-455

Ibs, K.H. and Rink, L. (2003). Zinc-altered immune function. *J Nutr.* **133** (5 Suppl 1): 1452S-1456S

Jones, D.P., Eklow, L., Thor, H. and Orrenius, S. (1981). Metabolism of hydrogen peroxide in isolated hepatocytes: relative contributions of catalase and glutathione peroxidase in decomposition of endogenously generated H2O2. *Archives of Biochemistry and Biophysics* **210**: 505-516

Knight, J.A. (1998) Free radicals: Their history and current status in aging and disease. *Annals of the Clinical and Laboratory Sciences* **28**: 331-346

Larsen, C.T., Pierson, F.W. and Gross, W.B. (1997). Effect of dietary selenium on the response of stressed and unstressed chickens to Escherichia coli challenge and antigen. *Biological Trace Element Research* **58**:169-176

Marklund, S.L. (1982). Human copper-containing superoxide dismutase of high molecular weight. *Proceedings of the National Academy of Science of the USA* **79**: 7634-7638

Marklund, S.L., Holme, E. and Hellner, L. (1982). Superoxide dismutase in extracellular fluids. *Clinica Chimica Acta* **126**: 41-51

Mates, J.M. and Sanchez-Jimenez, F. (1999). Antioxidant enzymes and their implications in pathophysiologic processes. *Frontiers in Bioscience* **4**: D339-D345

McCord, J.M. and Fridovich, I. (1969). Superoxide dismutase: An enzymatic function for erythrocuprein (hemocuprein). *Journal of Biological Chemistry* **244**: 6049-6055

Michalski, W. (1992). Resolution of three forms of superoxide dismutase by immobilized metal affinity chromatography. *Journal of Chromatography, Biomedical Applications* **576**: 340-345

Nath, R. (1997). Copper deficiency and heart disease: Molecular basis, recent advances and current concepts. *International Journal of Biochemistry and Cell Biology* **29**: 1245-1254

Niki, E. (1996). a-Tocopherol, In: *Handbook of antioxidants, Edited by* Cadenas E. and Packer L, Marcel Dekker, New York-London, pp. 3-25

Nordberg, J. and Arner, E.S. (2001), Reactive oxygen species, antioxidants, and the mammalian thioredoxin system. *Free Radical Biology and Medicine* **31**: 1287-1312

Percival, S.S. (1998). Copper and immunity. *Am J Clin Nutr.* 67(5 Suppl):1064S-1068S.

Pfeifer, H., Conrad, M., Roethlein, D., Kyriakopoulos, A., Brielmeier, M., Bornkamm, G.W. and Behne, D. (2001). Identification of a specific sperm nuclei selenoenzyme necessary for protamine thiol cross-linking during sperm maturation. *FASEB Journal* **15**:1236-1238

Singal, P.K., Khaper, N., Palace, V. and Kumar, D. (1998). The role of oxidative stress in the genesis of hart disease. *Cardiovascular Research* **40**: 426-432

Sinclair, S. (2000). Male infertility: nutritional and environmental considerations. *Altern Med Rev.* **5**: 28-38.

Spears, J.W. (2000). Micronutrients and immune function in cattle. *Proc Nutr Soc.* **59**: 587-594

Surai, P.F. (1999). Vitamin E in avian reproduction. *Poultry and Avian Biology Review* **10**: 1-60

Surai, P.F. (2002). *Natural Antioxidants in Avian Nutrition and Reproduction.* Nottingham University Press, Nottingham

Surai, P.F. (2003). Selenium-vitamin E interactions: Does 1 + 1 equal more than 2?. In: *Nutritional Biotechnology in the Feed and Food Industries*. Proc. of Alltech's 19th Annual Symposium (T.P.Lyons and K.A. Jacques, eds.). Nottingham University Press, Nottingham, UK, pp.59-76

Surai, P.F. and Dvorska, J.E. (2002). Strategies to enhance antioxidant protection and implications for the well-being of companion animals. In: *Nutritional Biotechnology in the Feed and Food Industries*. Proceedings of Alltech's 18th Annual Symposium, pp.521-534 (T.P.Lyons and K.A. Jacques, editors). Nottingham: Nottingham University Press.

Surai, P.F., Speake, B.K. and Sparks, N.H.C. (2003). Comparative Aspects of Lipid Peroxidation and Antioxidant Protection in Avian Semen. In: *Male Fertility and Lipid Metabolism*, pp. 211-249. [Stephanie DeVriese and Armand Christophe, editors] Champaign: AOCS Press.

Surai, K.P., Surai, P.F., Speake, B.K. and Sparks, N.H.C. (2003a). Antioxidant-prooxidant balance in the intestine: Food for thought. 1. Prooxidants. Nutritional *Genomics and Functional Foods*. 1: 51-70

Surai, K.P., Surai, P.F., Speake, B.K. and Sparks, N.H.C. (2004). Antioxidant-prooxidant balance in the intestine: Food for thought. 1. Antioxidants. *Current Topics in Neutraceutical Research* **2**: 27-46.

Weiss, G. (2002). Iron, infection and anemia—a classical triad. *Wien Klin Wochenschr.* **114:** 357-367

Werling, D. and Jungi, T.W. (2003). TOLL-like receptors linking innate and adaptive immune response. *Veterinary Immunology and Immunopathology* **91**: 1-12

Wong, W.Y., Thomas, C.M.G., Merkus, J. M.W, Zielhuis, G.A., and Steegers-Theunissen, R.P.M. (2000). Male factor subfertility: possible causes and the impact of nutritional factors. *Fertility and Sterility* **73**: 435-442.

Youn, H.D., Kim, E.J., Roe, J.H., Hah, Y.C. and Kang, S.O. (1996). A novel nickel-containing superoxide dismutase from Streptomyces spp. *Biochemical Journal* **318** (Pt 3): 889-896

Yu, B.P. (1994). Cellular defences against damage from reactive oxygen species. *Physiological Reviews* **74**: 139-162.

Zelko, I.N., Mariani, T.J. and Folz, R.J. (2002). Superoxide dismutase multigene family: a comparison of the CuZn-SOD (SOD1), Mn-SOD (SOD2), and EC-SOD (SOD3) gene structures, evolution, and expression. *Free Radical Biology and Medicine* **33**: 337-349

Novel approaches to improving poultry meat production: do organic minerals have a role?

Kenneth I. Bruerton
Protea Park Nutrition Services, Qld. Australia

Introduction

As time passes more and more constraints are placed on intensive animal production. Nutritionists now look for new approaches to improving performance. In the past we have concentrated on improving efficiency through increased growth and reduced feed intake. Now producers must strive to improve efficiency whilst also considering factors such as the impact on the environment, food safety, anti-biotic resistance and constraints on ingredient usage. These challenges have forced us to look in new directions and to revisit and question established dogma. This paper considers some of the issues surrounding trace mineral nutrition in broilers, and how this is changing in respect to poultry production.

Current practice

Nutritionists have many sources of advice with regard to trace mineral nutrition in broiler diets. Experiments defining requirements were conducted several decades ago on broilers with limited growth potential compared to the birds of today (Leeson, 2003). Typical levels of trace mineral addition to Australian broiler diets are shown in Table 1, sources of these minerals predominantly being inorganic salts and oxides.

Table 1. Some average commercial additions of inorganic trace minerals (ppm) for poultry

Diet (ppm)	Zn	Mn	Cu	Fe	I	Co	Mo	Se
Starter	60-100	80-100	10-150*	20-80	1-2	0.5	1-1.25	0.25-0.3
Finisher	40-60	70-90	5-10	20-80	1	0.4	1-2	0.2

* Some nutritionists use up to 150 ppm of Cu in Starter and 100 ppm in Grower, reverting to 5-10 ppm for Finisher and Withdrawal. The ranges shown were taken from commercial premixes supplied to the Australian broiler industry.

179

The major reason for supplementing diets with trace minerals is to prevent known deficiencies. As trace minerals are relatively cheap most nutritionists introduce safety factors over minimum requirements (such as those published by the NRC (Table 2)), to cope with the extra stresses of intensive production. The tendency for commercial nutritionists to ignore the trace mineral levels found in the macro ingredients of the diet, such as the grains and protein meals, have probably been prompted by the NRC recommendations, which quotes Kratzer and Vohra's (1986) claims that bioavailability of trace minerals in natural ingredients is typically low. Whether standard commercial levels of inorganic trace mineral supplementation allow modern broilers to reach their genetic potential is, however, a moot point.

Table 2.
Trace mineral
requirements of
broilers (mg/kg)
(after NRC 1994)

Diet (ppm)	Zn	Mn	Cu	Fe	I	Co	Mo	Se
Starter	40	60	8	80	0.35	N/A	N/A	0.15
Finisher	40	60	8	80	0.35	N/A	N/A	0.15

Challenges facing broiler performance

New factors must be considered when deciding the nutrient levels in poultry feed formulations. One important and far reaching constraint is that governments are placing limits on the output of waste from poultry production systems. In the near future the level of macro and trace minerals in poultry manure will be regulated in Europe, Japan and the USA. The current challenge is to reduce output of Zn, Cu, Mn and Fe whilst maintaining economic performance. Reducing the levels of supplemental inorganic minerals is one option, but it is uncertain if performance is maximized by current supplementation practices, so reduction may not be productive.

Currently the difference between levels that nutritionists consider adequate now and NRC minimum is not great. Nutritionists have therefore begun to investigate more readily available organically complexed forms of trace minerals to solve this problem. The question being: how low can we go with organic mineral supplementation and maintain performance? Furthermore, greater emphasis will be placed on the contribution of minerals from the major dietary ingredients – the grains and protein meals, in order to limit additional mineral use.

Another aspect is that there may be beneficial effects from increasing the levels of organically complexed minerals, above those required to prevent deficiency. Kidd and co-workers (1993) showed that a corn-soy diet, when fed to broiler breeder hens, gave equivalent egg output and hatchability as a diet supplemented with 40 ppm of Zn from either ZnO or Zn-methionine. Progeny of the birds fed the Zn-met diet were shown to have increased immunocompetence, as measured by cutaneous basophil hypersensitivity (CBH), compared to those hatched from eggs produced by hens fed the basal diet or that supplemented with ZnO. There was no effect of Zn supplementation on hatchability, fertility and embryo mortality.

The question arises as to what other advantages can be gained by increasing organic mineral supplementation over levels required to prevent deficiencies and maintain performance. Furthermore, can that be reconciled with the need to reduce excretion?

The role of the basal diet on the responses to organic mineral supplementation

In Australia and New Zealand poultry diets routinely contain animal by-products such as meat and bone meal (MBM) and blood meal. Both of these materials contain high levels of Fe and the former contains a relatively high level of Zn (NRC, 1998). In contrast, vegetable protein meals and grains contain lower levels of trace minerals and therefore contribute less to the overall intake of animals. Estimates of the levels of trace minerals in common ingredients taken from published values have been summarized in Table 3.

Table 3. General guideline values for trace minerals ranges (mg/kg) in common ingredients. (De Mol, 1992)

Feedstuff	Zn	Mn	Cu	Fe	I	Co
Yellow corn	10-25	3-9	2-4	25-40	0.05-0.3	0.02-0.1
Soft wheat	20-40	20-50	0.6-8	30-70	0.04-0.9	0.01-0.1
Soybean meal	50-61	27-80	15-36	120-250	0.09-0.5	0.08-0.3
Meat and bone meal	70-125	12-37	1.5-28	500-900	0.7-1.3	0.05-1.3
Canola meal	55-70	40-73	5-7.2	80-380	0.6	0.1-0.23
Fish meal anchovy	100-105	9-20	5-10	220-370	3	0.07-0.17
Corn gluten meal	30-40	3-8	7-26	120-280	0.02	0.05-0.1

Calculations of naturally occurring trace mineral levels for corn/soy diets containing 30% soybean meal, 65% corn and 5% additives and for wheat based diets containing 67% wheat, 8% MBM, 20% soy and 5% additives are shown in Table 4. These represent typical Asian diets and typical Australian/NZ respectively.

Table 4. Ranges of possible trace mineral levels in typical diets

ppm	Zn	Mn	Cu	Fe	I	Co
Corn/soy	22-35	10-30	6-13	46-101	0.06-0.3	0.04-0.2
Wheat/mbm	29-49	20-52	4-15	80-169	0.3-0.8	0.06-0.2

The data in Table 4 suggest that diets containing exclusively vegetable protein ingredients are likely to be lower in Zn, Mn and Fe than those containing MBM, although the extremes of their ranges may overlap. On that basis it is tempting to speculate that there may be better responses to organic mineral supplementation in diets lacking animal byproduct meals. Evidence exists for some species that minerals from animal protein meals may be more bioavailable than those from plant sources. In a human balance experiment a diet based on soybean protein containing 14 mg/kg of Zn resulted in a negative Zn balance whilst a diet containing 12 mg/kg of Zn based on animal protein resulted in a positive Zn balance (O'Dell 1984).

Analyses of trace minerals in ingredients sampled in Australia are shown in Table 5 (Bao and Choct 2004, personal communication). These data are compatible with published values and indicate that diets based solely on vegetable sources are lower in trace minerals. As a model to test the efficacy of organic trace mineral supplementation for broilers, a diet based on rice (65%) and soy protein isolate (30%) fails to meet NRC requirements for Fe, Mn and Zn, yielding levels of 39.8, 10.1 and 21.2 mg/kg respectively for those minerals. Cu, however, may be adequate at 6.6 mg/kg. It is planned to use such diets in testing the responses of modern broilers to graded levels of supplementation of Bioplex Zn, Fe, Mn and Cu.

Sample	Cu (mg/kg)	Fe (mg/kg)	Mn (mg/kg)	Zn (mg/kg)
Soybean meal (US)	19.5	140.4	45.4	81.6
Sorghum grain	2.3	29.2	11.7	14.3
Wheat grain	5.9	35.4	37.5	26.4
Barley grain	7.8	42	12.2	26.5
Canola grain	6.9	158.7	65.4	64.7
Soy protein isolate	14.05	125.2	7.1	41.9
Amaroo milled white rice	3.8	3.6	12.4	13.3
Amaroo milled white large broken	3.7	5	12.9	12.9
Amaroo Brown Rice	4.6	12.8	51.8	20.5
Amaroo Paddy Rice	14.1	49.2	129.1	19.6

Table 5.
Levels of trace minerals in Australian grains

After Bao and Choct (2004)

One of the hurdles faced by nutritionists interested in using organic forms of minerals is that there remains a good deal of uncertainty in the magnitude of improvement in bioavailability offered by these compounds. The literature on this subject is considerable, and a review is not within the scope of this paper. It is more practical to give a commercial assessment of what a nutritionist might consider in a commercial trial or test diet. Estimates of bioavailability vary considerably. Some of this is due to methodology and basal diet, and some is due to differences in the quality of organic trace mineral sources. Generally, however, estimates of the advantage of organic versus inorganic sources of minerals are of the order of 25-30% (Table 6).

Cu Cu-proteinate:not reported for poultry - In rats, proteinate was more bioavailable than Cu-lys in one experiment and the reverse in another. Studies in pigs indicate better utilization of Bioplex Cu compared to $CuSO_4$

I No information on organic sources except EDDI, which is equivalent in bioavailability to the inorganic sources of I, and DIS (di-iodo-salicylic acid) which is unavailable to cattle but available to rats

Fe Sulphates (mono and hepta hydrates) are rated as 100% bioavailable. No data presented on proteinate or Fe-amino acid chelates for poultry. Fe-fumarate reported at 100%. Proteinate in pigs reported as 130% bioavailable; Fe-met as 185% bioavailable

Mn There are a number of studies on Mn-proteinate bioavailability for chicks relative to MnO and $MnSO_4$. Estimates, taking $MnSO_4$ as 100%, are 90% for MnO and 120% for Mn-proteinate in 21 day old broilers. This experiment also reported that heat stress magnified the differences between sources to 100:82:145 for $MnSO_4$, MnO and Mn-proteinate respectively

Zn Estimates of the relative bioavailability of inorganic sources varies where $ZnSO_4$ is regarded as 100% bioavailable. Some experiments estimate ZnO to be equal in bioavailability to $ZnSO_4$, in others it is less. Amongst the organic sources estimates vary and seem dependent on diet formulation. There seems little consistency. Proteinates have been rated as more bioavailable in some experiments and less bioavailable than Zn-amino acid chelates in others. A PARC Inst. Experiment (PARC Inst, 1994) showed that Zn Propionate and Zn methionine were more effective at increasing broiler tibia Zn concentration than $ZnSO_4$ by about 25%.

Table 6.
Summary of trial findings comparing different mineral sources

A recent literature review (Ammerman et al,1998) summarized the relative bioavailabilities of essential trace minerals (Figure 1).

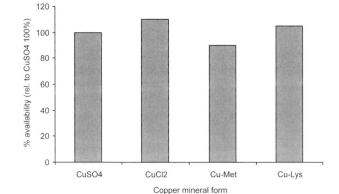

Figure 1.
Relative bioavailabilities of copper (Ammerman et al,1998)

The contribution of diet composition

Diet structure has a major effect on measurements of apparent bioavailability. Fly *et al* (1987), quoted in a review (Nelson, 1988), suggested that Mn-Met had a bioavailability of about 130% compared to MnSO4 in a low phytate ration. The relative bioavailability of Mn-met increased to 175% in a high phytate diet. Such effects have been shown with organic Zn as well. Allowances of organic minerals can be further decreased when phytase is added to the diet, as many key minerals are bound by phytate.

What are the chances of success?

The literature contains many examples of successful reductions in mineral excretion when organic mineral sources are used in place of inorganic salts. Burrell at al (2004) fed broilers increasing levels of Zn as either inorganic or organic forms. They found that the cumulative excretion of Zn over a 45 day feeding period was significantly lower ($p = 0.02$) in birds fed the organic source of Zn. These researchers also reported that increasing levels of Zn up to 80 mg/kg improved growth but there was no significant difference between Zn sources. In this case the basal diet contained 28 mg/kg so the level of Zn giving the fastest growth (101 mg/kg by analysis) was well above the NRC requirement of 40 mg/kg.

Similar results have been demonstrated in pigs using organically complexed Cu. Smits and Henman (2000) reported that entire male pigs fed diets containing 50 ppm of Cu from organic Cu (Bioplex Cu, Alltech Inc.) excreted significantly lower levels of Cu in the faeces whilst growing at a rate not different from pigs fed 160 mg/kg of Cu from CuSO4.

Summary

Gaps exist in our knowledge about the responses of broilers to diets supplemented with organically complexed trace minerals. Anecdotal reports and company trials carried out in commercial situations indicate that positive economic responses have been recorded in broilers (Caskey 2003, personal communication). However, these data have not been published in the scientific literature. A need exists to test the responses of broilers in controlled conditions to organically complexed trace minerals. Negative controls need to be included as well as positive controls containing inorganic minerals at commercial levels of supplementation. We now have enough evidence to be confident that organic minerals will reduce mineral excretion whilst maintaining performance, although the optimum balance and levels need to be determined. However, we also need to explore the upper levels of supplementation for metabolic effects on immunity, reproduction and other physiological effects. Knowing the limits of supplementation and their effects on production should ultimately lead to economic improvements in broiler production

Research recently started at the University of New England is attempting to answer some these questions.

References

Ammerman, C.B., Henry, P.R., and Miles, R.D. (1998) Supplemental organically bound mineral compounds in livestock nutrition. In *Recent Advances in Animal Nutrition*. Eds Garnsworthy, P.C., and Wiseman, J. Nottingham University Press, Nottingham, England.

Bao, Y., and Choct, M. (2004). Personal communication.

Burrell, A.L., Dozier III, W.A., Davis, A.J., Compton, M.M, Freeman, M.E., Vendrell, P.F. and Ward, T.L. (2004). Responses of broilers to dietary Zn concentrations and sources in relation to environmental indications. *British Poultry Science* **45**:(2) 255-263.

Caskey, S. (1993) Personal communication.

De Mol, J. (1992) Raw Material Compendium. Novus Corporation, USA.

Fly, A.D., Izquierdo, O.A., Lowry, K.R. and Baker, D.H., (1987) Manganese (Mn) bioavailability in a Mn-methionine chelate. *Federal Proceeding*. **46**: 911

PARC Inst (1994): Kemin Industries Asia Pte Ltd, Singarpore.

Kidd, M.T., Anthony, N.B., Newberry, L.A., and Lee, S.R. (1993). Effect of supplemental Zinc in either a corn-soybean or a milo and corn-soybean meal diet on the performance of young broiler breeder hens and their progeny. *Poultry Science* **72**: 1492-1499.

Kratzer, F.H. and Vohra, P. (1986) Chelates in Nutrition. Boca Raton Fla. CRC Press.

Leeson, S., 2003. A new look at trace mineral nutrition of poultry: Can we reduce the environmental burden of poultry manure. In: *Nutritional Biotechnology in the Feed and Food Industries*. 125-129. Lyons,T.P. and K.A. Jacques (Eds), Nottingham University Press, Nottingham, England.

Nelson, J. (1988) Bioavailability of trace minerals, In profitable animal nutrition for the future, *American Feed Ingredients Association Nutrition Symposium Proceedings.*, Kansas City Mo, USA.

Nutrient Requirements of Poultry: Ninth revised edition (1994). National Academic Press, Washington, DC, USA

Nutrient Requirements of Swine: Tenth revised edition (1998). National Academic Press, Washington, DC, USA.

O'Dell, B.L. (1984). Bioavailability of trace elements. *Nutrition Review* **42**(9): 301-308.

Paton, N.D., Cantor, A.H., Pescatore, A.J., Ford, M.J., and Smith, C.A., (2000) Effect of dietary selenium source and level of inclusion in selenium content of incubated eggs. *Poultry Science* **79** (Suppl. 1): 40.

Smits, R.J. and Henman, D.J. (2000). In: *Nutritional Biotechnology in the Feed and Food Industries*. 293-300. Lyons, T.P. and K.A. Jacques (Eds), Nottingham University Press, Nottingham, England.

Surai, P.F. (2000). Effect of selenium and vitamin E content of the maternal diet on the anti-oxidant system of the chick. *British Poultry Science* **41(2)**: 235-243

Eggs to chicks: optimising hen performance

Sally E. Solomon
Senior Research Fellow, University of Glasgow Veterinary School, Bearsden, Glasgow G61 1QH

Introduction

Egg production, whether for table eggs or hatching, is highly dependant upon correct mineral uptake and availability. Our understanding of how eggs are formed and the processes that determine egg quality and hatchability are essential if we are also to understand the impact of nutrition. The following chapter outlines the processes involved in egg production, hatchery practice and factors determining the quality of eggs, and considers how certain key trace minerals such as zinc and manganese affect egg production.

Producing eggs

It is tempting to treat the first part of the title of this chapter in its literal sense; thus the programme of events from egg to chick is fairly routine as follows: Eggs are collected from supply farms, sorted in "on- farm" cool rooms and disinfected with a subsequent microbiological check for pathogens. The eggs are then moved to the hatchery, disinfected and weighed. They then go through a pre-warming process before final disinfection. Eggs are 'set' (*i.e.* incubated) and are 'candled' (analysed for fertility) prior to transfer the hatchery. Once the egg has hatched the chick is sexed at day old and transported to broiler producers.

However in the light of the succeeding statement "optimising hen performance", it is more pertinent to consider the production of a "top grade" quality product, how mineral nutrition of the layer can impact both egg quality and hen welfare. It is also important to consider whether current techniques used to measure quality are sufficiently rigorous, and what should be recorded as a more accurate reflection of improved performance. In the routine egg preparation and hatching procedure outlined above, cleanliness and weight are the only criteria that could be interpreted as quality control measures.

Egg formation

In its progress from the ovary to the cloaca, the yolk mass becomes enveloped in the viscous albumen, with its complement of structural and antibacterial proteins. During these events, the paired shell membranes, each comprising a protein core surrounded by a carbohydrate mantle, wind themselves around the egg white and give the descending mass its characteristic shape. The inner surface of the membrane adjacent to the albumen is amorphous, however the outer surface of the membrane, onto which the calcium salts 'seed' is chemically modified at specific sites to encourage the nucleation process.

The shell is a multi-layered bio-ceramic complex comprising (from its inner surface) a mammillary layer, cone layer, palisade layer, vertical crystal layer and cuticle. The morphological variations that occur within the shell have been the subject of numerous publications (Solomon, 1991; Bain, 1990) and have been correlated with a variety of environmental and dietary influences. To date 12 structural variations have been described at the level of the mammillary layer. The last decade has seen an increase in interest with regard to the protein matrix *i.e.* the scaffolding within the shell that facilitates the elastic response when the egg is under load.

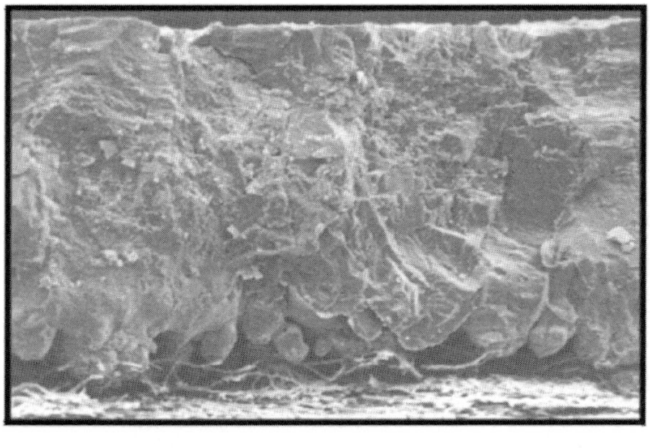

Figure 1.
Cross section of egg shell and membranes

Cuticle
VCL

Palisade

Mammillary layer
Outer membrane

Shell matrix proteins

When the eggshell is decalcified, a delicate web remains, which, at ultra-structural level, has a fibrous appearance interspersed with numerous vesicular holes. The distribution of the vesicles varies within the depth of the shell and with increasing bird age, demonstrating changes in the gross morphology of this complex protein network. It is of oviducal origin with all regions distal to

188

and including the magnum involved in the synthesis of the protein moiety.

To date several protein components including Ovocleidin-17, 23, 116, Ovocalyxin-21, 25, 32, 36, Ovotransferrin, Ovalbumin, Osteopontin, Lysozyme and Clusterin; have been isolated and identified using a variety of chromatographic techniques including anion exchange and gel filtration (Hincke *et al.*, 2000). Several of these proteins are derived from egg white. Others, like clusterin and osteopontin, are ubiquitous, but the ovocleidins and ovocalyxins are specific to the shell gland pouch. The functions of these proteins are as diverse as their type. For example, the egg white protein lysozyme is implicated in bacterial defence, as is the shell gland specific protein ovocalyxin–36. Others affect the process of mineralisation and are responsible for changes in the direction of crystal growth and hence uniformity of shell. Recent technology such as Microfocus Small Angle X-ray Scattering (SAXS), makes it possible to view the highly ordered bio-ceramic complex at the nanometer level. SAXS is a technique capable of providing information about the size, shape, arrangement and internal porosity of nanostructures.

In a series of experiments conducted at the University of Glasgow in 2002, both specialised and non- specialised measures of quality were used to isolate from a larger batch of eggs, a group of 30 classified as "good quality". Using both SAXS and the complementary wide–angle x- ray diffraction data, variations have been observed in both crystal size and angular distribution. It is hypothesised that these are a measure of nano-inclusions within the crystals resulting from the incorporation of matrix proteins (Lammie *et al.*, 2004). Existing as they do, both within and between the calcite crystals, the proteins modulate crystal nucleation and growth and thereby influence the shape and strength of the final egg structure (Hincke *et al.*, 1995).

The hatching egg and the table egg

The reproductive effort that goes into the construction of the egg as an embryonic chamber is identical to that resulting in the formation of the table egg. If there are differences in structure then they reflect the dietary regimes of breeder birds and layers and, more significantly, the lower numbers of eggs produced by the breeder bird. Within the shell and at ultra-structural level, this manifests itself as a reduction in the incidence of shell defects, particularly at the mammillary layer level.

During the growth process, the embryo utilises nutrients supplied by the yolk and albumen, including micro-minerals. As with other egg components, micro-minerals are transferred across the perivitelline membrane for inclusion within the yolk mass. This semi-permeable membrane consists in part of fine proteinaceous rodlets arranged in a staggered fashion. From a morphological point of view this organisation gives the membrane a high degree of integrity and strength, and serves to restrict the outward migration of yolk products.

Prior to chick emergence the shell must thin enough to allow the chick to break through ('pipping'). The shell membranes lose continuity with the "true" shell and erosion of the mammillary layer and part of the cone layer facilitate pipping. If the bond between shell membranes and the shell has not been adequately engineered because of mammillary malformation, then dissolution of the calcite complex will be hindered. Therefore a well-structured shell is essential not only for hatching, but also for embryo growth.

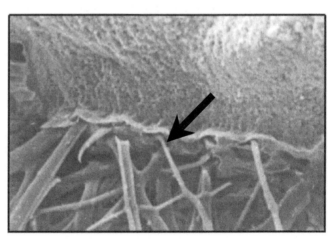

Figure 2.
Micrograph showing shell membrane attachment

Selecting eggs for hatchery and table

The process of selection differs between hatching and table eggs. The main problems associated with egg quality are the presence of excreta on the eggs, malformation, cracks, colour and texture. Hatching eggs are costly to produce but the selection process for setting is fairly rudimentary with cleanliness, intactness and the absence of gross malformation being the prime measures of quality. Not so for the table egg whose ultimate destination is the kitchen. It is graded according to weight and size, selected for colour and texture, and rejected on account of its standard of cleanliness. With the proposed move to more extensive (e.g. free range) bird housing, 'dirty egg' numbers are set to escalate, and in the absence of egg washing within the EU, will represent a further economic loss to the poultry industry.

Despite the years of effort devoted to improving shell quality, seconds persist and on a global scale account for in excess of 8% annually. This is not entirely unexpected as the egg is the end product of a 24-hour biological process in which integration between the nutritional, environmental and health status of the bird, in conjunction with the influence of its genetic background, come together to form the embryonic chamber and its contents. Cracked and malformed eggs are caused by different problems. No two eggs are the same, and within the shell subtle changes occur in crystal form and structure. When these variations dominate regions such as the mammillary layer, the likelihood of cracking increases. In terms of specific protein type, these abnormalities, by virtue of their location, implicate an imbalance in, or absence of, the protein ovocleidin-17, which is concentrated in the mammillary bodies (Hincke *et al.*,1995).

When the bird is under stress, the surface epithelium lining the oviduct undergoes patchy de-ciliation followed by cell breakdown in extreme circumstances. In this condition, the synthesis and transfer of matrix proteins will be impaired, and although recovery can follow, the process can take in excess of 15 days (Watt, 1989). During this time calcium transfer is also interrupted and the eggs produced are characteristically wrinkled and thin–shelled.

Measuring shell quality

If optimising bird performance means encouraging the production of top quality eggs, then the literature devoted to bird nutrition is a formidable source of information. However, given the fairly basic nature of the tests used to measure quality, it is pertinent to ask whether many of the results are at best incomplete, and at worst invalid. Consider the following statements; in a paper entitled 'Effect of supplementation of two different sources of phytase on egg production parameters in laying hens and nutrient digestibility,' Jalal and Scheideler (2001) state that 'there were no significant differences in egg production, egg weight, specific gravity *etc.*'. In a communication concerned with organochlorine and heavy metal contamination in the eggs of the Spanish Imperial Eagle, Gonzalez and Hiraldo (1988) reported a 12.6% decrease in egg shell thickness in conjunction with a slight decrease in the degree of crystallisation. Um and Paik (1999) in their paper on the use of microbial phytase supplementation provide data on 'changes in egg weight, specific gravity and shall thickness''. More recently Renema (2003) used egg and shell weight to demonstrate effects of selenium source on the shell quality of broiler breeders. According to Bain (personal communication), the key points to improving shell quality include:

1. Eliminate extremes in egg shape and egg size.

2. Improve the effective thickness of the shell; defined as the distance between the points of fusion of the palisade columns and the outer surface of the shell. The spaces between the palisade columns do not contribute to shell performance.

3. Improve the ultra-structural integrity of the shell.

The most commonly used methods of quality evaluation typically include; deformation, shell thickness, specific gravity and shell weight. With respect to values for deformation, the lower the value the stiffer the shell, and by implication the stronger the shell, BUT stiffness and strength are two different properties which do not always synchronise. In terms of shell thickness, only the effective thickness makes a meaningful contribution to shell performance under load. Thus it is possible to have two shells of the same total thickness, one of which is effectively thicker than the other. With all other aspects of good quality in place, the effectively thicker shell will be more resistant to breakage. Specific gravity provides an indirect measure of % shell or shell thickness, but increasing total shell thickness does not necessarily make for a stronger shell. As for shell weight, it provides no indication either of the functional or structural properties of the shell.

Specialised measures of shell quality

The shell is multi-layered, but not all layers contribute to shell stiffness. Bain (1990) demonstrated by the sequential removal of the cuticle, vertical crystal layer and palisade layer, that they all played a significant role in measured stiffness values. By contrast, removal of the mammillary layer had no obvious effect on shell stiffness. Using Finite Element Analysis, Bain (1990) redefined values for the Elastic Modulus of the egg. Also known as Young's Modulus, it describes the unique relationship that exists between the stresses and strains that are produced when the shell is subjected to moderate loads. She also commented on the fact that the fracture toughness value provides a quantitative relationship between the applied force necessary to cause failure, and the size of any defect that might be present. Fracture toughness can be used as an indicator of the degree of defects within a specified region, and with reference to the egg the mammillary layer provides a quantifiable source of data. In 1998 Coucke created and defined a new eggshell strength parameter termed "dynamic stiffness". Bain *et al.* (2003) have since shown that this property has some degree of heritability.

Mineral nutrition and egg formation

According to Kidd (2003), mineral deficiencies in the adult bird

192

can cause embryonic defects leading to mortality. In their paper of 1993, Kidd et al. highlighted the role of micro-minerals in the immune response. Zinc oxide is acknowledged to improve humoral immunity, while chelated zinc improves cellular immunity, manganese improves liveability, and selenium is recognised as an important part of the egg antioxidant system.

The following examples discuss the results of two trials designed to extract data from eggshells with regard to both their organic and inorganic aspects. The ability to absorb and utilise trace elements diminishes with increasing bird age and health status. The role of minerals in general bird well-being and embryo development is well documented (Kidd, 2003), however less is known about their specific involvement in the actual process of shell formation. Both zinc and manganese act as co-factors in the enzyme systems needed for calcium metabolism, i.e. zinc and carbonic anhydrase. With reference to manganese, Abdallah et al. (1994) reported a reduction in shell weight when this mineral was removed from the diet. Within the eggshell, the shell membranes contain a variety of trace elements viz. manganese (0.03773 mg/g), zinc (0.07889 mg/g), selenium (0.00301mg/g) (Solomon, unpublished data)

Phytate is known to strongly bind inorganic charged forms of minerals, which could particularly affect zinc and manganese availability and hence egg production in layers. A trial was designed to compare mineral source, level of phytase inclusion and age effects on egg production. The assumption was that phytase addition would improve the bio-availability of trace minerals from phytic acid and hence shell quality versus a di-calcium phosphate control diet. Albumen height, shell weight, egg weight, deformation, breaking strength, elastic modulus and ultra-structural score were all measured during the trial.

The trial data demonstrated that the phytase enzymes were efficient at 50% of the manufacturer's dose for laying hens. The elastic modulus decreased with increasing bird age in all groups, but shell structure deteriorated at the level of the mammillary layer .The poorest shell quality was observed in the eggs from phytase source C at the beginning of the trial, but at the second period of analysis a significant improvement was observed, thereafter quality resumed its original level. No effects of phytase source or level were observed with respect to shell weight or Haugh units. Eggs from phytase source B deformed less in the first two periods of the trial i.e. they were significantly stiffer at these times.

From such findings several conclusions can be drawn. If shell weight had been the only measure of quality made then it would have been assumed that source and level were irrelevant. The other data indicate otherwise; whether directly or more likely indirectly, phytase has influenced the organic matrix. In so doing it has altered the pattern of mineralisation to a certain degree within the basal layers of the shell. The effect was not ubiquitous thereby underlining the importance of carefully sourcing feed additives.

In another trial (Tucker *et al.*, 2003), the benefits of supplementing layer diets with a mineral supplement (Eggshell 49, Alltech Inc., Nicholasville, USA) were examined. The trial was carried out on 2 sites, one of which was the University of Glasgow. Two diets were compared, one supplemented with dicalcium phosphate (DCP), and the other with DCP and phytase. Each diet was fed as a control and also with the addition of "shell quality enhancing" mineral feed ingredients. The experiment was designed with 6 replicates of 10 birds per treatment monitored over 12 weeks of laying. Feed intake, egg numbers, FCR, egg weight, egg mass, % cracks, % dirties, shell thickness and shell density were all measured during this period. Additional specialised measures were carried out at the University to investigate shape index, breaking strength, stiffness, effective thickness, elastic modulus and shell ultra-structure.

Trial results showed that feeding the organic mineral supplement;

1. Reduced the percentage of cracked eggs.
2. Increased shell thickness (including effective thickness).
3. Increased shell density.
4. Reduced total ultra-structural score (*i.e.* fewer abnormalities in the mammillary layer).
5. Gave higher values for elastic modulus.

Within the context of the trial, the inclusion of organic minerals has resulted in a more brittle shell type, this indicates a change in the nature and/or distribution of the organic matrix, but probably not at the level of the mammillary layer since this is structurally sound.

Importance of feed formulation for egg quality

Feed formulation is a highly sophisticated practice matched only within the context of this chapter by the wealth of detailed information now available on shell structure and function. So does diet assist in optimising bird performance? The answer is a "qualified" yes. With proper management and the provision of a diet that takes account of the changes which egg production imposes on the oviduct, there is no reason why the reproductive effort should not proceed unchecked. BUT "downgrades" are part of egg production and only an accurate and full assessment of their structural status can aid in the targeting of remedial action.

References

Abdallah, A. G., Harms, R. H., Wilson, H. R., El-Husseiny, O. (1994) Effect of removing trace minerals from the diet of hens laying eggs with heavy or light weight shell. *Poultry Science* **73**(2): 295-301.

Bain, M. M. (1990) *Eggshell strength: A mechanical / ultrastructural evaluation*. PhD Thesis, University of Glasgow, Scotland.

Bain, M. M., Dunn, L. C., Edmond, A., Wilson, W., Joseph, N., Waddington, D., Solomon, S., De Ketelaere, B., De Baerdemaeker, J., and Preisinger, R. (2003) Marker assisted selection to improve shell quality: establishing the association between egg phenotypic traits and "candidate genes". *Proceedings of the WPSA Conference,* Ploufragan, France pp.126-131.

Coucke, P. (1998) *Assessment of some physical egg quality parameters based on vibration analysis*. PhD Thesis, Katholieke Universiteit Leuven, Belgium.

Gonzalez, L. M., and Hiraldo, F. (1988) Organochlorine and heavy metal contamination in the eggs of the Spanish Imperial Eagle (Aquila (heliaca) adalberti) and accompanying changes in eggshell morphology and chemistry. *Environmental Pollution* **51**(4): 241-258.

Hincke, M. T., Gautron, J., Panheleux, M., Garcia-Ruiz, J., McKee, M. D., Nys, Y. (2000) Identification and localisation of lysozyme as a component of eggshell membranes and eggshell matrix. *Matrix Biology* **19**(5): 443-453.

Hincke, M. T., Tsang, C. P., Courtney, M., Hill, V., Narbaitz, R. (1995) Purification and immunochemistry of a soluble matrix protein of the chicken eggshell (ovocleidin 17). *Calcified Tissue International* **56**(6): 578-583.

Jalal, M. A., and Scheideler, S. E. (2001) Effect of supplementation of two different sources of phytase on egg production parameters in laying hens and nutrient digestibility. *Poultry Science* **80**(10): 1463-1471.

Kidd, M. T. (2003) A treatise on chicken dam nutrition that impacts on progeny. *World's Poultry Science Journal* **59**: 475 - 494.

Kidd, M. T., Anthony, N. B., Newberry, L. A., and Lee, S. R. (1993) Effect of supplemental zinc in either a corn- soybean or a milo and corn-soybean meal diet on the performance of young broiler breeders and their progeny. *Poultry Science* **72**: 1492-1499.

Lammie, D., Solomon, S. E., Bain, M. M., and Wess, T. J. (2004) Microfocus small angle x-ray scattering study of the avian eggshell. *Proceedings of the XX11 World's Poultry Congress,* Istanbul.

Renema, R.A. (2003) Effects of dietary selenium source on egg production, fertility, hatchability and shell quality of broiler breeders. *Proceedings of the Annual Meeting of the Poultry Science Association* **82** (suppl. 1).

Solomon, S.E. (1991) *Egg and Eggshell Quality.* Manson Publishing Ltd. London.

Tucker, L.A., Kenyon, S., and Wilson, S. (2003) Benefits of organic minerals in commercial laying hen performance and egg quality. *Proceedings of the XVI European Symposium on the Quality of Poultry Meat,* Ploufragan, France.

Watt, J.M. (1989) *The effect of stress on the reproductive tract of the domestic fowl.* PhD Thesis, University of Glasgow, Scotland.

Um, J.S., and Paik, I. K. (1999) Effects of microbial phytase supplementation on egg production, eggshell quality and mineral retention of laying hens fed different levels of phosphorus. *Poultry Science* **78**(1)**:** 75-79.

The role of peptides in absorption pathways

K. E. Webb, Jr., E. A. Wong, Y-X. Pan, H. Chen, C. A. Poole, L. Van, and J. E. Klang
Department of Animal and Poultry Sciences, Virginia Polytechnic Institute and State University, Blacksburg, VA 24061-0306, USA

Introduction

An important body of literature, primarily from biomedical research, has accumulated over the last 15 years that is helping to define the physiological relevance of peptide absorption. No longer are we limited to simply suggesting that peptide absorption occurs; now we are aware of the existence of special proteins that are responsible for transmembrane movement of peptides. The mRNA for some of these proteins has been cloned and the structural and functional characteristics of the encoded proteins are being determined. As the basis for understanding peptide absorption has grown, so also has the interest of Animal Scientists. Different from the biomedical community, the interest of Animal Scientists is to explore the appropriate dietary foundation of nutrient absorption that will result in the desired growth, development, and production in animals. Important in this regard is understanding peptide absorption from the gastrointestinal tract. Also, knowing what, if any, role peptides may have as sources of amino acids for protein synthesis in different tissues and how they might be involved in controlling this process is of interest. Understanding how intestinal transport of peptides may be regulated is also important. These and other issues will be addressed in this paper.

Peptide transport: cellular and molecular aspects

It was not until the mid 1990's that the structures of the peptide transporters became clear. In 1994, two groups simultaneously reported the identification of a rabbit oligopeptide transporter designated PepT1 (Fei *et al.*, 1994; Boll *et al.*, 1994). This was the beginning of a new era of peptide transport studies. The reported size of rabbit PepT1 cDNA was 2.7 kb (Fei *et al.*, 1994), and it codes for a protein consisting of 707 amino acid residues. The amino acid sequence indicates that PepT1 is a membrane protein with 12 membrane-spanning domains. The protein has a large hydrophilic loop between domains 9 and 10 and this makes the protein different from transporters reported previously. Based on the information from *in vitro* translation, this loop is the target for N-linked glycosylation, and the authors believe it to be an extracellular portion of the protein. Other features, including a protein kinase C site and a cAMP-dependent phosphorylation site, appear also to be present on the protein. Others have cloned human (Liang *et al.*, 1995) and rat (Saito *et al.*, 1995) PepT1. Human PepT1 cDNA is 2.2 kb long with an open reading frame encoding for a protein composed of 708 amino acids (Liang *et al.*, 1995). Rat PepT1 cDNA is 2.9 to 3.0 kb long with an open reading frame encoding a 710 amino acid protein (Saito *et al.*, 1995; Miyamoto *et al.*, 1996). Results from studies on PepT1 indicate that peptide substrates are transported by an electrogenic, H^+-coupled cotransporter that is independent of the peptide's physicochemical characteristics (*i.e.*, size, charge; Daniel *et al.*, 1996; Wenzel *et al.*, 1996).

Functional characteristics of a peptide transporter

Absorption of Met-Gly and carnosine (ß-Ala-His) was observed to occur across ruminal and omasal epithelia (Matthews and Webb, 1995). At the substrate concentrations tested, absorption appeared to be primarily non-mediated, and the omasal epithelium appeared to have a greater capacity than ruminal epithelium to absorb and translocate these peptides. In a subsequent study, *Xenopus laevis* oocytes injected with poly(A)$^+$ RNA extracted from omasal epithelium absorbed more Gly-Sar than did oocytes injected with water (Matthews *et al.*, 1996b). This expressed peptide transport was Na^+-independent and pH-dependent.

In order to determine the structural features of peptides that might influence their affinity for the peptide transporter, *Xenopus laevis* oocytes were injected with ovine omasal epithelium poly(A)$^+$ RNA, and uptake at pH 5.5 of several peptides was examined (Pan *et al.*, 1997). Oocytes injected with poly(A)$^+$ RNA showed transport ability for dipeptides (Gly-Sar, Gly-Leu, Gly-Pro, Phe-Leu, and Leu-Leu) and tripeptides (Leu-Ser-Phe, Leu-Gly-Phe, Lys-Tyr-Lys, Ala-Pro-Gly, Met-Leu-Phe, and Leu-Leu-Tyr). The tetrapeptides, Met-Gly-Met-Met, Val-Gly-Asp-Glu, Ala-Gly-Ser-Glu and Val-Gly-Ser-Glu were transported, but Pro-Phe-Gly-Lys and Val-Ala-Ala-Phe were not. No uptake occurred with the penta- (2), hexa- (1), septa- (1), and octapeptides (1) examined.

When *Xenopus laevis* oocytes were injected with cRNA for an ovine peptide transporter, oPepT1 (Pan *et al.*, 2001), peptide uptake by the oocytes was observed to be concentration-dependent, electrogenic, and pH-dependent, but independent of Na^+, Cl^-, and Ca^{2+}. External pH was varied by bathing the oocytes in buffers ranging from pH 5.0 to 7.0. Uptake of Glu-Glu and Met-Met was greatest at pH 5.0, uptake of Gly-Sar was greatest at pH 5.0 to 6.0, and uptake of Lys-Lys was greatest at pH 7.0. These results agree with previously published reports indicating that an inwardly directed H^+ gradient as well as the charge on the peptide both influence transport (Fei et al., 1994). The oPepT1 displayed broad substrate specificity for transport of neutral and charged dipeptides and tripeptides. All dipeptides and tripeptides examined evoked inward currents in a saturable manner, with an affinity constant (K_t) ranging from 27 μmol/L to 3.0 mmol/L (Table 1). No responses were detected from tetrapeptides or free amino acids. Northern blot analysis demonstrated that oPepT1 was expressed in the small intestine, omasum, and rumen, but was not expressed in the liver and kidney.

To investigate the kinetics of peptide transport by oPepT1 when expressed in mammalian cells, Chinese hamster ovary cells (CHO) were transfected with an expression vector containing our cloned oPepT1 cDNA (Chen et al., 2002a). Transport was assessed by uptake studies using the radiolabeled dipeptide, [^{3}H]-Gly-Sar. Expression of oPepT1 was detected at 8 to 24 h post-transfection with an optimal time of 16 to 24 h. Uptake of Gly-Sar by oPepT1 was pH-dependent with an optimal pH of 5.5 to 6.0, concentration-dependent, and saturable with an apparent K_t value of 1.0 $\pm$ 0.1 mmol/L, and a maximum velocity of 14.3 $\pm$ 0.4 nmol·mg protein^{-1} 40 min^{-1}. Competition studies with non-radiolabeled peptides and [^{3}H]-Gly-Sar showed that all di- and tripeptides inhibited uptake of [^{3}H]-Gly-Sar (Table 1). In addition, three tetrapeptides (Met-Gly-Met-Met, Pro-Phe-Gly-Lys, and Val-Gly-Ser-Glu) also showed inhibition of [^{3}H]-Gly-Sar uptake. There was no inhibition of [^{3}H]-Gly-Sar uptake detected in the presence of non-radiolabeled free amino acids. Treatment of the cells with staurosporine, an inhibitor of protein kinase C (PKC), resulted in a significant increase of the transport system. This increase was specific and could be blocked if treatment was done in the presence of phorbol 12-myristate-13-acetate (PMA), an activator of PKC. The staurosporine- and PMA-induced changes in peptide transport activity were not affected by co-treatment with cycloheximide, an inhibitor of cellular protein synthesis. These data demonstrated that the transport of peptide substrates by oPepT1 in transfected mammalian cells was similar to that in microinjected Xenopus oocytes, and PKC phosphorylation plays a regulatory role in oPepT1 function.

Substrate	cPepT1			oPepT1		
	IC_{50} (mmol/L)[1,4]	K_t (mmol/L)[1,5]	I_{max} (nA)[1,5]	IC_{50} (mmol/L)[2,4]	K_t (mmol/L)[3,5]	I_{max} (nA)[3,5]
Dipeptide						
Glu-Glu	—	—	—	—	0.03	51
Gly-Met	0.07	0.10	126	—		
Gly-Sar	—	0.47	206	—	0.61	50
Leu-Val	—	—	—	—	0.16	39
Val-Leu	—	—	—	—	0.14	38
Leu-Trp	0.02	0.06	110	—	—	—-
Lys-Lys	7.9	6.3	183	739.8	0.07	33
Lys-Met	0.11	0.16	304	50.6	—	—-
Lys-Phe	0.11	0.15	70	23.9	—	—-
Lys-Trp	—	0.03	61	—	—	—-
Met-Glu	0.02	0.06	94	36.6	0.05	43
Met-Gly	0.27	0.08	166	15.6	0.18	44
Met-Leu	0.04	0.13	271	20.6	0.07	37
Met-Lys	0.07	0.17	160	123.0	0.45	33
Met-Met	0.02	0.08	113	24.0	0.03	41
Trp-Ala	0.04	0.07	119	—	—	—-
Trp-Gly	0.06	0.06	88	—	—	—-
Trp-Phe	0.02	0.03	62	—	—	—-
Trp-Leu	0.02	0.12	64	—	—	—-
Tripeptide						
Leu-Gly-Gly	0.08	0.25	179	126.7	0.65	42
Leu-Ser-Phe	—	—	—	70.7	—	—-
Lys-Trp-Lys	5.9	6.9	124	3,732	3.02	38
Lys-Tyr-Lys	—	—	—	2,028	—	—-
Met-Leu-Phe	0.04	0.55	331	13.6	0.15	48
Thr-Ser-Lys	—	—	—	3,012	0.68	33
Tetrapeptide						
Met-Gly-Met-Met	3.9	NR	NR	—	NR	NR
Pro-Phe-Gly-Lys	4.3	NR	NR	—	NR	NR
Val-Gly-Ser-Glu	27	NR	NR	—	NR	NR
Val-Gly-Asp-Glu	—	NR	NR	—	NR	NR

Table 1. Kinetics of peptide transport in *Xenopus* oocytes and Chinese hamster ovary (CHO) cells expressing cPepT1 or oPepT1.

NR = no response
[1]Chen *et al.*, 2002b.
[2]Chen *et al.*, 2002a.
[3]Pan *et al.*, 2001.
[4]In CHO cells expressing cPepT1 or oPepT1, inhibition studies were performed using 20 µmol/L [³H]-Gly-Sar (50 mCi/mmol) as the radiolabeled substrate and five concentrations (0.001 to 10 mmol/L) of peptides as inhibitors to calculate the concentration at 50% inhibition (IC_{50}).
[5]The two-electrode voltage-clamp technique was used to characterize peptide transport activity in oocytes injected with cPepT1 or oPepT1 cRNA. Oocytes were treated with various concentrations of substrates and inward currents induced were measured to calculate K_t and I_{max}.

To study peptide absorption in chickens, an intestinal peptide transporter cDNA (cPepT1) was isolated from a broiler duodenal cDNA library (Chen *et al.*, 2002b). The cDNA was 2,914-bp long and encoded a protein of 714 amino acid residues with an estimated molecular size of 79.3 kDa and an isoelectric point (pI) of 7.48. The cPepT1 protein is approximately 60% identical to PepT1 from rabbits, humans, mice, rats and sheep. Sixteen dipeptides, three tripeptides, and four tetrapeptides that contained the essential amino acids Met, Lys, and (or) Trp were used for functional analysis of cPepT1 in *Xenopus* oocytes and CHO cells. For most di- and tripeptides tested, the substrate affinities were in the micromolar range, indicating that cPepT1 has high affinity for these peptides (Table 1). Lys-Lys and Lys-Trp-Lys were exceptions with substrate affinities in the millimolar range. Neither free amino acids nor tetrapeptides were transported by cPepT1. Northern blot analysis using a full-length cPepT1 cDNA as the probe, demonstrated that cPepT1 mRNA is expressed strongly in the duodenum, jejunum and ileum, and at lower levels in kidney and caeca. The present study demonstrated for the first time the presence and functional characteristics of a peptide transport system from an avian species.

A cDNA clone encoding a turkey intestinal peptide transporter, tPepT1, was isolated from a turkey small intestinal cDNA library by screening with our chicken PepT1 (cPepT1) cDNA probe (Van *et al.*, 2005). The tPepT1 cDNA is 2,921-bp long and encodes a 79.4 kDa protein of 714 amino acids with 12 predicted transmembrane domains. The isoelectric point (pI) of tPepT1 is 5.9, which is much lower than that of PepT1 cloned from chicken (pI = 7.5) and other species. The amino acid sequence of tPepT1 is 94.3% identical to cPepT1 and approximately 60% identical to PepT1 from rats, sheep, rabbits, and humans. Using a two-electrode voltage-clamp technique in *Xenopus* oocytes expressing tPepT1, Gly-Sar transport was observed to be pH-dependent, but independent of Na^+ and K^+. For the dipeptides Gly-Sar and Met-Met, the evoked inward currents indicated that the transporter was saturable and had a high affinity for these substrates. However, transport of the tetrapeptide, Met-Gly-Met-Met, exhibited a possible substrate inhibition.

Screening of a porcine intestinal cDNA library with an oPepT1 cDNA probe resulted in the identification of a porcine PepT1 (pPepT1) cDNA encoding for a protein of 708 amino acids (Klang *et al.*, 2005). For functional analysis, pPepT1 was expressed in CHO cells. The transporter showed optimal uptake at a pH of 5.5 to 6.0. Eighteen different unlabeled dipeptides and tripeptides were found to inhibit the uptake of [^{3}H]-Gly-Sar in competition studies. The IC_{50} of 13 of the dipeptides and two tripeptides ranged from 0.015 to 0.53 mmol/L. Much greater IC_{50} values (1.37 mmol/L) were observed for Lys-Lys, Arg-Lys, and Lys-Trp-Lys, indicating that these are poor substrates for pPepT1. All three of the tetrapeptides examined showed very high IC_{50} values and inhibition of the uptake of Gly-Sar was too small to measure even at a 10mM concentration.

While results from our initial research with sheep indicated that absorption might be largely by non-mediated processes, it is obvious that a mechanism for mediated transport of peptides in the ruminant stomach is present in the form of oPepT1. As discussed above, we have shown that oPepT1 can transport a wide variety of peptides. Therefore, it is expected that when multiple peptides are present, they will compete with each other for transport via oPepT1. To measure the uptake of Gly-Sar in the presence of other peptides, omasal epithelium was collected from sheep and mounted in parabiotic chambers (McCollum and Webb, 1998). To our surprise, co-incubating high levels of potentially competing peptide substrates with Gly-Sar resulted in a stimulation and not a depression in Gly-Sar uptake. Even though our previous results clearly indicate that mRNA for oPepT1 is present in omasal epithelium, these results are certainly not consistent with mediated transport being the only mechanism involved in peptide transport across omasal epithelium. Madara and Pappenheimer (1987) discussed paracellular transport through intestinal epithelia and showed that a prerequisite for this process is the mediated uptake of the substrate (e.g., peptides via oPepT1). It may be that paracellular transport is the mechanism that was responsible for what appeared to be a non-mediated uptake of peptides by epithelial tissues mounted in parabiotic chambers (Matthews and Webb, 1995).

From the evidence that is accumulating, it seems reasonable to suggest that multiple mechanisms may be involved in the transport of peptides across gastrointestinal epithelia. Validation of the presence of, and the clarification of the relative importance of each of these mechanisms will increase our understanding of peptide absorption, and the contribution this may make to the overall nutritional status of the animal.

Stoichiometry and proton-dependence of peptide transporters

Peptide transporters are dependent on the presence of protons for transport activity. At a luminal pH of 7.4, dipeptides with a net charge of -1 (Phe-Glu) and +1 (Phe-Lys) were transported at substantially slower rates than the neutral dipeptides, Phe-Ala and Phe-Gln, in isolated rat jejunal loops (Lister *et al.*, 1997). At a pH of 6.8, transmural transport of Phe-Ala and Phe-Gln was increased by 61% and 49%, respectively. The lower pH increased the rate for negatively charged Phe-Glu by 306% and decreased the rate for positively charged Phe-Lys by 46%. Increasing luminal pH to 8.0 inhibited Phe-Ala transport by 60%, whereas Phe-Lys transport was increased 60%. These results demonstrate that the transport of neutral and negatively charged peptides is linked to the cotransport of protons, whereas that of the positively charged peptide is not.

Brandsch et al. (1997) studied the effect of protons on the affinity and V_{max} of Gly-Sar uptake by Caco-2 cells at an outside pH of either 6.0 or 7.0. The V_{max} was much greater (13.7 vs. 5.8 nmol × 10 min^{-1} mg^{-1} protein) at pH 6.0, but the pH did not affect the affinity of the transporter for the substrate.

The stoichiometry of peptide transport is variable and depends on the net charge carried by the substrate. The proton-peptide coupling ratio for anionic (Phe-Glu), neutral (Phe-Ala) and cationic (Phe-Lys) dipeptides was reported to be 2:1, 1:1, and 0:1, respectively (Temple et al., 1995). Steel et al. (1997) expressed PepT1 in Xenopus oocytes and observed a proton-peptide coupling ratio of 1:1, 2:1, and 1:1 for neutral, acidic, and basic dipeptides, respectively. The results also indicated that at a pH of 5.5 to 6.0, PepT1 favoured substrates in the neutral and acidic forms. However, Temple et al. (1998) found that the transport of the cationic peptide (Gly-Lys) was pH-dependent with a coupling ratio of 1:1. These results suggest that the peptide transporter prefers neutral substrates compared with charged peptides under physiological pH conditions.

The binding and dissociation of ions near the extracellular surface of PepT1 is thought to evoke a pre-steady-state current that results in a conformational change and leads to a translocation of the charged empty carrier (Mackenzie et al., 1996). However, results from Nussberger et al. (1997) indicated a symmetry of H$^+$ binding in response to either intra- or extracellular acidification, which suggested that PepT1 has only one proton-binding site that can be accessed from either side of the membrane.

Substrate specificity of peptide transporters

Transport studies have shown that cloned peptide transporters are capable of taking up a broad range of di- and tripeptides and peptidomimetics. Substrate specificity of rabbit PepT1 was examined in Xenopus oocytes injected with rabbit PepT1 cRNA (Amasheh et al. 1997). At each pH (8.0, 7.4, 6.5, or 5.5), Gly-Gln (zwitterionic) strongly inhibited the uptake of [^{3}H]-Phe-Ala. The Gly-Asp (anionic) inhibited the uptake of [^{3}H]-Phe-Ala at a pH of 7.4 or lower. Gly-Lys (cationic) inhibited uptake only when the pH was at, or higher than 6.5.

Results from the examination of the transport of the anionic cefixime and zwitterionic cefadroxil in Xenopus oocytes expressing rabbit PepT1 and in Caco-2 cells have been reported (Wenzel et al., 1996). In both oocytes and Caco-2 cells, zwitterionic cefadroxil was transported more rapidly at a pH equal to or higher than 6.0. The anionic cefixime was absorbed more efficiently when the pH was equal to or lower than 6.0 (Wenzel *et al.*, 1996). The authors calculated the percentage of the charged or zwitterionic forms of the substrates at each pH. For instance, the relative proportion of the neutral form of cefixime increased as the pH was lowered below 6.0.

In a study conducted by Ganapathy *et al.* (1997), the anionic peptidomimetics cephalosporins (cefixime, ceftibuten, and cefdinir) were used as substrates to study substrate interactions with PepT1 in Caco-2 cells. At pH 6.0, cefixime and ceftibuten are dianionic, and cefdinir is monoanionic. Uptake of [^{14}C]-Gly-Sar was inhibited by cephalosporins in the order of ceftibuten > cefixime > cefdinir. The same results were obtained when PepT1 was expressed in Hela cells. In a subsequent study, *Xenopus laevis* oocytes were injected with PepT1 mRNA. Oocytes incubated with the negatively charged ceftibuten at pH 7.5 showed a small outward current. At a pH of 6.0, addition of ceftibuten (dianionic) to the buffer induced a huge inward current.

The results from these several studies suggest that, under physiological conditions, the affinity of PepT1 for the zwitterionic or anionic substrates is greater than for cationic substrates.

Structural requirements for substrate recognition by PepT1

To investigate the functional role that the α-amino group of substrates has on affinity to PepT1, inhibition of radiolabelled Gly-Sar uptake was measured in the presence of a number of di- and tripeptides along with some non-peptide substrates (Terada *et al.*, 2000). In LLC-rPepT1 cells, Gly-Sar uptake was greatly inhibited by di- and triglycine, but not by Gly or tetraglycine. Most cyclic dipeptides tested, which lack free amino and carboxyl groups, showed no inhibitory effect on Gly-Sar uptake. This finding supports the hypothesis that the free amino and (or) carboxyl groups play an important role in substrate interaction with the peptide transporters (Döring *et al.*, 1998a; b; Ganapathy *et al.*, 1998; Sawada *et al.*, 1999a).

Inhibition studies were performed in PepT1 transfected cells using various di- and tripeptides (Terada *et al.*, 2000). Dipeptides with a modified α-amino group such as N-methyl-glycylglycine and N-formyl-methionylalanine, showed much lower affinity for PepT1 than their original counterparts (Gly-Gly for N-methyl-glycylglycine and Met-Ala for N-formyl-methionylalanine).

A study was conducted that focused on the N-terminal half of PepT1 (Chen *et al.*, 2000). Mutations were generated for histidine residues at amino acid positions 57 (H57), 111 (H111), and 121 (H121) of rabbit PepT1 that are predicted to be in the transmembrane segments, as well as tyrosine residues (Y56 and Y64) adjacent to H57. The H57 mutation showed little transport activity. Mutations of Y56 and Y64 from tyrosines to phenylalanines caused a slight decrease in transport activity, whereas mutations of these tyrosine residues into alanines resulted in no measurable transport activity. Therefore, comparisons between functions of wildtype and mutant PepT1 revealed that not only the H57, but also the aromatic residues near it were essential for the normal function of PepT1. The results support the concept (Fei et al., 1997) that the histidine participates in H^+-binding and the flanking aromatic residues stabilise the charge on H^+ when interacting with the histidine. Mutations of H111 did not cause substantial changes. In contrast, the mutation at H121 (H121R, histidine to arginine) decreased the substrate affinity for Gly-Leu, Gly-Glu, and Gly-Lys by 5-, 22-, and 13-fold, respectively. The affinity of mutation H121C (histidine to cysteine) decreased by 1.5-, 7-, and 4-fold for Gly-Leu, Gly-Glu, and Gly-Lys, respectively. The negatively charged Gly-Glu requires protonation to be transported. The above result then suggests that H121 is involved in the protonation of acidic substrates. The 13-fold decrease in affinity for Gly-Lys in mutation H121R was probably due to electrostatic repulsion between R121 and Gly-Lys. When H121 was replaced by the neutral residue cysteine (H121C), the change in affinity appeared to be less dramatic for Gly-Lys. Taken together, H57 and H121 are closely associated with the coupling of the H^+ and the recognition of transportable substrates, respectively.

In conclusion, these results from these investigations indicate that the free amino and (or) carboxyl groups of substrates play an important role in substrate interaction with the peptide transporters. The α- or ß-amino carbonyl group may be the key structure in determining the affinity to PepT1; and the H^+-binding site of PepT1 is located in the N-terminal half of the transporters and is associated with histidine residues at amino acid positions 57 and 121.

Tissue distribution of PepT1

PepT1 is mainly expressed in the small intestine and is responsible for intestinal absorption of protein digestion products (Miyamoto et al., 1996). In addition to its presence in the digestive tract, trace amounts of PepT1 mRNA were observed in the kidney of the rabbit, rat, and human, the liver of the rabbit and human, the brain of the rabbit, and the placenta and the pancreas of the human (Fei et al., 1994; Liang et al., 1995; Saito et al., 1995; Meredith and Boyd, 2000). In rat kidney, PepT1 mRNA was expressed in the early regions of proximal tubules (Meredith and Boyd, 2000). The role of PepT1 in the reabsorption of peptides from the nephron appears to be as a low-affinity, high-capacity transporter, and its activity accounts for the majority of peptide uptake from the ultrafiltrate.

Although it has been reported that the absorptive capability for small peptides is greater in the proximal small intestine than in the distal small intestine (Ganapathy *et al.*, 1994), the PepT1 mRNA distribution along the small intestine varies among species. An even distribution profile of PepT1 mRNA was observed along the longitudinal axis of rat and mouse small intestine (Erickson *et al.*, 1995; Miyamoto *et al.*, 1996). In rabbits and pigs, PepT1 mRNA abundance was higher in the duodenum and jejunum than in the ileum (Fei *et al.*, 1994; Chen *et al.*, 1999). In White Leghorns and broilers, the strongest hybridisation was found in the duodenum, and the jejunum and ileum showed only faint bands, whereas in sheep and lactating Holstein cows, the abundance of PepT1 was observed mostly in the jejunum and ileum of the small intestine (Chen *et al.*, 1999).

In monogastric animals, PepT1 mRNA was only detected in the small intestine, whereas in ruminant animals such as sheep and cattle, PepT1 mRNA was also observed in the omasum and rumen, although the expression was lower compared with the small intestine (Chen *et al.*, 1999). The results confirm the peptide transport capabilities of omasal and ruminal epithelial cells in ruminant animals, which had been demonstrated previously (Matthews and Webb, 1995; Matthews *et al.*, 1996b). So far, no PepT1 expression in the colon, caecum, skeletal muscle, heart, spleen, lung, or mammary gland has been found in any of these animals (Fei *et al.*, 1994, Chen *et al.*, 1999; Meredith and Boyd, 2000).

PepT1 is only located on the apical microvillus plasma membrane of the absorptive epithelial cells of the small intestine (Ogihara *et al.*, 1999). PepT1 mRNA became detectable at the villus/crypt junction and reached a maximum 100 to 200 μm from this point (Meredith and Boyd, 2000). Immunolocalisation of PepT1 confirmed this, showing that expression of the PepT1 protein was regulated, and that only as cells leave the crypt and migrate towards the tip of the villus do they express the peptide transporter (Meredith and Boyd, 2000). Results from a recent study of expression and cellular distribution of PepT1 during development in rat small intestinal epithelium, indicated different PepT1 cellular distribution patterns dependent upon age (Hussain *et al.*, 2002). The results of the immunocytochemical studies showed that, although the distribution of PepT1 protein was exclusively in the brush border membrane of the intestinal absorptive epithelial cells from both prenatal and mature animals, immediately after birth, PepT1 was found in the subapical cytoplasm, in basal cytoplasm, and in the basolateral membrane.

The existence of poly(A)$^+$ RNA transcript(s) is strong evidence for the presence of a peptide transport protein(s). Thus, peptide absorption from the small intestine of many species, and from the stomach of ruminants, appears to be a physiologically relevant process.

Regulation of intestinal peptide transporter activity and expression

Luminal nutrient transport activity varies in response to many factors, such as development, dietary nutrients, and luminal hormonal or neuronal signals (Shiraga et al., 1999; Meredith and Boyd, 2000). The cloning of the intestinal peptide transporters has led to a surge of studies on cellular mechanisms regulating intestinal peptide transport.

Developmental regulation

The gut faces two abrupt shifts in the functional demands placed on it (Tolza and Diamond, 1992). First, at birth or hatching, the gut suddenly takes over the entire burden of nutrient acquisition from the placenta or yolk sac. Second, mammals make a major qualitative change in diet as they grow, such as the shift from milk to the adult diet at the time of weaning. Thus, the digestive system of animals undergoes dramatic structural and functional change during development. However, ontogeny and developmental regulation of intestinal nutrient transport has received little attention.

Intestinal glucose and amino acid transporters were observed to be present prenatally in humans, guinea pigs, sheep, rabbits, and rats (Pácha, 2000). The intestinal peptide transporter was also observed to be present prenatally. In the rat, PepT1 mRNA and protein were present as early as d 20 of foetal life in intestinal tissue (Shen et al., 2001).

In the rabbit, Gly-Pro influx in both the jejunum and ileum increased from an early foetal stage to d 6 of postnatal life (Guandalini and Rubino, 1982), and then declined continually, reaching minimum values as an adult (> 3 mo). Further, the uptake of Gly-Gly was substantially higher than that of glycine in foetal (25 to 30 d gestational age), newborn (1 to 6 d old), and suckling or weaned (10 to 50 d old) rabbits, indicating the preferential uptake of small peptides over their free amino acids in newborns and infants (Guandalini and Rubino, 1982). It was also observed that Gly-Gly and Gly-Leu influx in isolated everted intestinal segments of guinea pigs were significantly greater in sucklings (3 to 4 d) than in weanlings (10 to 14 d), which, in turn, were greater than in adults (Himukai *et al.*, 1980). Kinetically, the developmental change in jejunal Gly-Gly influx was related to a decrease in maximal transport capacity.

Intestinal PepT1 mRNA levels were highest in 4-d-old rats, and then decreased reaching the adult level by d 28 after birth (Miyamoto *et al.*, 1996). Results from another recent study in rats confirmed this result, and indicated that expression levels of PepT1 mRNA and protein were maximal 3 to 5 d after birth in the duodenum, jejunum, and ileum, and then declined rapidly (Shen *et al.*, 2001). Expression of PepT1 was also observed to increase transiently at d 24, most notably in the ileum, but to a moderate extent (70% of that observed on d 3 to 5). Interestingly, significant PepT1 expression was observed in the colon during the first week of life, but levels were undetectable shortly thereafter through adulthood. The transport ability of the colon to absorb peptides and amino acids was suggested as compensation for the temporary low capacity of the small intestine to absorb nutrients.

The ontogenic development of PepT1 along the vertical and horizontal axes of the rat small intestine was evaluated using semiquantitative reverse transcriptase-polymerase chain reaction (RT-PCR) and immunohistochemistry. The results indicated that the regionalisation of PepT1 in the small intestine of rats was unchanged from birth (postnatal d 4) to adulthood (d 50; Rome *et al.*, 2002). On the cellular level, distribution of PepT1 along the enterocyte differed markedly on the day of birth in the small intestine of the rat as shown by immunocytochemistry (Hussain *et al.*, 2002). In both prenatal and mature animals, distribution of PepT1 was exclusively in the apical brush border of enterocytes. Immediately after birth, PepT1 immunoreactivity was increased, and was no longer confined to the brush-border membrane, but also was present in the subapical cytoplasm, basal cytoplasm, and the basolateral membrane. Although specific transport activity decreased with age and development, the total activities of the transporters actually increased because of the dramatic increase in intestinal length and surface area (Iji *et al.*, 2001).

In broilers, PepT1 mRNA was detected at embryonic d 18, although in very low abundance (Chen *et al.*, 2005). By d 0 (day of hatch), there was a 50-fold increase in cPepT1 mRNA abundance. In broilers fed a normal level of protein, an increase in cPepT1 mRNA abundance was observed with time. Most of the increase occurred during the first 2 weeks.

To study developmental regulation of PepT1 in broiler and turkey embryos, Nicholas turkey or Cobb × Cobb broiler embryos were sampled daily from 5 d before hatch to d 0 (Van et al., 2005). The abundance of PepT1 mRNA in the small intestine was quantified densitometrically from northern blots after hybridisation with full-length cPepT1 and tPepT1 cDNA as probes. There was a quadratic increase in PepT1 mRNA abundance with age in turkey and broiler embryos. The relative increase in abundance of PepT1 mRNA in intestinal tissue from 5 d before hatch to d 0 was much less in the turkey than in the broiler (3.2-fold vs. 14-fold). The dramatic increase in PepT1 mRNA abundance indicates a developmental regulation of the PepT1 gene and that there may be a crucial role for PepT1 in the neonatal chick and poult.

Developmental regulation of oPepT1 expression in the dorsal rumen, ventral rumen, omasum, duodenum, jejunum, and ileum of lambs was studied at 2, 4, 6, and 8 wk of age (Poole et al., 2003). The oPepT1 mRNA was present in all tissues studied at 2 wk, and age did not significantly influence the abundance of oPepT1 mRNA in the small intestine or stomach. In the small intestine, abundance of oPepT1 mRNA was greatest in the jejunum. Abundance was 56% greater than in the duodenum and 46% greater than in the ileum. Differences observed between the duodenum and ileum were not significant. In the stomach, the abundance of oPepT1 mRNA was approximately 68% greater in the dorsal rumen than in the omasum. Abundance of oPepT1 mRNA in the ventral rumen did not differ significantly from abundance in the dorsal rumen or omasum. This is in keeping with previous observations in our laboratory showing the distribution of oPepT1 mRNA in the gastrointestinal tract of sheep (Chen et al., 1999).

Dietary regulation

Substrate levels in the intestinal lumen regulate transport rates of most nutrients in the small intestine. Ferraris and Diamond (1989) offered a general scenario for nutrient regulation of transport. They suggested that metabolisable non-toxic nutrients, such as sugars, non-essential amino acids, and short-chain fatty acids should be up-regulated with increasing dietary substrate levels, and transporters for essential nutrients, which are toxic in large quantities, such as water-soluble vitamins and minerals, should be down-regulated by their substrates. Further, for essential amino acids that are potentially toxic but also yield calories, there are various responses.

Substrates can regulate nutrient transport specifically and non-specifically. Non-specific regulation involves mechanisms that are not specific for a single nutrient and includes changes in mucosal surface area, transcellular electrochemical gradient, paracellular permeability, and plasma membrane lipid composition and fluidity (Ferraris, 1994, 2000). Specific regulation includes a change in site density of transporters in enterocytes as a result of changes in protein synthesis or degradation rate or an increased insertion of preformed cytoplasmic transporters into the brush border membrane (Ferraris and Diamond, 1989). Dietary regulation of nutrient transport can be independent and (or) in concert with neural and hormonal control (Bates *et al.*, 1998; Matosin-Matekalo *et al.*, 1999).

Intestinal dipeptide absorption *in vivo* and *in vitro* increases with dietary protein and peptide level. Jejunal uptake of carnosine increased by 30% in mice fed a high-protein (72%) compared with a low protein (18%) diet (Ferraris *et al.*, 1988). Changing of dietary protein from 4% casein to 50% gelatin resulted in a 1.5- to 2-fold increase in rPepT1 mRNA abundance in rat intestine (Erickson *et al.*, 1995). Addition of Gly-Sar in the Caco-2 cell culture medium for 24 h increased the V_{max} of Gly-Gln transport and PepT1 mRNA abundance and PepT1 protein by increasing *de novo* synthesis (Thamotharan *et al.*, 1998). Walker *et al.* (1998) suggested that the dipeptide-induced increase in hPepT1 and hPepT1 mRNA abundance in Caco-2 cells was due to an increase in hPepT1 mRNA half-life as well as an increase in hPepT1 transcription. In that study, the magnitude of the increases in hPepT1 activity, mRNA, and protein levels were in the range 1.6 to 1.9 times basal values, demonstrating that control of mRNA accumulation rather than translation or post-translational modification was the primary mechanism of regulation.

A low-protein diet was observed to decrease PepT1 gene expression while starvation increased PepT1 expression and activity (Ogihara *et al.*, 1999). Starvation markedly increased the amount of peptide transporter present as determined by immunoblotting, whereas dietary administration of amino acids reduced it. The maximal Gly-Gln uptake (V_{max}) increased twofold without changing the K_t in brush-border membrane vesicles prepared from the jejunum of 1-d fasted rats (Thamotharan *et al.*, 1999). Both the amount of intestinal PepT1 protein in the brush-border membrane and PepT1 mRNA abundance in the intestinal mucosa increased by threefold, indicating starvation induced gene expression.

There is a direct interplay in amino acid and peptide transport in intestinal cells. PepT1 synthesis may be induced by certain amino acids and (or) peptides (Shiraga *et al.*, 1999). Feeding casein, Gly-

Phe, and Phe diets stimulated Gly-Sar transport activity and rPepT1 mRNA and protein abundance compared with feeding a protein-free diet. In contrast, Gly-Gln, Gly, and Gln diets did not increase intestinal dipeptide transport activity. Preincubation of Caco-2 cells with 10 mM of selected neutral, mono- or dicationic dipeptides increased the influx of L-Arg up to fourfold (Wenzel et al., 2001). Preloading with the corresponding free amino acids and dipeptides increased L-Arg influx, but dipeptides always proved to be more efficient (Wenzel et al., 2001). Other studies, however, showed that protein, protein hydrolysates, and free amino acid diets are equally effective at stimulating brush border amino acid and dipeptide transporters (Karasov et al., 1987).

The effect of dietary protein on chicken intestinal cPepT1 mRNA abundance was examined in a recent study (Chen et al., 2005). In one experiment, intestinal samples were obtained at d 0, 1, 3, 5, 7, 10, 14, 21, 28, and 35 from broilers fed diets containing 12, 18, or 24% crude protein (CP). Feed intake was equalised among the three diets. In a second experiment, a fourth group with free access to the 24% CP diet was added. In this study, intestinal samples were obtained at d 0, 1, 3, 5, 7, 10, 14, and 35. In chickens fed the 12% CP diet, cPepT1 mRNA abundance decreased throughout the experiment. Chickens fed restricted 18 or 24% CP diets showed an increase in cPepT1 mRNA abundance with time. Most of the increase occurred during the first 2 wk. In chickens with free access to the 24% CP diet, cPepT1 mRNA decreased until d 14, but returned to an intermediate level at d 35.

A group of 32 crossbred lambs were divided into two groups at birth and assigned to have access to, or not have access to a creep diet, and all lambs were allowed to nurse (Poole et al., 2003). Epithelial tissues were taken from the dorsal rumen, ventral rumen, omasum, duodenum, jejunum, and ileum at 2, 4, 6, or 8 wk of age. Lambs that did not have access to the creep diet had a greater abundance of oPepT1 mRNA in the rumen, particularly the dorsal rumen. Because no dry feed and little or no milk entered the rumen when no creep was fed, it is possible that a stimulus for development from the non-luminal direction, possibly blood-borne, may be involved in the ontogenesis of oPepT1. Access to creep feed did not influence the abundance of oPepT1 mRNA in the intestine. That PepT1 mRNA was present indicates that peptide transport occurs in the young lamb and the rumen and omasum appear to be involved in this process.

It is clear that expression of PepT1 in the gastrointestinal tract is influenced by both developmental and dietary factors. That PepT1 mRNA is present in intestinal tissues before birth or hatching and increases markedly at birth or hatching suggests that transport of peptides is an important physiological phenomenon even at a very early age. The importance of providing the proper diet is reflected in the fact that the regulation of peptide transport is influenced by the diet.

Peptide absorption

It is of interest to know the magnitude of peptide absorption under various physiological conditions. A number of experimental approaches have been used to examine the absorption of peptides including both *in vitro* and *in vivo* methodologies.

In vitro characterisation of gastrointestinal absorption of peptides

Casein, soybean meal, and distillers' dried grains were incubated in a buffered ruminal fluid inoculum for 8 h (Jayawardena, 2000). Following incubation, cell-free supernatants were obtained by centrifugation and these were used as the mucosal fluids in parabiotic chambers containing either ruminal or omasal epithelium. Serosal appearance of peptide amino acids was greater than serosal appearance of free amino acids in both tissues. Movement through omasal epithelium was much greater than through ruminal epithelium, especially for peptides.

Uptake of Gly-Sar by sheep jejunal and ileal brush border membrane vesicles (BBMV) in a study conducted in this laboratory showed that these membranes have the capability of translocating this dipeptide (Bowers, 1997). Uptake was greater in BBMV from jejunal tissue than from ileal tissue. Uptake of 0.3 mM Gly-Sar was not stimulated by an inwardly directed H^+ gradient (pH 6.4 outside, pH 7.5 inside) in either jejunal or ileal BBMV.

Portal flux of peptides

One of the more controversial issues regarding peptide transport revolves around the issue of the quantitative aspects of portal flux of peptides. Our suggestion many years ago that there may be a sizeable flux of peptides across portal-drained viscera (PDV) is the origin of this controversy. The fact that we suggested that the ruminant stomach may be involved in this process served only to heighten the controversy. This single issue, more than any other, likely has been responsible for stimulating laboratories other than ours to initiate investigations into peptide transport in ruminants. These aspects have been previously and extensively reviewed by myself and colleagues (Matthews *et al.*, 1996a; Webb, 1986, 1990;

Webb and Bergman, 1991; Webb *et al.*, 1992, 1993; Webb and Matthews, 1994, 1998).

In the first study that we conducted, we attempted to quantify the flux of free and peptide-bound amino acids across the PDV of calves (Koeln *et al.*, 1993). Through quantifying peptide-bound amino acids as the difference between total amino acids in the protein-free filtrate (following acid hydrolysis), and free amino acids (following sulfosalicylic acid precipitation), we observed that there was a much greater flux of peptide-bound amino acids than free amino acids across the PDV. Subsequently, we reported that not only did peptide-bound amino acids constitute a major fraction of PDV flux of amino acids, but that non-mesenteric tissues contributed substantially to this (Webb *et al.*, 1992, 1993).

A recent study was conducted to measure net fluxes of free and peptide-bound amino acids across PDV of lactating Holstein cows (Tagari *et al.*, 2004). Cows were fed alfalfa-based total mixed rations containing 40% steam-flaked (SFC) or steam-rolled corn (SRC) grain. The PDV flux of total essential free amino acids was greater in cows fed SFC. The PDV flux of essential peptide-bound amino acids was 69.3 $\pm$ 10.8 and 51.5 $\pm$ 13.2 g/12h for cows fed SFC and SRC, respectively. These fluxes were significantly greater than zero, but rarely differed between treatments.

Evidence suggests a net appearance of peptide-bound amino acids in portal and possibly mesenteric blood plasma. Methodological differences are likely contributors to variations in reports of observed differences in the magnitude of portal appearance of peptide-bound amino acids. The more recent reports indicate a much lower PDV flux of peptide-bound amino acids than the earlier ones, and likely represent more reasonable estimates of this flux. Continued efforts in this area will provide further clarification regarding the absolute magnitude of the contribution of peptide-bound amino acids to amino acid flux across PDV.

Utilisation of circulating peptides

It is clear from the preceding discussion that mechanisms are present in the gastrointestinal tract for the transport of peptides. Further, there is evidence that at least a portion of the transported peptides appear in the hepatic portal circulation. If transported peptides are in fact absorbed and appear intact in the hepatic portal circulation, the question arises as to the fate of these peptides and whether they contribute to the supply of amino acids for tissues. The potential for utilisation of the amino acids contained in circulating peptides will be addressed in this section.

Peptide utilisation by cultured myogenic cells

L-Methionine-containing peptides were evaluated as sources of methionine to support protein accretion in C_2C_{12} myogenic cells from mouse muscle (Pan *et al.*, 1996). Expressed as a percentage of the response to free methionine, growth of C_2C_{12} cells differed due to the type of dipeptide (11% to 108%). Met-Met, Met-Val, and Leu-Met were utilised as efficiently as free methionine. Pro-Met and Gly-Met were poorly utilised by C_2C_{12} cells. Met-Pro, Phe-Met, Met-Phe, Met-Leu, Met-Gly, Ala-Met, and Met-Ala were utilised at a rate of about 62 to 86% of the rate of free methionine, and Met-Ser, Ser-Met, and Val-Met were utilised at 26 to 43% of the rate of free methionine.

Primary cultures of ovine myogenic satellite cells were evaluated for their ability to use peptide-bound methionine as a source of methionine for protein accretion and cell proliferation after isolation from skeletal muscle (Pan and Webb, 1998). The cultured myogenic cells were able to utilise all the methionine-containing dipeptides tested for protein accretion with responses ranging from 49 to 95% of the response for free methionine. This is consistent with the concept that peptide-bound amino acids can serve as amino acid sources for protein accretion in sheep skeletal muscle. In some cases, the molecular arrangement of the dipeptides with the same amino acid composition influenced the relative ability of the dipeptides to serve as methionine sources. For all peptides studied, however, only Ala-Met was utilised to support protein accretion as well as free methionine.

Peptide utilisation by cultured mammary cells

L-Methionine-containing peptides were evaluated for their ability to be a source of methionine to support protein accretion in MAC-T, bovine mammary epithelial cells (Pan *et al.*, 1996). All of the methionine-containing dipeptides examined were able to support protein accretion in cultured MAC-T cells with the response ranging from 35 to 122% of the free methionine growth response. Met-Val, Met-Leu, Met-Met, and Leu-Met supported greater protein accretion than did free methionine. Phe-Met, Met-Phe, Ala-Met, Met-Ala, Met-Ser, and Met-Gly were utilised as effectively as free methionine. Gly-Met, Pro-Met, and Ser-Met were the least utilised peptides in MAC-T cells. Dipeptides with methionine at the N-terminus were preferred substrates to those with methionine at the C-terminus.

Regulation of the use of peptides as amino acid substrates for protein accretion and cell proliferation in MAC-T cells by serum factors was examined (Pan *et al.*, 1998). Results indicated that adult animal sera from humans, horses, chickens, pigs, and rabbits promote the utilisation of most methionine-containing peptides. By themselves, neither insulin nor serum lipids were able to facilitate peptide utilisation.

Cultured MAC-T bovine mammary epithelial cells were used to study the ability of methionine-containing peptides to substitute for free methionine in the synthesis of secreted proteins (Wang, 1994). All of the methionyl peptides examined were utilised by the MAC-T cells as sources of methionine for the synthesis of both secreted and cellular proteins. Most of the methionine-containing peptides were as efficient as free methionine in promoting protein synthesis. These results indicate that MAC-T mammary epithelial cells are able to utilise small methionine-containing peptides as sources of methionine to support cellular protein accretion and the synthesis of secreted proteins.

Peptide utilisation by mammary tissue explants

Mammary tissue explants from lactating (10 to 11 d) CD-1 mice were used to study the effect of methionine-containing peptides on the synthesis of secreted proteins (Wang *et al.*, 1996). Mammary tissue explants were able to utilise methionine from all peptides studied. Expressed as a percentage of the response to free methionine, eleven of the peptides promoted 115 to 176% the synthesis of secreted proteins. Dipeptides containing either valine or serine promoted the greatest synthesis. The remaining six peptides were not different from free methionine in promoting synthesis of secreted proteins.

Mammary explants were able to utilise lysine from all lysyl peptides examined for the synthesis of secreted proteins (Wang, 1994). These lysyl peptides generally were similar to free lysine in promoting synthesis of secreted proteins. The synthesis of proteins promoted by Gly-His-Lys was about 117% that promoted by lysine. The other peptides were not different from lysine in promoting protein synthesis that ranged from 91 to 108% of the synthesis promoted by lysine. Within each of the three peptide pairs, Asp-Lys and Lys-Asp, Gly-Lys and Lys-Gly, and Val-Lys and Lys-Val, location of the lysyl residue at either the N- or C-terminal position did not affect protein synthesis.

These results are consistent with those previously discussed for cultured MAC-T mammary epithelial cells. Together, these studies indicate that a wide range of peptide-bound methionine and lysine substrates can support the synthesis of milk proteins by mammalian epithelial cells, at least as well as free methionine and lysine.

Peptide flux across the mammary gland *in vivo*

Use of free- and peptide-bound amino acids by the mammary gland of lactating goats was investigated by Backwell *et al.* (1994). They observed that Phe from Gly-Phe and Leu from Gly-Leu were incorporated into casein in the mammary gland. It is obvious that the incorporation of Phe and Leu from these peptides into casein was an intracellular process. The authors were unable to determine whether there was transport of intact peptides into the cell or whether extracellular hydrolysis preceded transport of the amino acids. Shennan *et al.* (1998) concur that amino acids of peptide origin are utilised by the mammary gland (rat), but their data indicate that peptides are probably not transported but are hydrolysed prior to the constituent amino acids entering the cell. We cannot rule out the possibility that a peptide transporter other than PepT1 may be involved, but data from our laboratory supports their claims because we were unable to detect mRNA for PepT1 in the mammary gland of lactating cows (Chen *et al.*, 1999).

Estimates of the extent of incorporation of Phe, Met, Lys, and Tyr arriving at the mammary gland of lactating goats in peptide form have been recently reported (Bequette *et al.*, 1999). They report that 5 to 11% of Phe, 8 to 18% of Met, 4 to 13% of Lys, and 13 to 25% of Tyr incorporated into casein is of peptide origin. This confirms earlier work from the same laboratory indicating that peptides can contribute amino acids for milk protein synthesis (Backwell *et al.*, 1996).

Net fluxes of free- and peptide-bound amino acids across mammary tissues and the milk amino acid output of lactating Holstein cows were quantified in a recent study (Tagari *et al.*, 2004). Cows were fed alfalfa-based total mixed rations containing 40% steam-flaked (SFC) or steam-rolled corn (SRC) grain. Mammary uptake of essential peptide-bound amino acids was significantly greater than zero for half of the peptide-bound amino acids. It was observed that peptide-bound amino acids provided a substantial proportion of amino acids taken up by the mammary gland.

It appears certain from the results of the studies discussed above, that peptides contribute their constituent amino acids for the synthesis of milk proteins. In magnitude, these amino acids may account for only a small portion of the total amino acids incorporated into milk proteins. This source, however, may be critical and may play a role in controlling milk protein synthesis. Additionally, amino acids of peptide origin may also serve to meet a portion of the needs for protein synthesis of both muscle and mammary tissue, but this appears to be of a lesser magnitude than use of the peptide-bound amino acids for milk protein synthesis.

Summary

That peptides play an important role in amino acid metabolism is certain. The presence of mRNA encoding a peptide transporter in the small intestine of sheep, cattle, broilers, turkeys, and pigs, and the rumen and omasum of sheep and cattle provides strong evidence that there is expression of a protein capable of peptide transport in these regions of the gastrointestinal tract of these agriculturally important animals. This protein seems to be similar, at least in some respects, to PepT1 that has been identified in laboratory species and humans. It will transport a variety of peptides and its function is enhanced by a proton gradient. Initial observations indicate that transport may be limited to di-, tri- and some tetrapeptides. Diffusion and paracellular absorption may also be involved in peptide uptake from the gastrointestinal tract. It is possible that the transport of peptides represents the primary way that amino acids are moved across the brush border membrane, and possibly the epithelial membranes in the rumen and omasum. Subsequent intracellular hydrolysis results in mostly free amino acids reaching the hepatic portal circulation. The relative contributions that free- and peptide-bound amino acids make to amino acid appearance in the portal circulation remain a central question. Portal appearance of peptide-bound amino acids is not as great as was first thought, but no doubt some intact peptides are absorbed into the blood. Data from several studies are supportive of the concept that peptides serve as sources of amino acids that are substrates for protein synthesis by mammalian tissues. The source of these peptides is certainly equivocal (e.g. absorption from the gastrointestinal tract, synthesis and release by tissues, products of protein turnover). Peptides may supply only a small portion of amino acids for protein synthesis, but the supply may be critical. Peptide-bound amino acids in general or specific peptides in particular may be involved in controlling protein synthesis. One thing is certain, a complete understanding of how amino acids are absorbed and distributed to tissues will aid in our being able to develop feeding regimens to assure the desired animal growth, development, and production. Further research efforts will contribute to the resolution of all of these issues.

References

Amasheh, S., Wenzel, U., Weber, W-M., Clauss, W., and Daniel, H. (1997). Electrophysiological analysis of the function of the mammalian renal peptide transporter expressed in Xenopus laevis oocytes. *Journal of Physiology* **504**: 169-174.

Backwell, F.R.C., Bequette, B. J., Wilson, D., Calder, A. G., Metcalf, J. A., Wray-Cahen, D., MacRae, J. C., Beever, D. E., and Lobley, G. E. (1994). Utilization of dipeptides by the caprine mammary gland for milk protein synthesis. *American Journal of Physiology* **267:** R1-R6.

Backwell, F.R.C., Bequette, B. J., Wilson, D., Metcalf, J. A., Franklin, M. F., Beever, D. E., Lobley, G. E., and MacRae, J. C. (1996). Evidence for the utilization of peptides for milk protein synthesis in the lactating dairy goat in vivo. *American Journal of Physiology* **271:** R955-R960.

Bates, S. L., Sharkey, K. A., and Meddings, J. B. (1998). Vagal involvement in dietary regulation of nutrient transport. *American Journal of Physiology* **274:** G552-G560.

Bequette, B. J., Backwell, F.R.C., Kyle, C. E., Calder, A. G., Buchan, V., Crompton, J. France, L. A., and MacRae, J. C. (1999). Vascular sources of phenylalanine, tyrosine, lysine, and methionine for casein synthesis in lactating goats. *Journal of Dairy Science* **82:** 362-377.

Boll, M., Markovich, D., Weber, W.-M., Korte, H., Daniel, H., and Murer, H. (1994). Expression cloning of a cDNA from rabbit small intestine related to proton-coupled transport of peptides, b-lactam antibiotics and ACE-inhibitors. *European Journal of Physiology* **429:** 146-149.

Bowers, S. H. (1997). *Characterization of glycyl-sarcosine uptake by ovine intestinal brush border membrane vesicles.* M.S. Thesis, Virginia Polytechnic Institute and State University, Blacksburg, VA.

Brandsch, M., Brandsch, C., Ganapathy, M. E., Chew, C. S., Ganapathy, V., and Leibach, F. H. (1997). Influence of proton and essential histidyl residues on the transport kinetics of the H^+/peptide cotransport systems in intestine (PepT1) and kidney (PepT2). *Biochimica et Biophysica Acta.* **1324:** 251-262.

Chen, H., Pan, Y-X., Wong, E. A., and Webb, K. E. Jr. (2005). Dietary protein level and stage of development affect expression of an intestinal peptide transporter (cPepT1) in chickens. *Journal of Nutrition* (accepted).

Chen, H., Pan, Y-X., Wong, E. A., and Webb, K. E. Jr. (2002a). Characterization and regulation of the cloned ovine gastrointestinal peptide transporter (oPepT1) expressed in vitro in a mammalian cell line. *Journal of Nutrition* **132:** 38-42.

Chen, H., Pan, Y-X., Wong, E. A., Bloomquist, J. R., and Webb, K. E. Jr. (2002b). Molecular cloning and functional expression of a chicken intestinal peptide transporter (cPepT1) in *Xenopus* oocytes and Chinese hamster ovary cells. *Journal of Nutrition* **132:** 387-393.

Chen, X-Z., Steel, A. and Hediger, M. A. (2000). Functional roles of histidine and tyrosine residues in the H^+-peptide transporter

PepT1. *Biochemica et Biophysica Research Communication* **272:** 726-730.

Chen, H., Wong, E. A., and Webb, K. E. Jr. (1999). Tissue distribution of a peptide transporter mRNA in sheep, dairy cows, pigs, and chickens. *Journal of Animal Science* **77:** 1277-1283.

Daniel H., Amasheh, S., Wenzel, U., Weber, W-M., and Clauss, W. (1996). Transport of charged substrates by the intestinal peptide carrier PepT1 expressed in *Xenopus laevis* oocyte. *FASEB Journal* **10:** A121 (Abstr.).

Döring, F., Walter, J., Will, J., Föcking, M., Boll, M., Amasheh, S., Clauss, W., and Daniel, H. (1998a.) Delta-aminolevulinic acid transport by intestinal and renal peptide transporters and its physiological and clinical implications. *Journal of Clinical Investigation* **101:** 2761-2767.

Döring, F., Will, J., Amasheh, S., Clauss, W., Ahlbrecht, H., and Daniel, H. (1998b). Minimal molecular determinants of substrates for recognition by the intestinal peptide transporter. *Journal of Biological Chemistry* **273:** 23211-23218.

Erickson, R. H., Gum, J. R., Lindstrom, M. M., McKean, D., and Kim, Y. S. (1995). Regional expression and dietary regulation of rat small intestinal peptide and amino acid transporter mRNAs. *Biochemica et Biophysica Research Communication* **216:** 249-257.

Fei, Y.-J., Kanal, Y., Nussberger, S., Ganapathy, V., Leibach, F. H., Romero, M. F., Singh, S. K., Boron, W. F., and Hediger, M. A (1994). Expression cloning of a mammalian proton-coupled oligopeptide transporter. *Nature* **368:** 563-566.

Fei, Y.-J., Liu, W., Prasad, P. D., Kekuda, R., Oblak, T. G., Ganapathy, V., and Leibach, F. H. (1997). Identification of the histidyl residue obligatory for the catalytic activity of the human H+/peptide cotransporters PEPT1 and PEPT2. *Biochemistry* **36:** 452-460.

Ferraris, R. P. (1994). Regulation of intestinal nutrient transport. In: *Physiology of the Gastrointestinal Tract.* (L. R. Johnson, D. H. Alpers, E. D. Jacobson, and J. H. Walsh, (eds). 3rd ed. Raven Press, New York. pp. 1821-1844.

Ferraris, R. P. (2000). Intestinal transport during fasting and malnutrition. *Annual Reviews of Nutrition* **20:** 195-219.

Ferraris, R. P., and Diamond, J. M. (1989). Specific regulation of nutrient transporters by their dietary substrates. *Annual Reviews of Physiology* **51:** 125-141.

Ferraris, R. P., Diamond, J. M., and Kwan, W. W. (1988). Dietary regulation of intestinal transport of the dipeptide carnosine. *American Journal of Physiology* **255:** G143-G150.

Ganapathy, V., Brandsch, M., and Leibach, F. H. (1994). Intestinal transport of amino acids and peptides. In: *Physiology of the Gastrointestinal Tract.* (L. R. Johnson, D. H. Alpers, E. D.

Jacobson, and J. H. Walsh, (eds). 3rd ed. Raven Press, New York. pp. 1773-1794.

Ganapathy, M. E., Prasad, P. D., Mackenzie, B., Ganapathy, V., and Leibach. F.H. (1997). Interaction of anionic cephalosporins with the intestinal and renal peptide transporters PepT1 and PepT2. *Biochimica et Biophysica Acta* **1324**: 296-308.

Ganapathy, M. E., Wei, H. , Wang, H. , Ganapathy, V. , and Leibach, F. H. (1998). Valacyclovir: A substrate for the intestinal and renal peptide transporters PEPT1 and PEPT2. *Biochemica et Biophysica Research Communication* **246**: 470-475.

Guandalini, S., and Rubino, A. (1982). Development of dipeptide transport in the intestinal mucosa of rabbits. *Pediatric Research* **16**: 99-103.

Himukai, M., Konno, T., and Hoshi, T. (1980). Age-dependent change in intestinal absorption of dipeptides and their constituent amino acids in the guinea pig. *Pediatric Research* **14**: 1272-1275.

Hussain, I., Kellett, G. L., Affleck, J., Shepherd, E. J., and Boyd, C. A. R. (2002). Expression and cellular distribution during development of the peptide transporter (PepT1) in the small intestinal epithelium of the rat. *Cell Tissue Research* **307**: 139-142.

Iji, P. A., Saki, A., and Tivey., D. R. (2001). Body and intestinal growth of broiler chicks on a commercial starter diet. 2. Development and characteristics of intestinal enzymes. *British Poultry Science* **42**: 514-522.

Jayawardena, V. (2000). *Ruminal and omasal absorption of ruminally derived amino acids and peptides in vitro.* Ph.D. Dissertation, Virginia Polytechnic Institute and State University, Blacksburg, VA.

Karasov, W. H., Solberg, D. H., and Diamond, J. M. (1987). Dependence of intestinal amino acid uptake on dietary protein or amino acid levels. *American Journal of Physiology* **252**: G614-G625.

Klang, J. E., Burnworth, L. A., Pan, Y. X., Webb, K. E. Jr., and Wong, E. A. (2005). Functional characterization of a cloned pig intestinal peptide transporter (pPepT1). *Journal of Animal Science* (accepted)

Koeln, L. L., Schlagheck, T. S., and Webb, K. E. Jr. (1993). Amino acid flux across the gastrointestinal tract and liver of calves. *Journal of Dairy Science* **76**: 2275-2286.

Liang, R., Fei, Y.-J., Prasad, P. D., Ramamoorthy, S., Han, H., Yang-Feng, T. L., Hediger, M. A., Ganapathy, V., and Leibach, F. H. (1995). Human intestinal H^+/peptide cotransporter cloning, functional expression, and chromosomal localization. *Journal of Biological Chemistry* **270**: 6456-6463.

Lister, N., Bailey, P. D., Collier, I. D., Boyd, C.A.R., and Bronk, J.

R. (1997). The influence of luminal pH on transport of neutral and charged dipeptides by rat small intestine, *in vitro*. *Biochimica et Biophysica Acta* **1324**: 245-250.

Mackenzie, B., Fei, Y. J., Ganapathy, V., and Leibach, F. H. (1996). The human intestinal H+/oligopeptide cotransporter hPEPT1 transports differently-charged dipeptides with identical electrogenic properties. *Biochimica et Biophysica Acta* **1284**: 125-128.

Madara, J. L., and Pappenheimer, J. R. (1987). Structural basis for physiological regulation of paracellular pathways in intestinal epithelia. *Journal of Membrane Biology* **100**: 149.

Matosin-Matekalo, M., Mesonero, J. E., Laroche, T. J., Lacasa, M., and Brot-Laroche, E. (1999). Glucose and thyroid hormone co-regulate the expression of the intestinal fructose transporter GLUT5. *Biochemical Journal* **339**: 233-239.

Matthews, J. C., Pan, Y. L., Wang, S., McCollum, M. Q., and Webb, K. E. Jr. (1996a). Characterization of Gastrointestinal Amino Acid and Peptide Transport Proteins and the Utilization of Peptides as Amino Acid Substrates by Cultured Cells (Myogenic and Mammary) and Mammary Tissue Explants. In: *Nutrient Management of Food Animals to Enhance the Environment*, (E. T. Kornegay (ed.) CRC Press, Inc., Boca Raton, FL.

Matthews J. C., and Webb, K. E. Jr. (1995). Absorption of L-carnosine, L-methionine, and L-methionylglycine by isolated sheep ruminal and omasal epithelial tissue. *Journal of Animal Science* **73**: 3464-3475.

Matthews J. C., Wong, E. A., Bender, P. K., Bloomquist, J. R., and Webb, K. E. Jr. (1996b). Demonstration and characterization of dipeptide transport system activity in sheep omasal epithelium by expression of mRNA in in *Xenopus laevis* oocytes. *Journal of Animal Science* **74**: 1720-1727.

McCollum, M. Q., and Webb, K. E. Jr. (1998). Glycyl-L-sarcosine absorption across ovine omasal epithelium during coincubation with other peptide substrates and volatile fatty acids. *Journal of Animal Science* **76**: 2706-2711.

Meredith, D., and Boyd, C.A.R. (2000). Structure and function of eukaryotic peptide transporters. *Cellular and Molecular Life Science* **57**: 754-778.

Miyamoto, K., Shiraga, T., Morita, K., Yamamoto, H., Haga, H., Taketani, Y., Tamai, I., Sai, Y., Tsuji, A., and Takeda, E. (1996). Sequence, tissue distribution and developmental changes in rat intestinal oligopeptide transporter. *Biochimica et Biophysica Acta* **1305**: 34-38.

Nussberger, S., Steel, A., Trotti, D., Romero, M. F., Boron, W. F., and Hediger, M. A. (1997). Symmetry of H+ binding to the intra and extracellular side of the H+-coupled oligopeptide cotransporter PepT1. *Journal of Biological Chemistry* **272:** 7777-7785.

Ogihara, H., Suzuki, T., Nagamachi, Y., Inui, K.-I., and Takata, K. (1999). Peptide transporter in the rat small intestine: Ultrastructural localization and the effect of starvation and administration of amino acids. *Histochemical Journal* **31:** 169-174.

Pácha, J. (2000). Development of intestinal transport function in mammals. *Physiology Review* **80:** 1633-1667.

Pan, Y., Bender, P. K., Akers, R. M., and Webb, K. E. Jr. (1996). Methionine-containing peptides can be used as methionine sources for protein accretion in cultured C_2C_{12} and MAC-T cells. *Journal of Nutrition* **126:** 232-241.

Pan, Y., Bender, P. K., Akers, R. M., and Webb, K. E. Jr. (1998). One or more serum factors promote peptide utilization in cultured animal cells. *Journal of Nutrition* **128:** 744-750.

Pan, Y., and Webb, K. E. Jr. (1998). Peptide-bound methionine as methionine sources for protein accretion and cell proliferation in primary cultures of ovine skeletal muscle. *Journal of Nutrition* **128:** 251-256.

Pan, Y.-X., Wong, E. A., Bloomquist, J. R., and Webb, K. E. Jr. (1997). Poly(A)$^+$ RNA from sheep omasal epithelium induces expression of a peptide transport protein(s) in *Xenopus laevis* oocytes. *Journal of Animal Science* **75:** 3323-3330.

Pan, Y-X., Wong, E. A., Bloomquist, J. R., and Webb, K. E. Jr. (2001). Expression of a cloned ovine gastrointestinal peptide transporter (oPepT1) in *Xenopus* oocytes induces uptake of oligopeptides *in vitro*. *Journal of Nutrition* **131:** 1264-1270.

Poole, C. A., Wong, E. A., McElroy, A. P., Veit, H. P., and Webb, K. E. Jr. (2003).Ontogenesis of peptide transport and morphological changes in the ovine gastrointestinal tract. *Small Ruminant Research* **50:** 163-176.

Rome, S., Barbot, L., Windsor, E., Kapel, N., Tricottet, V., Huneau, J-F., Reynes, M., Gober, J-G., and Tome, D. (2002). The regionalization of PepT1, NBAT and EAACi transporters in the small intestine of rats are unchanged from birth to adulthood. *Journal of Nutrition* **132:** 1009-1011.

Saito, H., Okuda, M., Terada, T., Sasaki, S., and Inui, K.-I. (1995). Cloning and characterization of a rat H$^+$/peptide cotransporter mediating absorption of b-lactam antibiotics in the intestine and kidney. *Journal of Pharmacological and Experimental Therapeutics* **275:** 1631-1637.

Sawada, K., Terada, T., Saito, H., Hashimoto, Y., and Inui, K.-I. (1999a). Recognition of L-amino acid ester compounds by rat peptide transporters PEPT1 and PEPT2. *Journal of Pharmacological and Experimental Therapeutics* **291:** 705-709.

Shen, H., Smith, D. E., and Brosius, F. C. III. (2001). Developmental expression of Pept1 and PepT2 in rat small intestine, colon, and kidney. *Pediatric Research* **49:** 789-795.

Shennan, D. B., Calvert, D. T., Backwell, F.R.C., and Boyd, C.A.R. (1998). Peptide aminonitrogen transport by the lactating rat mammary gland. *Biochimica et Biophysica Acta* **1373:** 252-260.

Shiraga, T., Miyamoto, K., Tanaka, H., Yamamoto, H., Taketani, Y., Morita, K., Tamai, I., Tsiko, A., and Takeda, E. (1999). Cellular and molecular mechanisms of dietary regulation on rat intestinal H+/peptide transporter PepT1. *Gastroenterology* **116:** 354-362.

Steel, A., Nussberger, S., Romero, M. F., Boron, W. F., Boyd, C. A. R., and Hediger, M. A. (1997). Stoichiometry and pH dependence of the rabbit proton-dependent oligopeptide transporter PepT1. *Journal of Physiology* **498:** 563-569.

Tagari, H., Webb, K. E. Jr., Theurer, B., Huber, T., Sadik, M., Alio, A., Lozano, O., Delgado-Elorduy, A., Santos, J. E. P., Simas, J., Nussio, L., Santos, F., Cuneo, P., and DeYoung, D. (2004). Portal drained visceral flux, hepatic metabolism, and mammary uptake of free and peptide-bound amino acids and milk amino acid output in dairy cows fed diets containing corn grain steam flaked at 360 or steam rolled 490 g/L. *Journal of Dairy Science* **87:** 413-430.

Temple, C. S., Bronk, J. R., Bailey, P. D., and Boyd, C. A. (1995). Substrate-charge dependence of stoichiometry shows membrane potential is the driving force for proton-peptide cotransport in rat renal cortex. *Pflugers Arch* **430:** 825-829.

Temple, C. S., Stewart, A. K., Meredith, D., Lister, N. A., Morgan, K. M., Collier, I. D.,Vaughan-Jones, R. D., Boyd, C.A.R., Bailey, P. D., and Bronk, J. R. (1998). Peptide mimics as substrates for the intestinal peptide transporter. *Journal of Biological Chemistry* **273:** 20-22.

Terada, T., Sawada, K., Irie, M., Saito, H., Hashimoto, Y., and Inui, K.-I. (2000). Structural requirements for determining the substrate affinity of peptide transporters PepT1 and PepT2. *Pflügers Arch -European Journal of Physiology* **440:** 679-684.

Thamotharan, M., Bawani, S. Z., and Zhou, X. (1998). Mechanism of dipeptide stimulation of its own transport in a human intestinal cell line. *Proceedings of the Association of American Physicians* **110**(4)**:** 361-368.

Thamotharan, M., Bawani, S. Z., Zhou, X-D., and Adibi, S. A. (1999). Functional and molecular expression of intestinal oligopeptide transporter (PepT-1) after a brief fast. *Metabolism* **48:** 681-684.

Tolza, E. M., and Diamond, J. M. (1992). Ontogenetic development of nutrient transport in rat intestine. *American Journal Physiology* **263:** G593-G604.

Van, L., Pan, Y. X., Wong, E. A., Bloomquist, J. R., and Webb, K. E. Jr. (2005). Developmental regulation of a turkey intestinal peptide transporter (PepT1). *Poultry Science* (accepted).

Walker, D., Thwaites, D. T., Simmons, N. L. Gilbert, H. J., and Hirst, B. H. (1998). Substrate upregulation of the human small intestinal peptide transporter, hPepT1. *Journal of Physiology* **507**: 697-706.

Wang, S. (1994). *Peptides as amino acid sources for the synthesis of secreted proteins by mammary tissue explants and cultured mammary epithelial cells.* Ph.D. Dissertation, Virginia Polytechnic Institute and State University, Blacksburg, VA.

Wang, S., Webb, K. E. Jr., and Akers, M. R. (1996). Peptide-bound methionine can be a source of methionine for the synthesis of secreted proteins by mammary tissue explants from lactating mice. *Journal of Nutrition* **126**: 1662-1672.

Webb, K. E., Jr. (1986). Amino acid and peptide absorption from the gastrointestinal tract. *Fed. Proc.* **45**: 2268-2271.

Webb, K. E., Jr. (1990). Intestinal absorption of protein hydrolysis products: A review. *Journal of Animal Science* **68**: 3011-3022.

Webb, K. E., Jr., and Bergman, E. N. (1991). Amino acid and peptide absorption and transport across the intestine. *Proceedings of the 7th International Symposium on Ruminant Physiology.* pp. 111-128.

Webb, K. E., Jr., DiRienzo, D. B., and Matthews, J. C. (1993). Recent developments in gastrointestinal absorption and tissue utilization of peptides - A review. *Journal of Dairy Science* **76**: 351-361.

Webb, K. E., Jr., and Matthews, J. M. (1994). Absorption of amino acids and peptides In: Amino Acid Nutrition of Ruminants. (J. M. Asplund (ed.)) CRC Press, Boca Raton, FL.

Webb, K. E., Jr., and Matthews, J. C. (1996). Peptide Absorption and Its Significance in Ruminant Protein Nutrition. In: *Peptides in Mammalian Protein Metabolism: Tissue Utilization and Clinical Targeting.* (G. Grimble and C. Backwell (eds.)) Portland Press Ltd., London.

Webb, K. E., Jr., and Matthews, J. C (1998). Peptide Absorption and Its Significance in Ruminant Protein Nutrition. In: *Peptides in Mammalian Protein Metabolism: Tissue Utilization and Clinical Targeting.* (G. Grimble and C. Backwell (eds.)) Portland Press Ltd., London. pp. 1-10.

Webb, K. E., Jr., Matthews, J. C., and DiRienzo, D. B. (1992). Peptide Absorption: A review of current concepts and future perspectives. *Journal of Animal Science* **70**: 3248-3257.

Wenzel, U., Gebert, I., Weintraut, H., Weber, W.-M., Claub, W., and Daniel, H. (1996). Transport characteristics of differently charged cephalosporin antibiotics in oocytes expressing the cloned intestinal peptide transporter PepT1 and in human intestinal Caco-2 cells. *Journal of Pharmacology and Experimental Therapeutics* **277:** 831-839.

Wenzel, U., Meissner, B., Doring, F., and Daniel, H. (2001). PepT1-mediated uptake of dipeptides enhances the intestinal absorption of amino acids via transport system $b^{0,+}$. *Journal of Cell Physiology* **186:** 251-259.

Fertility: why it is declining and the role of trace minerals to reverse this trend

A.M. Mackenzie
Animal Production and Science, Harper Adams University College, Newport, Shropshire, TF10 8NB, UK

Introduction

Fertility in medium to high yielding dairy cattle has been reported to be declining with major economic impact on herd viability & profitability. The aetiology of this sub-fertility is multifactorial, and Esslemont *et al.* (2001) have attributed it to inadequate feeding and poor husbandry. Dietary deficiencies of single or multiple trace elements are not the sole cause of sub-fertility, but they do exert profound effects on the fertility of dairy cattle and other species. The main trace elements likely to affect ruminant livestock in the UK are copper, cobalt and selenium, which will be the focus of this paper. However, there is increasing interest in other trace elements such as manganese, zinc and iodine as dietary supplements, even though the incidence of clinical deficiency is infrequent. One of the major problems associated with identifying the role and requirements for trace elements is the ability to determine the animal's mineral status. Furthermore, our poor understanding of mineral interactions that occur in the intestines, and in particular the rumen, hampers mineral research.

Copper

Copper (Cu) is required by animals for numerous enzymes that are involved in many important metabolic functions ranging from antioxidant activity, production of the pigment melanin and the cross linkage of collagen, to list but a few (Underwood and Suttle, 1999). Clinical Cu deficiency is a problem in many areas, and is regarded as the second most common mineral deficiency of cattle in the world (Wikse *et al.*, 1992). Cu deficiency has been acknowledged to occur either as a primary deficiency, where Cu intake is below metabolic requirements, or as a secondary deficiency due to antagonistic interactions with other minerals in the diet.

These interactions predominantly occur between Cu, molybdenum (Mo), sulphur (S) and iron (Fe), and take place in the rumen under anaerobic conditions. Although zinc (Zn) also reduces Cu absorption, it occurs via a different mechanism in the small intestine via the induction of metallothionine. Depigmentation of hair, poor growth rates, alterations in cardiac function, anaemia, fragile bones, impaired immune function and infertility are the commonly reported clinical manifestations of Cu deficiency (McDowell, 1992).

There is still considerable debate as to the precise role of Cu, and its associated metabolism on the reproductive performance of ruminant livestock (Suttle, 2002; Telfer *et al.*, 2004). Much of this uncertainty stems from our inability to adequately assess the Cu status of ruminants using plasma Cu concentrations as the set biochemical criteria (Mackenzie *et al.*, 1997a; b). Early reports provide contradictory evidence of a possible relationship between low Cu status and fertility in cattle. Littlejohn and Lewis (1960), and later Larson *et al.* (1980), concluded that there was no relationship between fertility of cattle and blood Cu status. Similarly, Phillippo *et al.* (1982) studied suckler cows with serum Cu ranges from 2.5 to 14.5 mmol/l within one month of mating, and reported conception rates between 37 and 65% respectively. Phillippo *et al.* (1982) concluded that there was no significant relationship between mean herd serum Cu concentration and conception rates. Rowlands *et al.* (1977) found that in cattle with low blood Cu status, fertility varied. More recently, Wentink *et al.* (1999) reported very low levels of Cu in the blood or liver of dairy heifers that were not associated with clinical abnormalities.

Evidence of a positive relationship between Cu and fertility in ruminants originated from studies on high M peat soils in East Anglia (England) where fertility was increased by Cu therapy (Blakemore and Venn, 1950; Munro, 1957). Studies where sub-fertility was induced using Cu antagonists, or where fertility was improved by Cu supplementation has now firmly established the relationship between Cu and fertility in cattle (Bremner *et al.*, 1983; Phillippo *et al.*, 1985; 1987; Hurley and Doane, 1989; Mackenzie *et al.*, 2001; Black and French, 2004). The most common symptoms of clinical Cu deficiency on fertility are prenatal mortality, particularly embryonic loss (O'Gorman *et al.*, 1987), reduced ovarian activity, delayed or depressed oestrus activity, and reduced conception rates (Phillippo *et al.*, 1987).

To understand the contrasting observations cited above, it is appropriate to investigate the aetiology of Cu deficiency in ruminants. The condition termed 'secondary Cu deficiency' is caused by a series of complex interactions between Cu, Mo and S in the rumen, and has been extensively reviewed (Suttle, 1991). Within the rumen, Mo and S form a series of di-, tri- and tetra-thiomolybdates that can bind to Cu to form Cu thiomolybdates that are not absorbed by the animal and are excreted in the faeces. This has the net effect of reducing Cu absorption, and Suttle (1976) proposed a regression equation to predict Cu availability of diets based on this interaction. However, research conduced at the Rowett Research Institute, demonstrated that cattle with extremely low Cu status did not necessarily show clinical signs of deficiency (Phillippo et al., 1987). However, this state of hypocupraemia without clinical signs was induced by Fe and not Mo. This led to the hypothesis that clinical Cu deficiency was due to the formation and absorption of thiomolybdates, and not primarily a lack of Cu in the blood.

In a further series of experiments, heifer diets were supplemented with high levels of Mo (5 mg/kg DM) or Fe (800 mg/kg DM) or a combination of the two, and growth rates and Cu parameters recorded (Humphries et al., 1983; Bremner et al., 1983). The authors reported that Cu status (as measured by plasma and liver concentrations) was decreased by Mo and Fe treatments, as well as in the combination treatment, compared to control heifers (no supplemental Mo or Fe). However, clinical signs such as reduced growth rates, skeletal lesions and alterations in hair texture and colour were only apparent in the Mo-treated heifers, and not the Fe-only supplemented heifers or the controls. These results suggest that clinical Cu deficiency was due to high Mo intakes rather then a low liver or plasma Cu concentration. Mason (1986) and Mason et al. (1988) reported that thiomolybdates were potent antagonists of Cu metabolism, and once absorbed reduced the activity of Cu-containing enzymes. Williams (2004) later reported that the inhibition of enzyme activity in sheep due to dietary Mo was not attributed to alterations in gene expression, and was therefore either a direct inhibition of the enzyme by thiomolybdate or a prevention of the incorporation of Cu prior to its release from the hepatocyte. Williams et al. (2004) concluded that there was a marked alteration in the speciation of Cu in plasma due to dietary Mo.

Phillippo et al. (1987) examined the effects of Fe or Mo intakes on fertility and Cu status in heifers. Heifers were supplemented with either a) 800 mg Fe /kg DM, b) 5 mg Mo /kg DM, c) 800 mg Fe /kg DM plus 5 mg Mo /kg DM or d) control; no Mo- or Fe-supplementation. In the Fe-, Mo- and combination-supplemented groups (treatment groups a, b & c), Cu status was decreased compared with the controls. However, it was only in the Mo-supplemented heifers that effects on fertility were observed. Age and liveweight at puberty were delayed in the Mo-supplemented group compared with the controls and Fe-supplemented heifers (Table 1). Additionally, the pulsatile release of lutenising hormone (LH) was reduced.

	Control	Iron	Molybdenum	Restricted control[a]
Liver copper (mg/kg)	59.1	5.9	4.5	74.0
Age at puberty (days)	285	296	344	275
Liveweight at puberty (kg)	313	310	283	268
Peak LH concentration[b] (ng/ml)	18.2	14.8	6.6	14.0

[a]Intake was restricted to produce similar weight gains to Mo fed heifers
[b]Following two prostaglandin injections

Similar effects on dairy heifers have also been reported by Telfer *et al.* (1998), where the oestrus cycle was extended by the addition of Mo, S and Fe (5.1 mg Mo /kg DM, 550 mg Fe /kg DM and 3.1 g S /kg DM) to a basal diet (4.9 mg Cu /kg DM) (Table 2). Mackenzie *et al.* (2001) reported that cattle grazing pasture (2.5 mg Mo /kg DM; 10.4 mg Cu /kg DM) had significantly improved fertility when supplemented with Cu compared with the untreated control cattle (Table 3). Although plasma Cu concentrations were significantly increased in the supplemented cattle, the plasma Cu concentrations of the control animals were all in the normal range (> 12 mmol /l) for the duration of the trial, and none of the cows could be classified as hypocupraemic. However, these affects have not always been consistent, as Xin *et al.* (1993) demonstrated that Mo did not affect the pulsatile release of LH, but pituitary concentrations were significantly lower in dairy steers.

	Length of cycle (days)				
Cycle	Control	SE mean	Treated	SE mean	Sig
1st cycle	20.9	0.7	20.6	0.4	NS
2nd cycle	21.8	0.8	22.4	1.4	NS
3rd cycle	20.4	0.7	22.6	1.3	NS
4th cycle	20.6	0.7	24.8	1.3	p<0.05
5th cycle	21.6	0.8	24.4	1.0	p<0.05

	Control	Cu treated	SE mean	Sig
Number of insemination	2.5	1.7	0.16	p<0.01
Calving interval (days)	397	372	9.2	p<0.05
Calving to conception (days)	117	95	9.3	NS

There have been numerous studies comparing different types of Cu supplements, whether it be the form of delivery (*i.e.* injection or oral bolus), or source of dietary Cu such as organic versus inorganic. Black and French (2004) reported that there was a large variation in the response to different Cu supplements. For example, cattle orally-supplemented with Cu conceived at a rate 1.8 times greater than those treated by Cu injection, and the calving to conception interval was 84 days compared with 114 days for the same animals. O'Donoghue and Boland (1995) reported that supplementing cows with Bioplex™ (Alltech Inc., Nicholasville, USA) (organic) minerals (Cu 100mg, Zn 300mg & Se 2mg / hd /d) results in fewer days to the appearance of the first follicle and ovulation, with an improvement in conception rate (Table 4). However, Muehlenbein *et al.* (2001) reported that there was no effect of Cu source on pregnancy rates.

Table 4. Effect of Organic Mineral Supplementation on Reproduction in Dairy Cows (O'Donoghue and Boland, 1995)

	Control	Bioplex*
Days to 1st dominant follicle	9.3	7.8
Days post partum to ovulation	25.3 ± 3.1	20.4 ± 3.8
Days to 1st service	75.4 ± 6.1	68.8 ± 3.8
Conception rate (%)	57.7	65.2

* Bioplex 100 mg Cu; 300 mg Zn; 2mg Se-yeast (Sel-plex® Alltech Inc. Nicholasville) / hd /d

The mechanism by which dietary Mo / thiomolybdate alters reproductive function in ruminants still remains unclear. However, there are several studies that have attempted to address this issue. For example, Kendall *et al.* (2003) reported that thiomolybdates depressed steroidogenesis in cultured bovine ovarian cells, together with a decreased production of oestradiol. Additionally, similar effects on androstenedione have now been observed (unpublished observation, Kendall and Campbell). The inhibition of steroidogenesis was partially reversed by the addition of Cu to the culture medium of cells. Williams (2004) reported that lambs supplemented with dietary Mo had increased Mo concentrations in their ovaries along with a decrease in Cu concentrations (Table 5).

Table 5. Effect of dietary Mo, S and Fe on trace element concentration in the liver of growing lambs (μg /g DM; Williams, 2004)

	Control	Iron	2 Mo	5 Mo	10 Mo	s.e.d	Sig
Cu	215.1[a]	82.5[b]	77.7[b]	29.4[c]	82.1[b]	26.64	P<0.001
Mo	3.76[a]	3.51[a]	4.21[a]	4.94[b]	6.77[c]	0.32	P<0.001
Zn	106.1	102.4	109.2	114.7	115.1	6.90	NS
Fe	203.0[a]	520.1[b]	201.2[a]	206.1[a]	189.0[a]	35.5	P<0.001
Mn	8.01	8.54	9.01	8.68	8.62	0.937	NS

[a,b,c] Means within row with different superscripts were significantly different (P<0.05)

Haywood *et al.* (2004) reported that ewes administered thiomolybdate parenterally, displayed gross alterations in the pathology and function of the pituitary gland with the cells showing a non-inflammatory atrophy or degeneration. This was associated with an accumulation of Mo in the pituitary. In studies to assess the effect of Mo on pituitary function, Williams (2004) using immunocytochemistry, stained the pituitary glands for adrenocorticotropic hormone (ACTH) in lambs supplemented with 2, 5 or 10 mg/kg DM Mo or 500 mg/kg DM Fe. ACTH levels were greater in all lambs receiving the Mo treatments, in a dose-dependent manner, when compared with negative control lambs (no supplementation) or lambs supplemented with Fe. This suggests that dietary Mo at levels as low as 2.0 mg/kg have a direct effect on the pituitary and endocrine system in ruminants. This effect appears to be partly due to a direct effect on the pituitary cells resulting in the prevention of hormone release. The mechanism of this has not yet been established. However, the Cu-dependent enzyme, peptidylglycine α-amidating monooxygenase (PAM) (Stevenson *et al.*, 2003) is essential for the secretion of numerous peptides, hormones and neurotransmitters from cells. Removal of Cu from this enzyme leads to its inhibition (Bolkenius and Ganzhorn, 1998), as does inhibiting the supply of Cu to the enzyme (Stevenson *et al.*, 2003). Therefore, there is speculation that some of the effects in ruminants brought about by dietary Mo or thiomolybdates may be due to the inhibition of PAM activity within the pituitary (Haywood *et al.*, 2004; Williams, 2004)

Clearly, from the literature discussed above, the initial inconsistent findings concerning the relationship between Cu status and fertility in ruminants has to be placed in context, as plasma Cu concentrations do not reflect Cu status (Mackenzie *et al.*, 1997a; b; Wentink *et al.*, 1999; Telfer *et al.*, 2004). The evidence cited in this paper clearly demonstrates that Mo does affect pituitary and ovarian function, and ultimately fertility in cattle, and it is supplemental Cu that is required to prevent the effects of dietary Mo. However, uncertainty in Cu analyses has led to the widespread use of Cu as a supplement to treat many cases of sub-fertility in cattle as a likely Cu-responsive condition. There has been a dramatic increase in the incidence of Cu poisoning in dairy cattle, with Livesey *et al.* (2002) reporting 33 herds affected between 1999 and early 2002 in the UK. Laven *et al.* (2004) also suggested that over-supplementation of Cu to dairy cattle may be occurring based on the determination of plasma glutamate dehydrogenase (GLDH) levels. This enzyme, which reflects hepatopathy, which is not specific to Cu toxicity, was reported to be elevated in a dairy herd receiving 1325 mg Cu/day, although there were no clinical signs of toxicity. There are also conflicting views concerning the use of different forms of Cu in the diet and their relative merits. However, this area has received little attention in terms of published research and is being driven by farm studies where the control of external factors is often compromised.

Cobalt

Cobalt (Co) is the prosthetic component of vitamin B_{12} that is synthesised by micro-organisms in the rumen. As such, ruminants require dietary Co. Deficiency of Co is common throughout the UK and other regions of the world. Clinical signs of Co deficiency in ruminants include anorexia and reduced growth rates with resultant loss of condition, emaciation and if untreated, eventually death (McDowell, 1992). Other clinical manifestations in ruminants include anaemia and fat accumulation in the liver (Underwood and Suttle, 1999).

Vitamin B_{12} is required as a coenzyme in several important metabolic pathways in ruminants, either in the form of methylcobalamin that assists in methyltransferase enzymes or as adenosylcobalamin, which directly influences glucose synthesis from propionate (Underwood and Suttle, 1999). Propionate is required to be converted to glucose via succinate in the liver. This pathway involves the conversion of methylmalonyl CoA to succinyl CoA by the enzyme methylmalonyl CoA mutase, a vitamin B_{12}-dependent enzyme. Deficiency of this enzyme leads to an increase of methylmalonic acid in urine, and a build up of blood propionate resulting in inappetence. It is also required for erythrocyte synthesis and maintenance of the nervous system (McDowell, 1992).

Reduced conception rates have been reported to be one of the most common clinical manifestations of Co deficiency in adult cattle (Hidiroglou, 1979). Some studies have reported calving intervals of 24 months in Co-deficient cattle rather than the usual 14. Hurley and Doane (1989) listed reduced oestrus activity, delayed onset of puberty and abortion resulting from Co deficiency. The mechanism by which Co influences fertility in ruminants has largely been attributed to alterations in energy metabolism. However, Judson *et al.* (1997) reported improvements in the fertility status of cattle that received Co-supplementation, compared with cattle that did not receive a supplement when there were no signs of ill-thrift.

Consistent with several of the other trace elements, the accurate determination of the Co status of dairy cattle is difficult. The current practice is to measure serum / plasma vitamin B_{12} concentrations, which for sheep and goats correlates well with Co intakes.

However, this is not the case for cattle as reported by Carlos *et al.* (1987). These authors reported incomplete release of vitamin B_{12} from the binding protein that resulted in an underestimation of true vitamin B_{12} concentrations. Additionally, rumen microbes synthesise analogues of vitamin B_{12} that are detected by the assays, but are biologically inactive. The latter source of error is more common in dairy cattle fed high levels of concentrates, where a lower rumen pH results in a reduction of total vitamin B_{12} synthesised with a higher proportion of inactive analogues being produced.

Selenium

The essential role of selenium (Se) in animal health and nutrition is primarily involved in the antioxidant enzymes, glutathione peroxidases (GSH-Px). This series of enzymes has a synergistic role with vitamin E and other antioxidants in removing toxic peroxides from tissue, and preventing oxidative damage to membranes. Since the early discovery of Se-dependent GSH-Px, numerous other Se-containing proteins have been discovered. The most notable being the iodothyronine deiodinases which are involved in thyroid function (Arthur and Beckett, 1994) converting thyroxine to triiodothryonine, a reaction that has been shown to be inhibited in Se-deficient cattle (Arthur *et al.*, 1988).

Clinical signs of Se deficiency in cattle are primarily a muscular dystrophy commonly called white muscle disease. This is characterised by stiffness, muscle degeneration and a general weakness together with the animal having difficulty in standing. Other clinical signs include impaired immune function and increased incidence of disease, particularly pneumonia (McDowell, 1992). These can all be deemed to be resultant from low GSH-Px activity. Poor growth and ill-thrift have also been regarded as characteristics of Se-deficiency which can now be explained partly through the role of Se in thyroid metabolism.

Se deficiency is known to adversely affect reproduction in both male and female animals. In the dairy cow, the effect of Se deficiency is primarily manifested by the occurrence of retained placenta or cystic ovaries. Harrison *et al.* (1984) reported that the incidence of retained placentas was 17.4% in control animals compared to zero in the Se / vitamin E-treated animals. Also, the incidence of cystic ovaries was 47% in the controls and 19% in the treated animals. Similar results were reported by D'Aleo *et al.* (1983) in cattle fed a low-Se diet during the dry period. One month prior to calving, one group was supplemented with 0.3 mg Se / kg and subsequent reproductive performance monitored (Table 6). There was a trend for the number of inseminations to conception to be greater in the control animals fed the low-Se diet compared with the supplemented group (2.05 and 1.54 respectively). Also, the incidence of retained placentas and cystic ovaries was significantly lower in the Se-supplemented group. The role of Se in the incidence of retained placentas was reviewed by Mee (2004), who concluded that in the majority of studies, supplementation with Se and vitamin E, alone or in combination, reduced the incidence of retained placentas. However, the majority of these studies involved parenterally administered Se and vitamin E in combinations, and not orally supplemented Se. Additionally, improvements in milk production and growth have been reported, together with improvements in immunity.

Table 6.
Effect of selenium on the fertility of dairy cattle (D'Aleo et al., 1983)

	Control	+Se
Inseminations to conception	2.05	1.54
Retained placentas	20%	0%
Cystic ovaries	9.5%	5.6%

Manganese

Manganese (Mn) deficiency has been reported in several species where it results in alterations in bone growth, fertility and carbohydrate metabolism (Underwood and Suttle, 1999). Wilson (1966) stated that the main symptoms attributed to Mn deficiency in cattle were anoestrus, weak oestrus behaviour and, upon rectal examination, decreased or sub-normal ovarian size. These conditions have also been reported in other farm species, however, Underwood and Suttle (1999) regarded their occurrence in all farm animal as rare. Absorption of Mn is generally considered to be very low from the diet (typically less than 1%) and can be further suppressed by antagonism from calcium and phosphorus (Wilson, 1966). However, forages such as pasture and grass silage, together with concentrate diets would supply levels of Mn above their required levels. Currently there is little or no evidence of increased performance either in terms of growth rates or fertility resulting from increased supplementation (Whitaker, 1999).

Conclusion

Optimum levels of trace mineral supplementation to improve fertility in ruminants are the subject of much debate. Evidence contained within the literature indicates that the most important elements relating to sub-fertility are Cu and Se. Organic mineral sources are considered more bioavailable than inorganic sources, and may therefore alleviate fertility problems at lower supplementation levels. The role of Cu in fertility is complex, and the effects of Mo within the diet are yet to be full elucidated. Further research in this area is required.

References

Arthur, J.R., and Beckett, G.J. (1994). New metabolic roles for selenium. *Proceedings of the Nutrition Society* **53**: 463 - 470.

Arthur, J.R., Morrice, P.C., and Beckett, G.J. (1988). Thyroid hormone concentrations in selenium-deficient and selenium-sufficient cattle. *Research in Veterinary Science* **45**: 122 - 123.

Black, D.H., and French, N.P. (2004). Effects of three types of trace element supplementation on the fertility of three commercial dairy herds. *Veterinary Record* **154**: 652 - 658.

Bolkenhuis, F.N., and Ganzhorn, A.J. (1998). Review. Peptidylglycine a-amidating monooxygenase: neuropeptide amidation as a target for drug design. *General Pharmacology* **31**: 655 - 659.

Blakemore, F., and Venn, J.A.J. (1950). Conditions associated with hypocupremia of bovine in East Anglia. *Veterinary Record* **62**: 756 - 761.

Bremner, I. Phillippo, M., Humphries, W.R., Young, B.W., and Mills, C.F. (1983). Effect of iron and molybdenum on copper metabolism in calves. In: *Trace Elements in Animal Production and Veterinary Practice* (Eds. N.F. Suttle, R.G. Gunn, W.M. Allen, K.A. Linklater and G. Wiener). BSAP Occasional Publication No. 7. pp. 136 - 137.

Carlos, G.M., Telfer, S.B., Johnson, C.L., Givens, D.I., Wilkins, R.J., and Newberry, R.D. (1987). Microbiological assay of blood-serum for the vitamin B12 status of dairy cows. *Journal of Dairy Research* **54**: 463 - 470.

D'Aleo, J., Shelford, A., and Fisher, L.J. (1983). Selenium-sulphur interactions and their influence on fertility in dairy cattle. *Canadian Journal of Animal Science* **63**: 999.

Esslemont, R.J., Kossaibati, M.A., and Allcock, J. (2001). Economics of fertility in dairy cows. In: *Fertility in the High-Producing Dairy Cow* (Ed Diskin, M.G.). Occasional Publication 26, British Society of Animal Science, Edinburgh. pp. 19-29.

Harrison, J.H., Hancock, D.D., and Conrad, H.R. (1984). Vitamin E and selenium for reproduction of the dairy cow. *Journal of Dairy Science* **67**: 123 - 132.

Haywood, S., Dincer, Z., Jasani, B. and Loughran, M.J. (2004). Molybdenum-associated pituitary endocrinopathy in sheep treated with ammonium tetrathiomolybdate. *Journal of*

Comparative Pathology, **130**, 21-31.

Hidiroglou, M. (1979). Trace element deficiency and fertility in ruminants: A review. *Journal of Dairy Science* **62**: 1195 - 1206.

Humphries, W.R., Phillippo, M., Young, B.W., and Bremner, I. (1983). The influence of dietary iron and molybdenum on copper metabolism in calves. *British Journal of Nutrition* **49**: 77 - 86.

Hurly, W.L., and Doane, R.M. (1989). Recent development in the roles of vitamins and minerals in reproduction. *Journal of Dairy Science* **72**: 784 - 804.

Judson, G.J., McFarlane, J.D., Mitsioulis, A., and Zviedrans, P. (1997). Vitamin B12 responses to cobalt pellets in beef cows. *Australian Veterinary Journal* **75**: 660 - 662.

Kendall, N.R., Marsters, P., Scaramuzzi, R.J., and Campbell, B.K. (2003). Expression of lysyl and effect of copper chloride and ammonium tetrathiomolybdate on bovine ovarian follicle granulosa cells cultured in serum-free media. *Reproduction* **125:** 657 - 665.

Larson, L.L., Mabruck, H.S., and Lowry, S.R. (1980). Relationship between early postpartum blood composition and reproductive performance in dairy cattle. *Journal of Dairy Science* **63**: 283 - 289.

Laven, R.A., Livesey, C.T., Offer, N.W., and Fountain, D. (2004). Apparent subclinical hepatopathy due to excess copper intake in lactating Holstein cattle. *Veterinary Record* **155**: 120 - 121.

Littlejohn, A.I., and Lewis, G. (1960). Experimental studies of the relationship between calcium phosphorous ratio of the diet and fertility in heifers: a preliminary report. *Veterinary Record* **72**: 1137- 1144.

Livesey, C.T., Bidewell, C.A., Crawshaw, T.R., and David, G.P. (2002). Investigation of copper poisoning in adult cows by the Veterinary Laboratory Agency. *Cattle Practice* **10**: 289 - 294.

Mackenzie, A.M., Moeini, M.M., and Telfer, S.B. (2001) The effect of a copper, cobalt and selenium bolus on the fertility and trace element status of dairy cattle. In: *Fertility in the High-Producing Dairy Cow* (Ed. M.G. Diskin). Occasional Publication 26, British Society of Animal Science, Edinburgh. pp. 423 - 427.

Mackenzie, A.M., Illingworth, D.V., Jackson, D.W., and Telfer, S.B. (1997a). The use of caeruloplasmin activities and plasma copper concentrations as indicators of copper status in ruminants. In: *Trace Elements in Man and Animal -9: Proceedings of the Ninth International Symposium on Trace Elements in Man and Animals.* (Eds. P.W.F. Fischer, M.R. L'Abbé, K.A. Cockell and R.S. Gibson). NRC Research Press,

Ottawa, Canada. pp. 137 - 138.

Mackenzie, A.M., Illingworth, D.V., Jackson, D.W., and Telfer, S.B. (1997b). A comparison of methods of assessing copper status in cattle. In: *Trace Elements in Man and Animal -9: Proceedings of the Ninth International Symposium on Trace Elements in Man and Animals.* (Eds. P.W.F. Fischer, M.R. L'Abbé, K.A. Cockell and R.S. Gibson). NRC Research Press, Ottawa, Canada. pp. 301 - 302.

Mason, J. (1986). Thiomolybdates: mediators of molybdenum toxicity and enzyme inhibitors. *Toxicology* **42**: 99 - 109.

Mason, J., Lamand, M., Tressol, J.C., and Mulryan, G. (1988). Studies of the change in systemic copper metabolism and excretion produced by the intravenous administration of trithiomolybdate in sheep. *British Journal of Nutrition* **59**: 289 - 300.

McDowell, L.R. (1992). *Minerals in Animal and Human Nutrition.* Academic Press, London.

Mee, J.F. (2004). The role of micronutrients in bovine periparturient problems. *Cattle Practice* **12**: 95 - 108.

Muehlenbein, E.L., Brink, D.R., Deutscher, G.H., Carlson, M.P., and Johnson, A.B. (2001). Effect of inorganic and organic copper supplemented to first-calf cows on cow reproduction and calf health and performance. *Journal of Animal Science* **79**: 1650 - 1659.

Munro, I.B. (1957). Infectious and non-infectious herd infertility in East Anglia. *Veterinary Record* **69**: 125 - 129.

O'Donoghue, G.G., and Boland, M.P. (1995). Effects of an organic trace mineral supplement on reproduction in dairy cows. *Journal of Dairy Science* **78** (Suppl. 1): 239.

O'Gorman, F., Smith, F.H., Poole, D.B.R., Boland, M.P., and Roche, J.F. (1987). The effect of molybdenum-induced copper deficiency on reproduction in beef heifers. *Theriogenology* **27**: 265.

Phillippo, M., Humphries, W.R., Lawrence, C.B. and Price, J. (1982). Investigation of the effect of copper status and therapy on fertility in beef suckler herds. *Journal of Agriculture Science,* **99**, 359-364.

Phillippo, M., Humphries, W.R., Bremner, I., Atkinson, T., and Henderson, G.D. (1985). Molybdenum-induced infertility in cattle. In: *Trace Elements in Man and Animals: TEMA-5,* (Eds. C. Mills, L. Bremner, and J. K. Chesters). pp. 176 - 180.

Phillippo, M., Humphries, W.R., Atkinson, T., Henderson, G.D., and Garthwaite, P.H. (1987). The effect of dietary molybdenum and iron on copper status, puberty, fertility and oestrus cycle in cattle. *Journal of Agricultural Science* **109**: 321 - 336.

Rowlands, G.J., Little, W., and Kitchenham, B.A. (1977).

Relationship between blood composition and fertility in dairy cows - a field study. *Journal of Dairy Research* **44**: 1 - 7.

Stevenson, T.C., Ciccatosto, G.D., Ma, X.-M., Mueller, G.P., Mains, R.E., and Eipper, B.A. (2003). Menkes protein contributes to the function of peptidylglycine a-amidating monooxygenase. *Endocrinology* **144**: 188 - 200.

Suttle, N.F. (1976). Predicting the effect of dietary molybdenum and sulphur on the availability of copper to ruminants. *Proceedings of the Nutrition Society* **35**: 22a.

Suttle, N.F. (1991). The interaction between copper, molybdenum, and sulphur in ruminant nutrition. *Annual review of Nutrition* **11**: 121 - 140

Suttle, N.F. (2002). Copper deficiency – how has the disease and its diagnosis changed in the last 15 years? *Cattle Practice* **10**: 275 - 278.

Telfer, S.B., Moeini, M.M., and Mackenzie, A.M. (1998). The effect of molybdenum, sulphur and iron on the oestrus cycle and copper status of Holstein Friesian heifers. *XX World Buiatrics Congress, Syndey*. pp. 1063.

Telfer, S.B., Kendall, N.R., Illingworth, D.V., and Mackenzie, A.M. (2004). Molybdenum toxicity in cattle: an underestimated problem. *Cattle Practice* (In Press).

Underwood, E.J., and Suttle, N.F. (1999). *The Mineral Nutrition of Livestock*. CABI Publishing, Oxon.

Wentink, G.H., Smolders, G., Boxem, Tj., Wensing, Th., Müller, K.E. and Van Den Top, A.M. (1999). Lack of clinical abnormalities in dairy heifers with low blood and liver copper levels. *Veterinary Record* **145**: 258 - 258.

Whitaker, D.A. (1999). Trace elements – the real role in dairy cow fertility? *Cattle Practice* **7**: 239 - 242.

Wikse, S.E., Herd, D., Fiald, R. and Holland, P. (1992). Diagnosis of copper deficiency in cattle. *Journal of the Veterinary American Medical Association* **200**: 209 - 211.

Williams, C.L. (2004). The effects of molybdenum, iron and sulphur on copper metabolism and physiology of sheep. PhD Thesis, Harper Adams University College.

Wilson, J.G. (1966). Bovine functional infertility in Devon and Cornwall: response to manganese therapy. *Veterinary Record*, **79**, 562-566.

Xin, Z., Silvia, W.J., Waterman, D.F., Hemken, R.W. and Tucker, W.B. (1993). Effect of copper status on luteinizing-hormone secretion in dairy steers. *Journal of Dairy Science*, **76**, 437-444.

Mastitis in the modern dairy cow and the role of nutrition and management

Jim Spain

Associate Professor, Animal Science Unit, University of Missouri-Columbia, USA

Introduction

Mammary gland health and milk quality are important issues for the dairy industry. Lowering the somatic cell count (SCC) in milk improves the overall quality of milk produced and consumed, while reducing the use of intramammary antibiotics. Reduced use of antibiotics is seen as a major step in preventing the development of antibiotic resistant bacteria. This outcome would also reduce the chances of antibiotic-contaminated milk leaving the farm. Thus, mammary gland health and milk quality are issues of animal health and animal productivity, as well as consumer confidence and consumer safety.

Globally, mastitis is recognized as the most costly disease facing the world's dairy industry (Dingwell et al., 2003). Increased efforts to monitor milk quality have resulted in reports from the National Dairy Herd Improvement Association (NDHIA) and the National Animal Health Monitoring System (NAHMS). The NDHIA data were based on state-level DHIA SCC linear scores of individual cows (Wells and Orr, 1995). In 1993, the NDHIA database included 28 percent of the US operations, 42 percent of the national's dairy cows, and 51 percent of the countries milk production. Somatic cell count linear scores weighted by cow numbers show states in the southeast, corn-belt, west coast, and Pennsylvania to have SCC linear scores of 3.5 or greater. The lost revenue calculated in dollars per cow was greatest in the southeast, and is connected with the high fluid milk production and associated higher farm level prices. Estimated losses exceeded 30 dollars per cow in more than forty states. These losses did not include added costs associated with treatment and milk discard. The National Mastitis Council estimates value of reduced milk yield exceeds $120 dollars. Defining the true economic impact of mastitis is difficult given each case differs in the treatment costs and the effects of the disease event on animal longevity, lifetime productivity, culling and genetic progress (Dingwell *et al.*, 2003). It is clear that mastitis control is economically important to the world's dairy producers.

Due to the effects of mastitis on milk quality and dairy farm economics, much effort of research scientists has been focused on improving udder health and milk quality. Most progress has been accomplished in reducing the incidence of contagious mastitis. However, mastitis infections in dairy cattle have not decreased. Instead, environmental mastitis has increased in many countries (Pyorala, 2002). Pyorala (2002) concluded that some consider antibiotics to be the most effective "fight against mastitis". However, the development and use of post milking teat dips, barrier teat dips, vaccinations and other udder health products, focused on preventing new infections, imply much of the focus of the dairy industry has been given to prevention of mammary gland infections. Indeed, a survey of 50 Ohio dairy farms reported in a review by Dingwell and colleagues (2003) found mastitis prevention comprised 48% of the cost of preventing diseases (2003). A comprehensive plan to achieve real and significant improvement in milk quality and udder health will include a complete management effort that improves the environment, nutrition and overall management of dairy cows (Pyorala, 2002).

Cow factors and mastitis

Anatomical factors

What factors predispose cattle to mastitis? These factors can be broadly categorized as animal factors and environmental factors. Animal factors have been evaluated in an effort to describe the ability to exercise genetic selection to reduce mastitis. Detilleux *et al.* (1995) reported "heritabilities for all mastitis indicators averaged 10%..." "Although heritablilty estimates were small, genetic variability was observed..." "Therefore selection against the occurrence of mastitis seems realistic." Similarly, Slettbak and co-workers (1995), evaluated the influence of milking characteristics and physical traits of udder and teats on clinical mastitis. The results of this study involving 565 matched pairs of Norwegian cattle showed decreasing teat-end-to floor distance and periparturient udder edema to be significant risk factors for clinical mastitis. Distance between the teat-end and floor would decrease the exposure of the teats to pathogens, while the animal is standing in the housing environment. Therefore, the selection of sustainable udder conformation should lead to improved udder health and animal longevity.

In addition to the exposure of the udder to the environment as controlled by udder support and distance between pathogens and teat ends, health and function of the teat end is important in determining udder health. Sordillo and Streicher (2002) described the defense mechanisms of the bovine mammary gland as having "two distinct categories" - the innate immunity and specific immune responses. Nickerson (1994) and Craven and Williams (1985) have provided excellent reviews of the mammary gland anatomy and the important defense features relative to the immune function of the bovine udder. In both reviews, the authors describe the first key defense mechanism of the bovine mammary gland as being the teat-end and teat canal. Indeed, the teat-end is defined in several reports as being the first line of defense of the mammary gland (Sordillo and Streicher, 2002; Kehrli and Harp, 2001; Zecconi *et al.*, 2000; Spain, 1993). Thus, the key to anatomical defense involved in the innate immunity of the mammary gland is the teat-end.

Zeconni *et al.* (2000) reported that the average length of the bovine streak canal is about 10 mm, and is the main entrance through which pathogens enter the mammary gland. These authors described the importance of the closure of the streak canal which is maintained by constant tension of the sphincter muscle via the autonomic nervous system. Nickerson (1994) reported that the streak canal may be dilated for up to 2 hours after milking as the sphincter muscles "re-contract" following the stretching associated with the milking machine vacuum and milk flow. Sordillo and Streicher (2002) reported that increased patency of the streak canal was correlated with increased rates of mastitis infections. Therefore, management strategies that promote animals standing after milking allow the sphincter muscle to recover while decreasing risk of exposure to pathogens while the teat end defense is compromised.

Another important feature of the streak canal is the keratin plug. Bitman and co-workers (1992) described the keratin lining of the teat canal as a physical and chemical barrier for the protection of the mammary gland. Teat keratin accumulates in the streak canal as it is produced by stratified squamous epithelium (Sordillo and Streicher, 2002). Capuco *et al.* (1992) suggested that the keratin lining may physically trap bacteria and prevent migration into the mammary gland. More recently, Zeconni and co-workers (2000) described keratin's mode of action as having three mechanistic functions: physical occlusion; adsorption of the pathogens in a "mesh-like matrix"; and elimination when keratin is flushed out of the streak canal during milking.

In addition to a physical barrier, streak canal keratin contains antimicrobial agents which have bacteriocidal and (or) bacteriostatic effects. Sordillo and Streicher (2002) reported the antimicrobial agents present in the keratin included esterified and non-esterified fatty acids (myristic, palmitoleic and linoleic acid) and cationic proteins. Capuco *et al.* (1992) found removal of the keratin lining the streak canal significantly increased the percentage of infected quarters by 13 to 15 percentage units. Harmon and Crist (1994) reported the highest rate of new infections occurs at dry off and at the end of that dry period. Dingwell and co-workers noted that 95% of all intramammary infections during the early dry period were the result of environmental pathogens (2003). In their review, Dindwell *et al.* (2003) also summarized research that showed that closure of the teat end by the keratin plug was significantly important in udder health during the early dry period. Indeed, over 80% of mastitis in the dry period occurred within 21 days after dry off, and over 95% of the cases occurred in quarters with teat ends classified as open. Thus, teat-end health and the presence of an adequate keratin plug influence teat-end "function" and will be key to preventing new infections as the udder is challenged by exposure to pathogenic microorganisms.

Metabolic factors

Dingwell *et al.* (2003) reported that the dry period is an important production phase relative to udder health. The incidence of mastitis occurs in two distinctive periods of the dry period. As previously noted, the dry cow has a period of high risk of intramammry infection during the first three weeks after dry off. The cow is also highly susceptible to mastitis during the last two weeks of gestation and early lactation. Chassagne *et al.* (1998) summarized reports that found the periparturient period of the dairy cow to be the period of greatest risk. The survey conducted over four years was a collaborative effort with producers, veterinarians, and research technicians who collectively gathered data from 47 herds and included 8,938 lactation records on 4,123 cows. Biological indicators included body condition scores, cleanliness scores and blood metabolic profiles. The herds had an average incidence of early clinical mastitis of 19.3% of lactations with a range of 7.1% to 50% across farms. The Early Lactation Clinical Mastitis (ECM) occurred in an average 9.3 days postpartum. Previous lactation last test day SCC was not different between diseased and non-diseased animals. Higher producing cows were at greater risk. The increased flow of milk would increase the removal of the keratin from the streak canal and increase the risk of infection.

The increased risk of mastitis during the periparturient period is associated with a period of decreased immune function. With the combined effects of high milk flow contributing to loss of keratin and high intramammry pressure causing teat ends to leak colostrum and milk, the risk of pathogenic bacteria gaining access to the gland cistern is greatly increased. In this situation, the health of the lactating mammary gland depends on the immune cells and soluble immune factors present in the secretions of the mammary gland.

The conclusion thus far is that that udder conformation influences the dairy cows' risk of developing mastitis. The significance of genetic influence on mammary gland health is small. Similar to traits associated with reproductive efficiency, the relatively small heritabilities indicate the large influence of the animal's environment on mammary gland health.

Cow environment and mastitis

The components of the environment that contribute to udder health include housing, milking center, ambient conditions (air temperature, wind speed, humidity, etc.). The health of the mammary glands is a balance between the anatomical defenses, the cellular defenses and the risk of exposure or challenge by the pathogens. Reduced exposure includes providing ideal conditions of a low stress with a clean and dry resting area for cows to lie down. Pankey (1990) pointed out that cattle spend the majority of their time lying down "between" milkings and emphasized the importance of animal housing and feeding environment relative to the control of clinical environment mastitis. Just as cow factors have been associated with mammary gland health; environmental factors also influence the risk of lactating dairy cows developing mastitis.

In well managed, high producing dairy herds, environmental mastitis is of primary concern and considered by some as the most important challenge in udder health. Clinical environmental mastitis infections are most common during periods of elevated ambient temperatures associated with summer heat stress. Housing and bedding systems are key variables as these components of the production system influence the exposure of the udder to coliform bacteria present in bedding material and/or feces that might contaminate bedding and resting areas. Harmon and Crist (1994) emphasized the importance of maintaining procedures used to prevent contagious mastitis. They suggested including therapy, in conjunction with other strategies to reduce the incidence of environmental mastitis.

Schukken *et al.* (1991) reported that cows housed inside with poor sanitation had increased incidence of environmental mastitis. Herlin (1998) surveyed 1,709 Swedish herds to determine factors associated with milk quality. Elite herds (herds with SCC < 250,000 cells/ml and no poor milk quality deductions) reported similar bedding and feeding practices compared to herds experiencing low milk quality. What were noted as being different were the design and cleanliness of the stalls, with elite herds having more properly designed and therefore cleaner stalls which contributed to cleaner cows (Herlin, 1998). Primiparous Swedish Fresian cows had an incidence rate of clinical mastitis of 15%, with the greatest risk occurring in cows calving in July and August. Physical trauma to the teat and udder also resulted in increased risk of clinical mastitis of 6 and 3 fold respectively. In addition, these investigators reported the cumulative effects of 200 kg less milk produced associated with an almost 3 times higher risk to be culled (Oltenacu and Ekesbo, 1994).

Lehenbauer *et al.* (1994) conducted a retrospective study of the differences in SCC between cows from different housing systems. The winter season corresponded with higher levels of rainfall and the authors suggested the conditions in the open lots would expose cows to a higher risk of environmental mastitis.

Immune function and mastitis

Once pathogenic bacteria invade past the initial defense structures of the teat end, the animal relies on a variety of immune responses including: non-specific humoral proteins, immune cells, and antibodies. A certain base level of immune protection is constantly present in the milk and mammary gland. If the macrophage and lymphocytes are able to clear the gland of the initial invasion of pathogens, clinical infection is prevented.

If the basal immune system is unable to successfully destroy the pathogens, an infection will result which may lead to clinical disease. As the disease develops in severity, neutrophils are attracted, through chemical signals, and migrate into the gland, thus causing an increase in the somatic cell count of the milk. The severity and duration of the infection is therefore affected by the animal's immune system as it relates to the level and quality of the immune response

As discussed earlier, Harmon and Crist (1994) discussed opportunities to enhance milk quality that included reducing exposure and enhancing immune function, which would include more recent management strategies of vaccinating the animal against mastitis-causing organisms. Other approaches to enhancing immune function include utilizing management strategies to improve nutritional status. Research has focused on the role nutrition plays as a component of the immune system's cell function and the impact on mammary gland health.

Nutrition, immune function and mastitis

Nutritional status of the animal has been shown to directly influence the animal's immune function. As presented earlier, the animal's immune function includes both anatomical resistance mechanisms of the teat-end and the cellular and soluble protective mechanisms (Sordillo and Streicher, 2002). In many discussions, the influence of nutrition on immune function focuses on the role of micronutrients such as selenium and Vitamin E in cellular immunity. The importance of nutrition on the anatomical defense is often not considered. However, given the important role the anatomical resistance of the teat-end serves, it is logical to explore the role nutrition serves in this component of the immune function of the dairy cow. Simply put, the skin is the first line of defense.

In the case of the mammary gland, teat and skin condition and health are essential for optimal resistance to environmental pathogens. Zinc is required for the maintenance of healthy skin. Moynahan (1981) reported nearly 20% of total body zinc is present in skin. Furthermore, application of topical zinc mixtures have been used to promote wound healing for centuries. More relevant to livestock, oral zinc-supplementation has been used in the control of foot rot in lambs housed under dry conditions (Cross and Parker, 1981). Zinc is associated with its role as a cofactor of DNA and RNA polymerases (Moynahan, 1981). A deficiency of zinc appears to alter amino acid incorporation required for the synthesis of keratins and collagen. Moynahan (1981) reported that zinc is required for the incorporation of cystine into skin protein which is essential for the production of keratin. Parakeratosis is the manifestation of this disruption of keratin synthesis and is the classical manifestation of zinc deficiency. As discussed earlier, keratin is removed from the streak canal during optimal anatomical defense barriers of the teat-end and the streak canal.

Kellogg (1990) summarized data on the use of organically-complexed zinc and showed a significant decrease in milk somatic cells. These data suggested that either the animal was more resistant to intramammary invasion post the teat-end defense, or that cellular immunity was enhanced. In a trial conducted at the University of Missouri, we found that dairy cows fed a chelated zinc had fewer new infections compared to control cows fed zinc oxide. In fact, during the feeding trial, cows fed zinc oxide experienced 11 new infections, while cows fed bioplexed zinc had only 5 new intramammary infections (Spain, 1993). There were no differences in the duration of infection indicating immune cell function was similar between the two groups. These results suggested an improved resistance with improved zinc status.

Nutrition has also been clearly shown to affect immune cell function of lactating dairy cattle. Sordillo *et al.* (1997) summarized more than 10 research reports concerning the immunomodulatory effects of specific nutrients. Most research has dealt with micronutrients that function as a component of immune cells. Selenium, vitamin E, B-carotene, copper and zinc have been shown to enhance the function of immune cells including leukocytes, lymphocytes, and neutrophils. However, before emphasis can be placed on the "micronutrients", energy and protein status of the high producing dairy cow must be considered.

Dairy cattle experience a period of negative energy balance during the periparturient period. This period of negative energy balance corresponds with a time at which dairy cows have been shown to be most susceptible to new infections, especially those due to environmental pathogens. As several authors have noted (for example, Harmon and Crist, 1994; Dingwell *et al.*, 2003), the dairy cow is most susceptible to clinical environmental mastitis during the periparturient period. This has led to much research on pre-partum nutrition and incidence of early lactation clinical mastitis.

Chandra (1992) summarized work that described the relationship between protein-energy status and immunocompetence (1992). Much of the research in this area deals with malnutrition in human subjects. However, the biological relationships between the nutritional status and immune function would be similar in cattle. Malnutrition, as reported in Chandra's summary, decreased the size and robustness of tissues responsible for producing components of the immune system. Furthermore, the malnourished have decreased activity of immune cells. The "soluble" components of the immune system including the antibody response were also adversely affected.

The relationship between body condition scores (Chassagne *et al.*, 1998) and ketosis (Oltenacu and Ekesbo, 1994) would imply that the energy and protein balance of the periparturient dairy cow might contribute to the animal's immune function and risk of early lactation mastitis. It is also important to recall that the periparturient dairy cow experiences large shifts in endocrine balance that may also impact upon immune function. As it relates to this transition phase and early lactation, milk production and flow is increasing at a rapid rate with a narrowing of the teat end. The result is a decreased thickness of this anatomical protective barrier. Concurrent to the thinning of the streak canal is an increased milk flow and the loss of keratin. The combined effects are an increased risk of early lactation clinical mastitis.

Dingwell and co-workers (2003) more recently summarized the direct impact of negative energy balance on immune function of dairy cows during early lactation. Negative energy balance is associated with a decrease in cytokine production which reduces the recruitment of immune cells to the site of infection. Chemotaxis is also reduced when leukocytes are exposed *in vitro* to ketone-enriched media. Furthermore, phagocytosis and bactericidal activity of PMN are decreased in media containing elevated concentrations of ketone bodies. Therefore, severe decreases in energy balance must be avoided during transition from pregnant, non-lactating to early lactation. Improved energy balance will enhance the benefits of antioxidants fed to enhance immune function.

Significant efforts in laboratories around the world have led to work focused on the feeding of the antioxidant micronutrients Cu, Se, Zn, and vitamins A,E, and beta-carotene on immune function of the dairy cow and udder health. Most recently, Scaletti *et al.* (2003) reported that cows fed diets containing 20 ppm copper had improved immune function compared with cows fed a copper-deficient diet. Following an intramammary *E. coli* challenge, cows in good copper status had fewer cfu in the milk by 12 and 18 hours post challenge. The copper-supplemented cows also had lower SCC, and the clinical score was also reduced. Cows fed copper-deficient diets had a peak body temperature of 40.8°C at 18 hours post-challenge in contrast to 40.0°C for cows fed the copper-adequate diet. These results illustrate the importance of copper in the immune response to an intramammary infection.

Malbe and co-workers (2003) recently reported the benefits of selenium on immune function of Estonian dairy cows. Cows were fed a selenium enriched yeast at 0.2 ppm. The supplemental selenium increased blood glutathione peroxidase with a concurrent increase in the number of pathogen free quarters. Numerous studies agree with the benefits of supplemental selenium on immune function and mammary gland health.

Summary and conclusion

Mammary gland health and milk quality management programs are multifactorial. Proper mammary gland conformation affects the risk of mastitis. The environment in which the udder is managed is also a significant variable, as are cleanliness and dryness. Proper function and operation of milking procedure and system can contribute to the success of the udder health program. Nutritional balance or status also impacts immunocompetence or immune function of the dairy cow. Macronutrients should be a priority with micronutrients supplemented in the diet to aid energy and protein metabolism and immune function. Strategies to prevent severe and prolonged periods of negative energy and protein balance should be in place for the periparturient cow. Sufficient micronutrients should also be provided in the diet throughout the transition phase in amounts to assure peak immunocompetence. Improving mammary gland health benefits not only the farm business, improved management associated with such a program also enhances the quality of the product available to dairy processors and consumers.

References

Bitman, J., Wood, D.L., Miller, R.H., and Botman, J. (1992) Increased susceptibility to intramammary infection following removal of teat canal keratin. *Journal of Dairy Science* **74:** 414.

Capuco, A.V., Bright, S.A., Pankey, J.W., Wood, D.L., Miller, R.H., and Bitman, J. (1992) Increased susceptibility to intramammary infection following removal of teat canal keratin. *Journal of Dairy Science* **75:** 2126.

Chandra, R.K. (1992) Protein-Energy malnutrition and immunological responses. *Journal of Nutrition* **122:** 597-600.

Chassagne, M., Barowin, J., and Chacornac, J.P. (1998) Biological predictors for early clinical mastitis occurrence in Holstein cows under field conditions in France. *Preventative Veterinary Medicine* **35:** 29-38.

Craven, S. and Williams, M.P. (1985) Defenses of the bovine mammary gland against infection and prospects for their enhancement. *Veterinary Immunology and Immunopathology* **10:** 71-127.

Cross, R.F. and Parker, C.F. (1981) Oral administration of zinc sulfate for control of ovine foot rot. *Journal of American Veterinary Medical Association* **178**(7): 704.

Detilleux, J.C., Kehrli, M.E., Freeman, A.E., Fox, L.K. and Kelley, D.H. (1995) Mastitis of periparturient Holstein cattle: a phenotypic and genetic study. *Journal of Dairy Science* **78:** 2285-2293.

Dingwell, R.T., Kelton, D.F. and Leslie, K.E. (2003) Management of the dry cow in control of peripartum disease and mastitis. *Vet Clinic – Food Animal.* **19:** 235-265.

Harmon, R.J. and Crist, W.L. (1994) Environmental mastitis in lactating and dry cows and prepartun heifers. In: Dairy Systems for the 21ˢᵗ century. *Proceedings of the Third International*

Dairy Housing Conference. American Society of Agricultural Engineering, St. Joseph, MI

Herlin, A.H. (1998) Production of Quality Milk: Housing and management factors. In: *Proceedings of the Fourth International Dairy Housing Conference.* pp 239-244.

Kehrli, M.E. and Harp, J.A. (2001) Immunity in the mammary gland. *Immunology* **17**(3): 495-516.

Kellogg, D.W. (1990) Zinc Methionine affects performance of lactating cows. *FeedStuffs.* **62**(35).

Lehenbauer, T., Jones, T. and Collar, L. (1994) The impact of free-stall housing on somatic cell counts. In: Dairy Systems for the 21st century. *Proceedings of the Third International Dairy housing Conference.* American Society of Agricultural Engineering, St. Joseph, MI.

Malbe, M., Klaassen, E., Kaartinen, L., Altila, M. and Atroshi, F. (2003) Effects of oral selenium supplementation on mastitis markers and pathogens in Estonian cows. *Veterinary Therapeutics* **4**(2): 145-154.

Moynahan, E.J. (1981) Acrodermatitis enteropathica and the immunological role of zinc in Immunodermatology. Ed. B. Safai and R.A. Good. Plenum Medical Book Co., N.Y., N.Y.

Nickerson, S.C. (1994) Bovine mammary gland: structure and function; relationship to milk production and immunity to mastitis. *Agri-Practice* **15**(6):8-18.

Oltenacu, P.A. and Ekesbo, I. (1994) Epidemiological study of clinical mastitis in dairy catle. *Veterinary Research* **25:** 208-212.

Pankey, J.W. (1990) Mastitis- Two different diseases: contagious and environmental. In: *Proceedings of the national mastitis council.* pp 167-173.

Pyorala, S. (2002) New strategies to prevent mastitis. *Reproduction in Domestic Animals* **37:** 211-216.

Scaletti, R.W., D.S. Trammell, B.A. Smith, and R.J. Harmon. 2003. Role if dietary copper in enhancing resistance to Escherichia coli mastitis. J. Dairy Sci. 26:1240 – 1249.

Schukken, Y.H., Grommer, F.J., VonDeGees, D., Erb, H.N., and Brond, A. (1991) Risk factors for clinical mastitis with a low bulk somatic cell count. 2. Risk factors for *E.coli* and *S. aureus*. *Journal of Dairy Science* **74:** 826.

Slettbakk, T., Jorstad, A., Farner, T.B., and Homes, J.C. (1995) Impact of milking characteristics on morphology of udder and teats on clinical mastitis in first and second lactation Norwegian cattle. *Preventative Veterinary Medicine* **24:** 235-244.

Sordillo, L.M., Shafer-Weaver, K. and DeRosa, D. (1997) Immunobiology of the mammary gland. *Journal of Dairy Science* **80:** 1851-1865.

Sordillo, Lorraine M. and Katie L. Streicher. 2002. Mammary gland immunity and mastitis susceptibility. J. o Mammary Gland Biology and Neoplasia l7(2):135-146.

Spain, J.N. (1993) Tissue Integrity: A Key defense against mastitis infection and the role of zinc proteinates and a theory for the mode of action. In: *Biotechnology in the Feed Industry.* Proceedings of Alltech's 9th Annual Symposium, Alltech Technical Publications, Nicholasville, KY. Page 53.

Wells, S.J. and Orr, S.L. (1995) Individual and bulk tank milk somatic cell count results: What's the quality of the U.S. milk supply? In National Mastitis Council Annual Meeting proceedings pp 11-22.

Zecconi, A., Hamann, J., Bronzo, V., Moroni, P., Giovannini, G. and Piccinini, R. (2000) Relationship between teat tissue immune defenses and intramammary infections. *Advances in Experimental Med. and Biology.* **480:** 287-293.

Organic selenium for supplementation of farm animal diets: it's influence on the selenium status of the animals and on the dietary selenium intake of man

B. Pehrson
Department of Animal Environment and Health, Swedish University of Agricultural Sciences, S-53223 Skara, Sweden

Introduction

Until 1957 selenium (Se) was simply considered to be a toxic element without any biological function in mammals. But that year Schwarz and Foltz discovered that Se could prevent hepatic necrosis in rats. Fifteen years later, Rotruck *et al.* (1973) and Flohe *et al.* (1973) identified a Se-containing enzyme, glutathione peroxidase (GSH-Px), as being responsible for this effect. For a few years, GSH-Px was then considered to be the only Se-substance with biological activity, but the epochal findings of the American researchers initiated a huge amount of research, which has made it increasingly obvious that Se is an essential nutrient of fundamental importance to all mammals. Today, more than 25 selenoproteins have been partially or fully characterised in mammalian tissues, and 14 of them have been found to have biological functions (5 types of GSH-Px, 3 deiodinases, 3 thioredoxin reductases, selenophosphate synthetase, selenoprotein P, and selenoprotein W).

Selenium is widely distributed in the crust of the earth (Oldfield, 1995). A few regions (*i.e.* South and North Dakota in USA, Venezuela and Colombia) have extremely high Se levels in soil and herbs. In such regions, the Se-status of animals and man might even be too high. In other regions, the Se-content in feeds and foods are adequate, *i.e.* in the central parts of North America, and no signs of Se-deficiency can be expected.

Of more importance in this context is, however, the fact that vast Se-deficient areas are spread all over the world, and in severely-deficient regions, health problems are, or have been, fairly common both in farm animals and humans. The Scandinavian countries have long since been found to be extremely Se-deficient (refer to Lindberg and Bingefors, 1970; Carlström *et al.*, 1979). During the last decade, many other countries in Europe have been found to be equally or almost equally deficient (Rayman, 2000), as has northwestern and

253

eastern parts of North America (Oldfield, 1995). Regions of China and New Zealand are well known for being even more deficient than Scandinavia.

Farm animals

Selenium-deficiency diseases

Nutritional muscular degeneration (NMD), sudden deaths, reduced weight gain, and impaired fertility have been related to Se-deficiencies in most farm animals (Radostits *et al.*, 1999). Increased incidence of retained placenta (Julien *et al.*, 1976), mastitis (Erskine *et al.*, 1989; Hogan *et al.*, 1990) and significant reductions in weight gain ("ill-thrift"; Andrews *et al.*, 1968), have been found in Se-deficient cattle. Hepatosis dietetica and mulberry heart disease are considered to be typical so-called "Se- and vitamin E deficient diseases" in swine (Radostits *et al.*, 1999), as is exudative diathesis, nutritional encephalomalacia and nutritional pancreatic atrophy in poultry (Surai, 2000).

The clinically manifest symptoms of these diseases appear most often due to severe Se-deficiencies. However, although no clear correlation has been proven between the Se-status of domestic animals and their ability to resist disease, there are many reports indicating that less pronounced Se-deficiencies might reduce the animals' resistance against infections and other challenges. It seems reasonable to suspect that this may be due to background effects on antibody responses, or neutrophil and / or lymphocyte functions that has been reported in 15 out of 21 studies in ruminants (Weiss, 2003), and in 13 out of 19 studies in other kinds of farm animals (Finch and Turner, 1996). As noted by Arthur *et al.* (2003), Se influences both the innate and acquired immune systems. It must, however, be emphasised that most of the evidence is based on *in vitro* studies: it should be questioned whether they can be fully applied to *in vivo* situations.

Sources of selenium for dietary supplementation

It is logical to assume that if farm animals from extremely Se-deficient regions are fed solely on home-produced feedstuffs, they will be highly Se-deficient. For example, in a Swedish study with heifers, 116 out of 122 grass-fed herds were found to be severely Se-deficient (Carlström *et al.*, 1979). As a consequence, today, most rations for farm animals are supplemented with Se, mainly through the mineral premix. Until now, inorganic Se as sodium selenite has routinely been used for the supplementation. However, recent research has demonstrated the benefits of using organic instead of inorganic Se-compounds since selenite has several disadvantages:

- it has prooxidative effects (Yan and Spallholz, 1993; Spallholz, 1997), and can then - at least theoretically - counteract itself as an antioxidant, and reduce the activity of other antioxidants during storing of feeds and foods, and also in the digestive system;

- it is not a naturally-occurring ingredient in any feedstuff or food; almost all natural Se is organic, predominantly as the amino acids selenomethionine and selenocysteine (Levander and Burk, 1990; Whanger, 2002);

- it has a low degree of retention in tissues (*i.e.* Whanger and Butler, 1998).

On the contrary, organic Se has several advantages:

- it is the natural form of Se found in feeds and foods (Levander and Burke, 1990);

- it is easily retained non-specifically into tissue proteins, from which it can be easily mobilised when required (Levander and Burke, 1990; Gerloff, 1992);

- it has a higher capacity than inorganic Se to increase the Se-concentration in foods of animal origin, as will be discussed later in this chapter.

It has been postulated that the high retention rate of Se from organic Se-compounds might imply the risk of gradual accumulation of Se to toxic levels. However, two recent trials indicate that such a risk is negligible (Ortman and Pehrson, 1997; Knowles *et al.*, 1999). After four to nine months of daily dietary supplementation of dairy cow rations with higher doses of Se than would be realistic in normal commercial practice (3 and 4 mg Se as selenium yeast), the Se-contents in the liver were 263 and 310 μg/kg wet weight, respectively. These levels are at the lower level of what is considered optimal, and far from the lowest toxic level of 4000 μg/kg (Rosenberger, 1978). In reality, inorganic Se should be more toxic than organic Se, because a surplus cannot be stored as tissue protein, but will be transferred to potentially toxic metabolites (mainly methylselenol; Figure 1).

Pure selenoamino acids (selenomethionine, selenocysteine) are far too expensive to be used for supplementation of farm animal diets. However, some selenium-yeasts have been found to be equally effective, but it must be emphasised that the following criteria must be fulfilled if a selenium-yeast is to be acceptable:

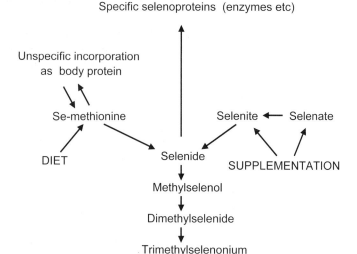

Specific selenoproteins (enzymes etc)

Unspecific incorporation
as body protein

Se-methionine   Selenite ← Selenate

DIET   Selenide   SUPPLEMENTATION

Methylselenol

Dimethylselenide

Trimethylselenonium

Figure 1.
Metabolic pathways
of organic and
inorganic Se sources
(adapted from
Whanger, 2003)

- it must have been produced by adding selenite (or selenate) to a living yeast cell culture. Only in this manner are the yeast cells able to transform the inorganic Se to selenoamino acids;

- it must have been documented to contain at least 95% organic Se - of which the majority should be selenomethionine - and must have been scientifically proven to have significant bioavailability and biopotency.

According to the author´s knowledge, there are today just two commercial products that fulfil both these criteria; one of which has been used in more than 90% of the published trials (Sel-Plex® Alltech Inc., Nicholasville), and is now approved by the FDA for use in North America. Other Se-yeast products that do not fulfil the aforementioned criteria have been found to contain levels of organic Se that are too low (Whanger, 2002).

Many different so-called "organic Se products" have also been commercially introduced. However, it is important to highlight the following facts:

- to simply mix dry yeast and selenite, and market it as "Se-yeast" is unacceptable;

- complexes between Se and amino acids do not contain selenoamino acids, and recent research (see Givens *et al.*, 2004) has revealed that they – as can be expected – are not more potent than selenite;

- Se-chelates are chimeras: Selenium cannot be chelated.

Dietary requirement and evaluation of selenium status

For many years, 0.10 mg of Se /kg DM diet (ppm) was considered to be adequate for all farm animals. However, this figure has recently been adjusted. The official requirement for all dairy cattle is now 0.3 ppm (NRC, 2001), while the requirement for beef cattle is still considered to be met by 0.1 ppm (NRC, 2000). According to NRC recommendations, for growing swine and sows, a dietary level of 0.15 ppm is recommended, and for weanling pigs 0.30 ppm (NRC, 1999). Food and Drug Administration (FDA) permits 0.3 ppm for poultry feed (Surai, 2002).

Quite often these levels cannot be reached in practice without dietary supplementation of Se. Therefore, FDA approved the incorporation of up to 0.3 ppm of Se to all livestock diets, originally just in the form of sodium selenite or sodium selenate (Mahan and Parrett, 1996), but recently also as certain Se-yeast products. No consideration has hitherto been taken into whether the source of the supplemented Se is inorganic or organic. This is unfortunate since there is a significant difference in the bioavailibility and biopotency between the sources, which has been revealed during the last decade. However, the recent BSAS publication does state; *"Account should be taken of any well-evidenced differences in availability in diet formulation"* (BSAS, 2003). Surai (2002) notes that most Se-related research in food animals has until recently been conducted using inorganic Se, and that more research conducted with organic Se sources is crucial.

The borderlines between sub-optimal and optimal Se-status based on blood measurements varies between animal categories, and data are often conflicting. For cattle, Ortman (1999), after having reviewed the literature, proposed that less than 50 μg/L whole blood should be considered to carry a risk that clinical signs of Se-deficiency diseases might develop, that concentrations between 50 and 100 μg/L might indicate a sub-optimal immune capacity, and that concentrations exceeding 100 μg/L should be considered as adequate, although several authors (for example, Smith *et al.*, 1988; Hogan *et al.*, 1993; Jukola, 1994; Olson, 1994), recommend at least 200 μg/L to obtain optimal preventative protection against mastitis and reproductive problems. For swine, the corresponding requirement figures are considered to be less than 60, 60-120 and more than 120 μg/L, respectively (Radostits *et al.*, 1999).

Inorganic vs. organic selenium: influence on selenium status

Although the dietary supplementation with selenite, that was introduced in many Se-deficient countries about 20 years ago, has improved the Se-status of animals, practising veterinarians report that typical Se-deficient diseases still exist. A more pronounced preventative effect on these diseases should be possible if organic Se in the form of Se-yeast is used instead of selenite. As an example, Pehrson *et al.* (1999) and Gunter *et al.* (2003), reported that suckling calves had insufficient blood-Se values when their mothers´ diet was supplemented with selenite, but adequate values when they were supplemented with Se-yeast at an equal dosage level. From these results it been postulated that NMD, which still is a fairly common disease amongst fast-growing calves, could be abolished if Se-yeast is routinely used for dietary supplementation of suckler cows.

There are reasons to believe that the supplementation with selenite has removed the most extreme Se-deficiencies. However, it can be suggested that a further improved Se-status will positively influence the resistance against those infectious diseases and other environmental challenges that are today common within intensive animal production systems. With reference to the data presented later in this chapter, such an improved Se-status can easily be achieved, and quantitatively controlled by a dietary supplementation with organic Se, but will be difficult, or even impossible through supplementation with inorganic Se.

Man

Selenium-deficiency diseases

In an excellent review article, Rayman (2000) presented different aspects of the importance of selenium to human health. Sudden deaths through cardiomyopathy in Chinese nursing babies ("Keshan disease"), a specific type of deforming arthritis ("Kachin-Beck disease"), mutation of viruses, reduced immune function, certain types of cancer, cardiovascular diseases and reduced fertility have been related to Se-deficiency. Although extremely low Se-intakes seem to be necessary for typical clinical signs to appear in several of the aforementioned problems, there is an increasing knowledge that less-overt Se-deficiencies may have adverse consequences for disease susceptibility, and for maintenance of optimal health (Rayman, 2000). For example, a reduced immunocompetence may contribute to health problems caused by physiological and environmental stressors and infections (Combs, 2001).

Selenium status in different countries

The official recommended daily intake of Se varies from 44 to 75 µg between countries. Irrespective of which level is most accurate, it is evident that the Se-intake is lower than required in many parts of Europe (Table 1), while it is most often adequate in USA. The intake in the UK has declined over the past 25 years, and is now just half of that recommended (Rayman, 2000; Jackson et al., 2003).

Table 1.
Recommended and real average daily selenium intake in different countries, μg. (From Rayman (2000) except [a] and [b]) [a] NNR, 1996 [b] Larsson and Johansson, 2002)

	Recommended intake		Real intake	
	Male	Female	Male	Female
Sweden	50[a]	40[a]	40[b]	27[b]
United kingdom	75	60	39	29
Europe	45-75		17-67	
USA	55	55	60-220	

The average Se-intake of Swedish omnivores has been reported to be 27 μg for females, and 40 μg for males (Larsson and Johansson, 2002), implying that the Swedish population is equally deficient as the British, although the official requirement figures are lower in Sweden.

Combs (2001) reviewed the literature concerning the estimated daily dietary Se-intake in 26 different countries, and also the Se-status - based on serum/plasma values - from 63 countries. On the assumption that a daily intake of less than 40 μg, and a serum concentration of less than 70 μg/L certainly indicates Se-deficiency[*], he estimated that the total number of Se-deficient individuals around the world is likely to be in the range of 500-1000 million. If that is correct, up to 15% of the people living on earth should have insufficient Se-status!

[*] Rayman (2000) has suggested the value of 100 μg/L serum as a criterion of nutritional adequacy)

Selenite vs. selenium yeast: research trials

The lowered Se-status among British people is considered to give cause for concern (Rayman, 2000). Therefore, the British Ministry of Agriculture, Fisheries and Food (MAFF) commissioned a research group to investigate different Se sources in dairy rations with a view to improving milk quality. The conclusion from a trial conducted by the group was that supplementation with Se-yeast, at doses that were safely within the maximum level permitted under EU regulations, significantly increased the Se-content in the milk (Givens et al., 2004). In contrast, the increase in milk-Se was just marginal after supplementation with selenite or a complex-bound Se-product, even at dosage levels that were considerably higher than permitted by the EU, thus confirming results earlier presented by Fisher et al. (1980).

The sulphur-containing amino acid methionine is of crucial importance to attain high productivity in all farm animals. Since animals are unable to distinguish between methionine and selenomethionine (Burk and Hill, 1993), a low supply of methionine can be compensated by selenomethionine. This is probably the principal reason for the convincing results of several other trials from the last decade other than that of Givens *et al.* (2004). The superiority of Se-yeast for increasing the Se-content in foods of animal origin has thus been documented for meat of cattle (Ortman and Pehrson, 1997; 1999, swine (Mahan and Kim, 1996; Mahan and Parret, 1996; Mahan *et al.*, 1999) and poultry (Downs *et al.*, 2000; Leng *et al.*, 2003), for liver of swine (Mahan and Parett, 1996; Mahan *et al.*, 1999) and cattle (Ortman and Pehrson, 1997), for egg (Surai, 2002), and for colostrum and milk of swine (Mahan, 2000), for cheese (Pehrson, 2004 unpublished) and for milk of dairy cows (Ortman and Pehrson, 1997; 1999; Knowles *et al.*, 1999; Pehrson and Arnesson, 2003; Givens *et al.*, 2004).

The difference in capability to influence milk-Se between Se from yeast and from selenite or selenate has been found to be particularly pronounced for milk of cows, as illustrated in Figures 2-6. It can thus be said to be well documented that:

- Se-yeast is much more potent than selenite (Figures 2-6);

- the capacity of selenite to increase the Se-level in milk is highly restricted at conventional dosages (Figures 2-6);

- even at very high dosage levels of selenite-Se, it is incapable to further increase the Se-content in milk, while the content can be increased in relation to the dosage level if Se-yeast is used (Figure 6);

- there is no difference between selenite and selenate (Figure 3), and between selenite and complexed-bound Se (Figure 6).

The results presented in Figures 4 and 6 warrant further comments. The unsteady levels of milk-Se in Figure 4 were probably caused by the fact that the cows were on grass, implying differences in feed intake and nutritional quality during the experimental period. The extremely high Se-content of approx. 100 μg/L in one of the groups supplemented with Se-yeast (Figure 6), can be considered higher than desirable. However, it must be emphasised that the Se in that group – and also in the group that received a diet with 0.76 mg Se - was supplemented at levels that significantly exceed the highest level of 0.55ppm Se in the total ration approved by the EU.

Figure 2.
Mean Se-
concentration in
milk from cows
supplemented with
3 mg Se as sodium
selenite, 3 mg as Se
yeast or 0.75 mg as
Se yeast daily (from
Ortman and
Pehrson 1997)

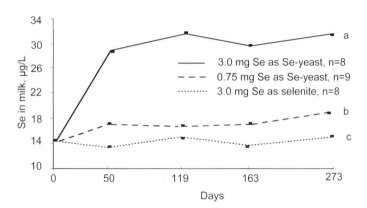

Figure 3.
Mean Se-
concentration in
milk from cows
supplemented with
3 mg Se as sodium
selenite, 3 mg as
sodium selenate, 3
mg as Se yeast or
unsupplemented
(from Ortman and
Pehrson, 1999)

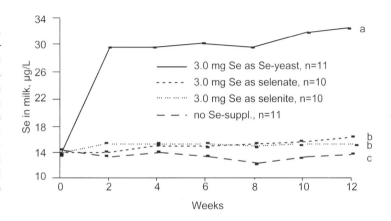

Figure 4.
Effects of dietary
supplementation
with 0.13 and 0.26
ppm of Se as
sodium selenate or
0.13 and 0.26 ppm
as Se yeast on milk
Se-concentration.
Each point
represents the mean
of 7 cows (adapted
from Knowles et
al., 1999)

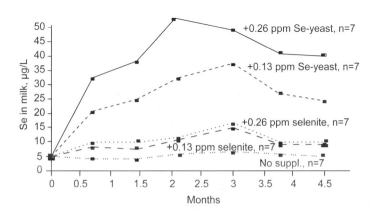

Figure 5.
Mean Se-
concentration in
bulk milk from 22
organic herds
supplemented
through the mineral
feed at two dosage
levels of Se yeast or
at dosage levels of
sodium selenite used
in commercial
mineral feeds (from
Pehrson and
Arnesson, 2003)

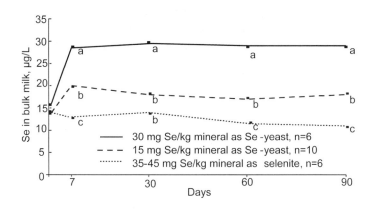

Figure 6.
Mean Se-
concentration in
milk after 8
weeks´supplementation
with Se yeast,
complex-bound Se
or sodium selenite at
three dosage levels.
Ten cows at each
compound and
dosage level
(adapted from
Givens *et al.*, 2004)

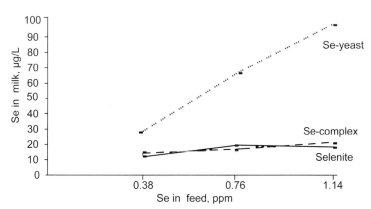

Figures 2, 3 and 5: [a,b,c] Means within day differ (p <0.05)

Consequently, these levels of supplementation are unrealistic for use in practice, not at least for economical reasons. According to Aspila (1991) a milk-Se concentration of at least 20 μg/L is desirable.

Influence of dietary selenium supplementation of farm animals on foods

Based on the results of the scientific reports referred to above (page 8 of this chapter, first paragraph), the author has calculated that a change from inorganic to organic Se for supplementation of farm animal diets, at a dosage level of 0.3 ppm in the dry matter diet, can be expected to result in an increased Se-content in milk of at least 100%, in cheese at least 150% in beef and pork meat about 75%, in chicken meat about 100%, in eggs at least 100%, and in liver about 25%.

Of the total dietary intake of Se for an average Swede, about 20% comes from milk and milk products, about 25% from meat, 10-15% from eggs, 20-25% from marine products, about 15% from grain products, about 4% from vegetables, and about 4 % from drinks, potatoes and fruits (calculated from Becker, 2000). Considering the eating habits in Sweden, the total daily Se-intake would increase by at least 50% after a change to organic Se in farm animal diets, implying that the Se-supply for an average Swede will change from being deficient or marginal to optimal. Givens *et al.* (2004) concluded that a similar change of the Se-source in dairy cow rations would increase the daily Se-intake of an average Briton by approx. 15% (excluding the effect on the Se-content in cheese and meat). In countries with different eating habits, the magnitude of the influence on the total daily Se-intake might be different from that in Sweden and the UK, but will certainly always be significant.

Conclusions

The positive influence of organic Se-compounds on the total Se-intake in man will depend on the eating habits in each individual country. In many parts of the world, the dominant food sources of Se are cereals, meats and fish, while dairy products and eggs only comprise a small proportion (Combs, 2001). However, it is clear that a switch from supplementation of farm animal diets with inorganic Se to organic Se as Se-yeast will give rise to a significant increase in the Se-intake in human beings. Such a change can be recommended in all Se-deficient countries, and can be expected to have positive health benefits.

A positive effect can also be expected on the health and productivity of farm animals. It seems reasonable that the dosage level of Se used today for dietary supplementation of farm animals can be reduced considerably, if organic Se in the form of an adequately produced Se-yeast is used instead of selenite. In this way, the risk of exceeding the maximal permitted Se-concentration of 0.55ppm in the total DM diet will be minimised.

References

Andrews, E.D., Hartley, W.J., and Grant, A.B. (1968). Selenium-responsive diseases of animals in New Zealand. *New Zealand Veterinary Journal* **16:** 3-17.

Arthur, J.R., McKenzie, R.C., and Beckett, G.J. (2003). Selenium and the immune system. *Journal of Nutrition* **133:** 1457s-1459s.

Aspila, P. (1991). Metabolism of selenite, selenomethionine and feed-incorporated selenium in lactating goats and dairy cows. *Journal of Agricultural Science in Finland* **63:** 1-74.

Becker, W. (2000). Vilka är källorna till våra näringsämnen? (The sources of our food substances). In Swedish. *Vår Föda* **51:** 16-20.

British Society of Animal Science (2003). Nutrient Requirement Standards for Pigs.

Burk, R.F. and Hill, K.E. (1993). Regulations of selenoproteins. *Annual Review of Nutrition* **13:** 65-81.

Carlström, G., Jönsson, G., and Pehrson, B. (1979). An evaluation of selenium status of cattle in Sweden by means of glutathione peroxidase. *Swedish Journal of Agricultural Science* **9:** 43-46.

Combs, G.F. Jr. (2001). Selenium in the global system. *British Journal of Nutrition* **85:** 517-547.

Downs, K.M., Hess, J.B., and Bilgili, S.F. (2000). Selenium source effect on broiler carcass characteristics, meat quality and drip loss. *Journal of Applied Animal Research* **18:** 61-72.

Erskine, R.J., Eberhart, R., Grasso, P. J., and Scholz, R. W. (1989). Induction of *Escherichia coli* mastitis in cows fed selenium-deficient or selenium-supplemented diets. *American Journal of Veterinary Research* **50:** 2093-2100.

Finch, J.M., and Turner, R.J. (1996). Effects of selenium and vitamin E on the immune responses of domestic animals. *Research in Veterinary Science* **60:** 97-106.

Fisher, L. J., Hoogendorn, C., and Montemurro, J. (1980). The effect of added dietary selenium on the selenium content in milk, urine and faeces. *Canadian Journal of Animal Science* **60:** 79-86.

Flohé, L., Güntzler, W.A., and Schock, H.H. (1973). Glutathione peroxidase: a selenoenzyme. *Federation of European Biochemical Society: Letters* **32:** 132-134.

Gerloff, B. (1992). Effect of selenium supplementation on dairy cattle. *Journal of Dairy Science* **70:** 3934-3940.

Givens, D.I., Allison, R., Cottrill, B., and Blake, J.S. (2004). Enhancing the selenium content of bovine milk through alteration of the form and concentration of selenium in the diet of the dairy cow. *Journal of the Science of Food and Agriculture* **84:** 811-817.

Gunter, S.A., Beck, P.A., and Phillips, J.M. (2003). Effects of supplementary selenium source on the performance and blood measurements in beef cows and calves. *Journal of Animal Science* **81:** 856-864.

Hogan, J. S., Weiss, W. P., and Smith, K.L. (1993). Role of vitamin E and selenium in host defence against mastitis. *Journal of Dairy Science* **76:** 2795-2803.

Jackson, M.J., Broome, C.S., and McArdle, F. 2003. Marginal dietary selenium intakes in the UK: are there functional consequences?

Journal of Nutrition **133:** 1557s-1559s.

Jukola, E. (1994). Selenium, vitamin E and beta-carotene status of cattle in Finland, with special reference to epidemiological udder health and reproduction data. *Thesis.* College of Veterinary Medicine, Helsinki.

Julien, W.E., Conrad, H. R., Jones, J.E., and Moxon, A.L. (1976). Selenium and vitamin E and incidence of retained placenta in parturient dairy cows. *Journal of Dairy Science* **59:** 1954-1959.

Knowles, S., Grace, N.D., Wurms, K., and Lee, J. (1999). Significance of amounts and form of dietary selenium on blood, milk, and casein selenium concentrations in grazing cows. *Journal of Dairy Science* **82:** 429-437.

Larsson, C.L., and Johansson, G.K. (2002). Dietary intake and nutritional status of young vegans and omnivores in Sweden. *American Journal of Clinical Nutrition* **76:** 100-106.

Leng, L., Bobzek, R., Kuriková, S., Boldizárová, K., Gresáková, L., Sevcíková, Z., Révajová, V., Levkutová, M., and Levkut, M. (2003). Comparative metabolic and immune response of chickens fed diets containing inorganic selenium and Sel-Plex ™ organic selenium. In: *Nutritional Biotechnology in the Feed and Food Industries.* Edited by T.P. Lyons and K.A. Jacques. Nottingham University Press, Nottingham UK, pp. 131-145.

Levander, O.A., and Burk, R.F. (1990). In: *Selenium: Present Knowledge in Nutrition.* Edited by M.L. Brown, International Life Sciences Institute, Washington DC, pp. 268-273.

Lindberg, P., and Bingefors, S. (1970). Selenium levels of forages and soils in different regions of Sweden. *Acta Agricriculturae Scandinavica* **20:** 133-136.

Mahan, D.C. (2000). Effect of organic and inorganic selenium sources and levels on sow colostrum and milk selenium. *Journal of Animal Science* **78:**100-105.

Mahan, D.C., Cline, T.R., and Richert, B. (1999). Effects of dietary levels of selenium-enriched yeast and sodium selenite as selenium sources fed to growing-finishing pigs on performance, tissue selenium, glutathione peroxidase activity, carcass characteristics, and loin quality. *Journal of Animal Science* **77:** 2172-2179.

Mahan D.C., and Kim, Y.Y. (1996). Effect of inorganic and organic selenium at two dietary levels on productive performance and tissue selenium concentrations in first-parity gilts and their progeny. *Journal of Animal Science* **74:** 2711-2718.

Mahan, D.C., and Parett, N.A. (1996). Evaluating the efficacy of selenium-enriched yeast and sodium selenite on tissue selenium retention and serum glutathione peroxidase activity in grower and finisher swine. *Journal of Animal Science* **74:** 2967-2974.

NNR (Nordic Nutrition Recommendations). (1996). *Scandinavian*

Journal of Nutrition **40:** 161-165.

NRC. (2001). *Nutrient Requirements of Dairy Cattle.* National Research Council, National Academy Press, Washington DC.

NRC. (2000). *Nutrient Requirements of Beef Cattle.* National Research Council, National Academy Press, Washington DC.

NRC. (1999). *Nutrient Requirements of Swine.* National Research Council, National Academy Press, Washington DC.

Oldfield, J.E. (1995). Selenium in maps. *The Bulletin of Selenium-Tellurium Development Association.* April, 7 pages.

Olson, J.D. (1994). The role of selenium and vitamin E in mastitis and reproduction of dairy cattle. *The Bovine Practitioner* **28:** 446-452.

Ortman, K. (1999). Organic vs. inorganic selenium in farm animal nutrition with special reference to supplementation of cattle. *Thesis.* Swedish University of Agricultural Sciences, Uppsala.

Ortman, K., and Pehrson, B. (1999). Effects of selenite as feed supplement to dairy cows in comparison to selenite and Se yeast. *Journal of Animal Science 77*: 3365-3370.

Ortman, K., and Pehrson, B. (1997). Selenite and selenium yeast as feed supplements for dairy cows. *Journal of Veterinary Medicine A* **44:** 373-380.

Pehrson, B., and Arnesson, A. (2003). Tillförsel av oorganiskt och organiskt selen till mjölkkor. (Supplementation with inorganic and organic selenium to dairy cows). In Swedish with an English summary. *Svensk Veterinär Tidning (Swedish Veterinary Journal)* **55:**17-23.

Pehrson, B., Ortman, K., Madjid, N., and Trafikowska, U. (1999). The influence of dietary selenium as selenium yeast or sodium selenite on the concentration of selenium in the milk of suckler cows and on the selenium status of their calves. *Journal of Animal Science* **77**: 3371-3376.

Radostits, O.M., Blood, D.C., Gay, C.C., and Hinchcliff, K.W. (1999). Selenium and/or vitamin E deficiences. In: *Veterinary Medicine.* WB Saunders Company Ltd, London, New York, Philadelphia, Sydney.

Rayman, M.P. (2000). The importance of selenium to human health. *The Lancet* **356:** 233-241.

Rosenberger G. (1978). In: *Krankheiten des Rindes.* Verlag Paul Parey, Berlin, Hamburg.

Rotruck, J.T, Pope, A.L., Ganther, H.E., Swanson, A.B., Hafeman, D.G. and Hoekstra, W.G. (1973). Selenium: Biochemical role as a component of glutathione peroxidase. *Science* **179:** 588-590.

Schwarz, K., and Foltz, C.M. (1957). Selenium as an integral part of Factor 3 against dietary necrotic liver degeneration. *Journal of the American Chemical Society* **79:** 3292-3293.

Smith, L.R., Hogan, J.S., and Conrad, H.R. (1988). Selenium in dairy cattle: its role in disease resistance. *Veterinary Medicine* **83:** 72-78.

Spallholz, J.E. (1997). Free radical generation by selenium compounds and their prooxidant toxicity. *Biomedical and Environmental Science* **10:** 260-270.

Surai, P. (2002). In: *Natural Antioxidants in Avian Nutrition and Reproduction.* Nottingham University Press, Nottingham UK.

Surai, P. (2000). Organic selenium: benefits to animals and humans, a biochemist´s view. *Biotechnology in the Feed Industry.* Edited by T.P. Lyons and K.A. Jacques. Nottingham University Press, Nottingham UK, pp. 205-260.

Weiss, W.P. (2003). Selenium nutrition of dairy cows: comparing responses to organic and inorganic selenium forms. In: *Nutritional Biotechnology in the Feed and Food Industries.* Edited by T.P. Lyons and K.A. Jacques. Nottingham University Press, Nottingham UK, pp. 333-343.

Whanger, P.D. (2003). Metabolic pathways of selenium in plants and animals and their nutritional significance. In: *Nutritional Biotechnology in the Feed and Food Industries.* Edited by T.P. Lyons and K.A. Jacques. Nottingham University Press, Nottingham UK, pp. 51-58.

Whanger, P.D. (2002). Selenocompounds in plants and animals and their biological significance. *Journal of the American College of Nutrition* **21:** 223-232.

Whanger, P.D., and Butler, J.A. (1998). Effects of various dietary levels of selenium as selenite or selenomethionine on tissue selenium levels and glutathione peroxidase activity in rats. *Journal of Nutrition* **118:** 846-852.

Yan, L., and Spallholz, J.E. (1993). Generation of reactive oxygen species from the reaction of selenium compounds with thiols and mammary tumor cells. *Biochemical Pharmacology* **45:** 429-427.

Dairy farming in the EU: is there a future?

David E Beever
Ruminations Ltd., Marlow, Bucks.

Introduction

The unequivocal answer to the title of this paper is 'Yes'. Despite continuing low milk prices, uncertainties over the Mid Term Review and an increasing number of dairy farmers seeing little future opportunity of their businesses providing acceptable returns on invested labour and capital, dairy farming in the EU will continue. However the type of industry that exists in 10 years time is likely to be quite different from that of today. Many factors can be identified that may affect the future shape of the EU dairy industry, but it is how these will interact that will have the greatest bearing on the eventual outcome.

The dairy farmer

It has been estimated that in 2002, over 60% of all milk produced on UK dairy farms was sold at a loss (Colman *et al.*, 2004). Recurring losses lead to a lack of suitable investment capital, and failure to improve this situation has led to an increasing number of herds, both large and small, being disposed of. It can be concluded that a similar situation with respect to lack of acceptable returns exists in many pre-enlargement member states, where milk prices remain depressed with little evidence of price increases in the immediate future. However, in the same survey, it was reported that over 80% of the UK farmers interviewed planned to remain in dairying, with many intending to increase the size of their herd and overall business.

The population

Europe has a large population to feed and food supplies are generally plentiful. Overall EU citizens enjoy increasing affluence, but whilst spending an increasing proportion of their income on non-food items, many show a growing discernment for wholesome food, including high quality milk products. At the same time, consumers are being constantly reminded by the media of possible health issues associated with the consumption of milk and dairy products. Despite this, it is reassuring that a large proportion of people still enjoy dairy products in their many different forms, whilst recognising their nutritional benefits as part of a balanced diet.

Increased wealth and awareness brings forward another issue, with consumers becoming increasingly concerned about the manner of production from animals, demanding livestock production systems that are more benign with respect to both animal welfare and the environment.

World trade

Against a background situation where the EU is more or less self-sufficient with respect to the production and consumption of milk and dairy products, recent and ongoing WTO agreements aim to remove most forms of import restrictions, thus increasing opportunities for imported dairy products from non EU countries at very competitive prices. This will inevitably interest those involved in the procurement and processing of milk and represents a significant threat to the long-term viability of the EU dairy industry. However, a number of counteractive forces must be taken into account. Firstly the quality of many dairy products originating from EU countries cannot be readily reproduced by outside competition. Secondly, many countries capable of supplying dairy products to the EU are unable to claim compliance with the high demands being placed on livestock farmers in respect of welfare and environment. Thus, whilst the supermarket buyer and consumer will always be interested in sourcing food at competitive prices, there remains a market for quality milk products that have been produced in a responsible manner with respect to animal welfare and the environment. Recent consumer trends show that the size of this market, over time, will increase. Thirdly (as seen with recent food scares associated with the BSE and FMD outbreaks, as well as Salmonella in poultry and dioxin contamination of feedstuffs) the public, when sufficiently motivated, make buying decisions that reflect their concerns over food safety.

For many non-EU countries to become serious net importers of dairy products to the EU, it will be necessary for them to improve and demonstrate compliance in terms of animal welfare, environmental considerations and food safety. New Zealand producers are already recognising the need to discontinue certain animal management practices (tail docking, induction of calving) that would simply not be acceptable on EU dairy farms.

EU landscape

There is another issue of great concern that has undoubtedly exercised the minds of politicians during the recent WTO negotiations: Europe has a large land mass well suited to growing forages which are an important feed resource for many classes of ruminants including the dairy cow. This land mass is a highly valued asset in terms of ruminant meat and milk production. Whilst few governments of member states appear to have concern for farm businesses, encouraging farmers, some times by draconic means, to become market orientated, a wholesale departure of animals from the rural landscape due to the collapse of dairying (as well as beef and sheep) would cause serious and largely irreversible damage to the countryside. Change beyond all recognition would result and almost certainly would become an issue that the general public would not find acceptable.

Increasing feed resources

In terms of feed resources there are certain issues, largely attributable to increased affluence of the population that need addressing. Changing lifestyles means that more food is processed outside the home, a response to increased affluence as well as time pressure on families. More food is also consumed outside home, and fast food consumption as well as the restaurant trade are both important outlets for agricultural products. These changes in lifestyle has lead to increasing availability of quality by-products arising from the human food industry, many of which make ideal feeds for ruminants. By-products of the potato, baking and confectionery industries are just some such products, adding to those from the brewing industry that have been long term favourites with many farmers. Ruminant animals make an ideal repository for such materials, especially when contrasted with other alternatives such as power generation or disposal in landfill sites.

Immediate and ongoing threats

The real effects of recent EU enlargement have not yet been realised, and the way low cost labour from the Eastern countries, leading to cheaper agricultural products, may threaten some of the more established dairy industries in the Northern and Western regions of the EU has yet to be analysed. The removal of trade disincentives allows countries such as New Zealand to see opportunities to expand their imports, and the recent expansion of dairying into the South Island, largely at the expense of sheep, is testament to the optimism that exists in that country. Similarly, other countries are seeing great opportunities for dairy production. Brazil is starting to emerge on the international stage as a serious dairy producer, where their annual milk yield of 14bn litres in 1995, exceeded 19bn litres in 2000 and is planned to reach 29bn by 2010. In contrast, the EU total milk production has remained more or less constant due to the continuation of production quotas.

A considerable proportion of the milk produced in Brazil will be exported as dairy products, especially to the USA where there is likely to be a discernable reduction in total milk production in response to increasing environmental concerns. It can not however be ruled out that some Brazilian products may ultimately reach the EU, and even if it doesn't, the sheer size of the increase in little over a decade is bound to have a downward pressure on world milk price, given the abundance of cheap labour and land available in Brazil.

Milk quotas were introduced in the EU in 1984 as a means of curbing milk production in order to reduce the Commissions budget supporting dairy production. In this respect they have been successful as they have certainly managed to limit milk surpluses but over time quota has become a major restriction to those progressive farmers wishing to expand. At its peak, milk quota traded in the UK for between four and five times the prevailing price of milk, with the quota (licence) to produce milk from an average yielding cow worth £4000 against a market value for the cow of less than £1000. Since those days, milk quota prices have fallen but farmers remain quota-conscious and are still prepared to acquire extra quota in line with any planned herd expansion. It is inevitable that this investment has led to an overall reduction in other investments that could have improved overall efficiency of individual farming businesses (e.g. milking, housing or feed storage and preparation facilities). It is strange that on the one hand the commission wishes Agriculture to be fully accountable in a free market economy yet it remains shackled by limits on production due to some historic intervention 20 years ago. Many now feel quotas should be abolished; yet the commission has indicated their continuation for another 6 to 10 years at least, perhaps not because of their overall support for them but rather lack of a suitable mechanism to abolish them without returning to the days of excess surplus in the late 1970s and early 1980s.

Against the backdrop of such issues in the EU, it is possible that relocation of the industry may occur. The real threat of dairying from the new EU member countries is currently unpredictable, but within original member states it is difficult, with declining support systems, to believe that some of the smaller as well as less efficient producers can survive. Based on the main milk producing countries of the EU, this paper will attempt to review current dairying practices, to identify the strengths and weaknesses of different systems and provide some possible scenarios for future dairy farming in the EU.

Current and possible future systems of milk production

The breeds

Undoubtedly many different systems of dairying are being practised within the EU but, with limited exceptions, the Holstein cow dominates herds. This is not intended to dismiss others such as the Brown Swiss and the Jersey and local breeds as being unimportant, but it has been the focussed selection of Holsteins for milk production that has made them so attractive to many dairy farmers. It is only 10-15 years since the Friesian was the dominant animal in many herds, such has been the pace of change. Most farmers are continually seeking higher yields, and the genetically improved Holstein is able to satisfy such demands. In contrast some farmers, particularly those supplying milk for processing, still recognise the value of cows that produce higher levels of milk solids, and in this respect there has been a renewed interest in Jerseys in some areas. In other countries, especially those based on extensive use of grazed grass such as Ireland, the last few years have seen considerable interest in the importation of New Zealand Holstein genetics. This initiative was based on the belief that the New Zealand cow was bred to be more suitable to efficient milk production from grass, thus offering a possible solution to the declining fertility common in modern high producing Holstein.

Cross breeding options have also been explored recently in Ireland. Norwegian red cattle have been extensively studied as a possible choice for cross breeding with the Holstein, on the basis of better fertility and improved feet traits, whilst others see potential in the Jersey for cross breeding with the Holstein. Cross breeding is popular within the beef industry, especially in the production of beef cattle from the dairy herd, and better conformation traits as well as higher feed conversion efficiencies are attractive for beef producers. There is also the possibility of heterosis (hybrid vigour) when cross breeding beef cattle. In most situations however the crossbred beef animal is used for meat production and not for the production of maternal replacements. Hybrid vigour will also occur when cross breeding dairy animals but evidence suggests that it is only likely to improve overall performance by 5% above the average of the two parental breeds and only in the initial cross. Secondly the issue remains as to how to breed the dairy F1 hybrid to produce the second generation. In the pig industry, the comparability in performance of the Landrace and the Large White has allowed reciprocal or criss-cross breeding to be adopted with success. In dairy cow breeds, only the Friesian comes anywhere close to the Holstein and such crosses could be quite successful. In all other situations, where extremes such as the Jersey and the Holstein have been bred, the advice is to outcross one further generation, perhaps using the Brown Swiss or even the Ayrshire, before breeding the F2 hybrid female back to either of the breeds represented in the first cross. Given each generation takes almost three years from conception to first calving, this represents a minimum of almost 7 years to complete the breeding cycle, when the off spring of the F2 heifer bred back to one of the original breeds would be first expected to produce milk. Not only is this a long commitment but will complicate breeding policy, reduce opportunities to take advantage of genetic development in more progressive breeds and could reduce the commercial value of all the dairy cows in the herd. It is not surprising therefore that cross breeding was seen as nothing more than a one-generation fix by Cunningham (2004).

The feeds

Grass

At the same time as breed changes have occurred, only relatively modest changes have occurred in the feed base available for many dairy farmers. Grass is still a major resource on most farms, and one that can be produced at relatively low cost. It can be utilised either by grazing or after conservation, normally as silage although in some countries hay is still popular. Fortunately for dairy farmers, cereal prices have been quite low for several years and this has provided important feed opportunities, whilst, as mentioned earlier, there is an increased availability of by-product feeds, especially for those dairy farms situated within access of urbanisation.

Whilst grass is a cheap source of nutrients, it does have serious limitations. Nutritional quality is unpredictable, being affected by seasonality as well as pasture management. Secondly, availability is weather dependant and without adequate supplies of rain, grass growth can be seriously affected making feed budgeting difficult on those farms prone to summer droughts. Thirdly, despite recent advances in silage methods, making grass silage of consistent quality can be difficult and poor ensiling conditions (weather at time of harvest, poor consolidation and inadequate sheeting) will affect silage quality with consequential reductions in silage intake and levels of animal performance. Levels of silage DM intake will never exceed those that can obtained with the same forage as grazed by livestock, and in such situations recourse to other feeds is essential if adequate levels of nutrition are to be provided. Equally, grazed grass has limitations in the amount that cows will consume.

The DM content of grazed grass varies according to weather and growth stage and can range between 12 and 20% or maybe even more. At best, a cow consuming 16kg grazed grass DM will need to consume 80kg fresh grass per day, equivalent to over 12% of her body weight whilst wet grass can increase these amounts to 130kg or more than 20% of body weight. This is a huge commitment for the cow and thus it is not surprising that maximum pasture intake rarely exceeds 17-18kgDM/day or 2.8 to 3.0% of cow bodyweight. Such levels of intake will only be achieved when all conditions are ideal, and will support no more than 27kg milk production per day. In contrast, cows in full lactation are capable of eating up to 4% of bodyweight each day. Thus for higher levels of milk production, it will be necessary to offer supplementary feeds. The usual practice is to provide a proprietary concentrate, fed in the parlour at the time of milking. In turn this will reduce total grass DM intake due to forage substitution, although choice of concentrate type can limit this effect.

The ultimate target of many who supplement cows at pasture with concentrates is to obtain an economic response to all purchased feeds. Without any substitution of grazed grass intake, every 1 kg of concentrate (DM) provided is capable of producing an additional 2.2 - 2.4 kg milk. Such returns are economic at current prices for milk and concentrates, but the resulting reduction in grazed grass intake generally reduces the overall response. A minimum response of 1.2kg milk/kg concentrates is still profitable whilst many would feel that at less than 1 kg/kg, feeding concentrates becomes questionable. What many farmers fail to see in such situations is the potential benefit as well as associated costs. Consuming less grass by grazing allows more to be conserved for winter feeding and whilst conserved grass will be more expensive per unit metabolisable energy (ME) than grazed grass, an increased supply of winter feed will bring associated cost reductions in terms of reduced reliance on purchased feeds for winter milk production. Secondly the cow at pasture may often fail to perform to expectations due to grass shortage and this will be rapidly detected in reduced milk yields and compromised milk composition. Periods of under nutrition in dairy cows can allow other problems, such as poor fertility through excessive body condition loss, to be manifested.

Poor and erratic intakes at pasture may predispose cows to displaced abomasums, a painful and costly problem. Recent work from Australia (Williams *et al.*, 2004) supported by Irish research (Sayers *et al.*, 2003) indicated that cows grazing lush spring pasture may experience prolonged periods of the day when the rumen pH is below 6.0. This is clearly due to the high content of soluble carbohydrates in spring grass, and rumen acidosis (considered to occur when rumen pH falls below 6.0) can lead to digestive upsets, compromising feed intakes and resulting in ill cows.

The role of supplementary feeding at pasture is complex and the potential benefits are likely to be more far reaching than simply the weight of extra milk per kg weight of concentrates supplied.

One final consideration with respect to those systems that rely heavily on the use of grazed grass to produce milk with reasonable margins is the issue of seasonality. Grass is usually plentiful during May and June but will mostly be available between April and September. Systems designed to exploit extended grazing aim to have significant amounts of grass available between February and November, certainly in many Northern EU countries. Clearly this will bring a glut of milk during the best grass months and lower prices during certain months reflect the pattern of production. However an increasing proportion of milk is being processed rather than consumed as liquid milk and milk processors need to ensure a more constant supply of milk. This is necessary for the efficient operation of processing plant whilst controlling transport costs.

A recent review of the impact of such seasonality on future milk prices (DIAL/FMG, 2004) concluded that further widening of the ratio between monthly peak and trough productions (which currently stands at 1.24:1 in the UK) should be resisted as all signals from milk buyers are for more level profiles of milk production. The report gave a significant number of findings including the prediction that average producers moving from level production to a spring season profile would gain approximately 0.2p/l in terms of reduced costs of production, only to lose 0.8p/litre due to increased transportation and processing costs. Benefits from increased spring milk production were difficult to establish. Only the top 25% producers (who moved from their current profile of 1.13:1 to more milk from grass with a ratio of 1.50:1) were predicted to have an improved margin, amounting to 0.68p/litre. Such findings suggest that moving to spring milk production will not provide the long term improved margins that most dairy farmers seek, and such a strategy is not to be recommended for average producers, although interestingly enough it is this class of farmer who is most tempted by cheap grass.

Mixed ration feeding

In contrast to those systems based extensively on grazed and ensiled grass, mixed ration feeding aims to exploit other feedstuffs available on the farm or that can be purchased at competitive prices. The aim is to supply cost effective rations that can achieve the lactation potential of the cows. Alternative forages such as forage maize or whole crop cereal silage provide highly suitable feeds that can be grown successfully on many farms. In mainland Europe maize silage has been an important part of dairy cow diets for many years, but it is the Northern climates where there has been a marked increase in production that is most relevant. Forage maize is now routinely grown on many farms in Northern England and is increasing in popularity in parts of Ireland, especially Southern Ireland. Fodder beet is also a highly nutritious crop that can be grown for dairy diets and has been popular for many years in certain mainland EU countries. It is a crop which farmers either like or hate, for whilst yields can be good, the need to wash the crop prior to feeding often deters growers.

Where maize cannot be grown successfully, then whole crop cereal silage is an alternative. It can be harvested at a wide range of DM contents and either fermented, urea treated or machine milled and treated with an enzyme or urea additive with advancing maturities respectively. Cereal crops may also be combined to provide highly nutritious feeds for dairy cows, with on-farm processing of the dry grain either by rolling, caustic treatment or crimping and ensiling of moist grain harvested at an earlier stage of maturity.

Other forage crops include legumes such as Lucerne or red clover that can be grown as pure crops or white clover which is usually grown in combination with grass. All legumes can be difficult to ensile or make into hay, and when producing silage it is advisable to use a suitable additive due to their high buffering capacity.

Equally legumes can be difficult to grow on some soils but the benefits in terms of improved feed intake and animal performance make them worthy of serious consideration. One recent initiative is the breeding of 'high sugar' containing grasses; the claim being that the additional water-soluble carbohydrate content will improve overall nitrogen utilisation in the rumen and support improved animal performance (Moorby et al., 2001). Closer examination of available research data suggests some of the claims may be excessive, as increased sugar content appears to be unpredictable and often only marginally better than that achieved with tetraploid varieties, whilst robust animal performance data is still not available. Furthermore, despite increased levels of water soluble carbohydrates in silages prepared from high sugar grasses, very high levels of fermentation acids (>190g/kgDM) have been reported and these are of concern in terms of possible effects on feed intake as well as overall conversion of energy from the harvested crop to the final animal product.

With a variety of home grown feeds as well as purchased straights, including protein sources (soya, rape or canola meal and maize gluten feed), energy sources (sugar beet feed, molasses and citrus pulp) and various by-products (brewery or distillery grains), dairy farmers who feed mixed rations have a wide range of feeds available for ration formulation. In such situations it is possible to feed less (or none) in the milking parlour and thus reduce the cost of the ration, or to modify feed ingredients in order to achieve more balanced rations. Mixed ration feeding normally requires some mechanisation with associated costs. However as ration requirements for today's dairy cow become more sophisticated, there is an increasing need to include adequate levels of physically effective fibre and balancing different forms of starch (with respect to their rumen fermentation characteristics) in the diet. Therefore the option to provide mixed rations on the farm is likely to become more attractive not only in terms of overall costs but resultant animal performance. Such systems also allow the fuller exploitation of grass silage, but can also be advantageous in providing buffer feeds during early turnout to pasture as well as when grazed grass quality or quantity may be limiting. Many farmers are reluctant to discontinue in-parlour feeding in the belief that cows need to be fed in order to achieve satisfactory milk letdown. Others see it as an option for providing additional feed to high yielders, thus avoiding the need to establish different groups of cows. It is interesting to note however that in the increasing number of herds which have discontinued in parlour feeding, some have now elected to feed one single mixed ration to all cows, with no adverse effects on animal condition.

It is likely that the benefits provided by mixed ration feeding will be realised by an increasing number of farmers over the next few years especially when depreciation of the mixer wagon over 10 years for a 100 cow herd receiving 60% of their annual feed requirement as a mixed ration can be as little as 0.4p(EU 0.6cents)/kg DM fed. For cows fed 20kgDM/day this amounts to 8p (11 cents)/day but when compared with possible daily feed costs of £2.00 (EU 2.85)/cow and milk sales of £5.40 (EU7.70)/cow it is not difficult to see where savings and improved production can easily cover such increased costs.

Another often cited problem with mixed rations is the need to store feed on the farm and to comply with Farm Assurance schemes as these become increasingly important to all dairy farmers. For the larger operator, dedicated shed storage is the easiest option at a cost that can be borne over many years of continued use. For smaller farmers such investments are not possible, but in such situations it is possible to purchase feed blends according to an agreed specification and to store these in dedicated feed hoppers.

Herd size

Latest survey data indicates over 19m dairy cows in the EU, a herd size that is highly variable, with larger herds being concentrated in the Northern states. In the UK the average herd size is more than 80 with many herds in excess of 300 and some herds milking over 1000 cows. Compared with some other EU countries such herd sizes may appear to be large, until US herd sizes (as reported by Hutjens, 2003) are taken into account. There are also some exceedingly large herds in Middle East countries including Saudi Arabia.

The last ten years has seen the total number of dairy farmers in the EU decline with a concomitant increase in herd size and such trends are likely to continue. At the same time total cow numbers have declined largely as a consequence of increased milk yields that can be achieved from genetically improved cows when fed well, thus requiring fewer cows to meet annual production quotas.

Larger herds are considered to be one way of covering fixed costs with increased milk sales, bringing savings through more efficient resource use. In contrast many herds, which are unable to expand, need to establish other sources of income regardless of milking efficiency. The possibility of an increased number of dairy farmers seeking part time paid employment off the farm now exists. These farmers will not be the providers of the majority of the milk produced by the EU, which in the last milk year amounted to 118bn litres.

At the same time as herd sizes are on the increase, the limited availability of skilled labour is becoming an important issue for many farmers. Less reliance can be placed on family labour with an increasing number of sons and daughters not wishing to pursue careers in agriculture where returns are modest in relation to total work effort. It is important that as herd sizes get bigger they are managed as efficient business units. In the UK the target is 750,000 litres milk produced per year per full time worker equivalent and whilst many farmers are failing to achieve this, it demonstrates the size and cost of the labour component involved in milk production. In a comparable analysis, Hutjens (2003) provided a target of 550-680 kg milk per unit of labour in the USA. With an increasing skill base and greater career expectations for those involved in dairy farming, as well as the declining availability of qualified staff, there will be an increasing need to improve on-farm mechanisation in order to make better use of the limiting labour resource, whilst at the same time improving overall working conditions. Undoubtedly working with dairy cows can be a rewarding career but aspirations can easily be affected when there is an excess of recurring menial tasks for the work force, that does not represent the most efficient use of qualified and expensive staff.

Increased investment in the farm could include replacement parlours to reduce milk staffing needs, as well as milking times, or the possible introduction of robotic systems to remove milking completely. Other areas include better cow housing with easier bedding and waste disposal, improved cow flow both within the farm and through the introduction of cow tracks (will also reduce incidence of lameness) umbilical spreading of slurry to avoid the annual chore of emptying slurry lagoons and more covered feed preparation space. Such investments are expensive but are already being contemplated by those farmers who intend to remain in the industry and make their businesses profitable but are usually related to an increase in herd size.

At the same time a recent economic analysis of the UK industry by Colman, (2004) revealed that small ($\sim$80 cow) herds, when run efficiently, had similar overall profits as larger herds operating via more average management practices with an average of 180 cows. This clearly indicates that it is not always necessary to increase herd size to achieve better profits. The analysis also showed that well-run small herds achieved higher yields per cow through better nutrition without compromising animal health, milk quality or herd fertility. Thus before contemplating major increase in herd size with the associated costs of more cows, more quota, more staff and more buildings, it is important to fully review the business, and identify where improvements in margins can be achieved. Only then when the business is considered to be operating at optimal efficiency should moves to increase herd size be contemplated.

In reviewing almost 400 herds in North West England, Colman *et al*, (2004) noted a difference in margin of 4.57p/litre between the 10% leading herds and those classified as 'average'. Of this 1.42p/litre was due to higher milk price, but most interestingly, the remaining 3.15p/litre was attributable almost entirely to better management of costs. In particular the better-managed herds had achieved such improvements through higher yields and, most importantly, with better attention to detail, thus not sacrificing animal health, fertility or milk quality.

Future issues for dairy farming in the EU

Within the confines of this paper it is not possible to provide a comprehensive review of all possible future issues and consequently three major ones have been identified. Market opportunities need to be considered if the value of milk to the producer in terms of margin can be improved. Environmental issues are becoming increasingly important from a legislative point of view, and dairy farmers now must respond to increasing pressures being placed on them to reduce environmental emissions. Finally, improved nutritional management must be considered. A number of different scenarios are discussed below that could improve the overall margins on milk production, and thus reduce some of the current excess wastage which erodes overall profitability.

Market opportunities

With little indication of any major increases in milk price over the foreseeable future, the options for dairy farmers to improve overall margins are relatively limited. Adding value to the milk produced on the farm through processing or production of high value products is a commendable route and those farmers who have done so are realising the benefits. However such opportunities are not available to all producers as there is a limit to the quantity of niche products that any one market will bear. Some dairy farmers have radically changed their faming practices in order that their milk could be sold as 'organic', for which initially the price differential was attractive. However the uptake of organic milk and dairy products by the public has failed to meet the predictions of buyers and processors. Despite repeated attempts to instil confidence in this sector of the industry, overall demands remain relatively static. In Denmark, where the period of conversion to organic production was only 12 months (unlike most other EU countries where conversion took 2 years) there has been a marked oversupply of milk in relation to demand, a situation evident in several other EU states. In the UK it is estimated that over 40% of organic milk supplied to OMSCo (Organic Milk Supply Cooperative) is currently being sold into conventional markets. Consequently the price differentials being offered between organic and conventional milk have reduced and the number of farmers starting conversion to organic production has fallen significantly. At the same time, some existing producers are abandoning organic systems of milk production, which aim to be more demanding next year, reverting to conventional milk production allows them to exploit cheaper purchased feeds and better farm cropping options, generating improved margins.

For the bulk of EU milk, it is inevitable that the Holstein will remain the dominant breed for some time to come, but as a greater proportion of milk production is being processed into dairy products, the obvious advantages of breeds that produce milk with higher solids contents is being recognised. In this respect Jersey cow numbers have increased in some countries, and this trend is likely to continue, especially when herds are genetically improved. American and Danish lines have superior milk compositions to the more typical Island cow, but the Jersey is not only capable of producing milk of higher solids contents than the Holstein, where due to lower cow maintenance costs and a reduced output of lactose in relation to fat and protein output, overall feed conversion efficiency (FCE) in Jerseys is higher compared to Holsteins (Beever, 2003). Taking the example of a herd of 100 Holsteins with an annual average milk production of 7500 litres (37g/kg fat; 31.5g/kg protein), it would require only 113 Jerseys (5100 litres, 49.5g/kg fat; 39.5g/kg protein) to produce the same annual yield of fat and protein (51.3 tonnes) To achieve this Holsteins were estimated to require a total of 543 tonnes feed DM (Av ME; 11.5MJ/kgDM) compared with only 500 tonnes for the Jerseys, a net saving of 43 tonnes, which would allow another 10 Jerseys to be kept, producing an additional 4.5 tonnes of milk fat and protein. The Holsteins had an estimated FCE of 94.5g milk solids (fat and protein)/kg feed DM, compared with 102.6g/kg for Jerseys, an overall improvement of more than 8%. In addition, the Jersey herd of 113 cows were estimated to produce 492 tonnes of water in their total milk sales, compared with 655 tonnes for Holsteins. This translates to an additional 163 tonnes water per annum which milk processors do not want due to extra costs associated with transportation and disposal after processing.

Environmental issues

Despite having fewer dairy cows in the EU than perhaps 20 years ago, the environmental impact of livestock production is now recognised by most Governments of EU countries. This will undoubtedly lead to increasing pressures being placed upon the industry to reduce total emissions. Of most concern are carbon, nitrogen and phosphorus and already legislation exists with respect to the application of nitrogen contained in natural and artificial manures in many areas.

Carbon is excreted by dairy cattle in several different forms, in faeces as undigested feed or gut microbial biomass, in urine as waste metabolites and in breath as carbon dioxide and methane. An average dairy cow yielding 25-30 litres milk per day will produce between 5-6000 litres carbon dioxide and up to 600 litres methane/

day. The higher global warming effect of methane compared with CO_2 is leading initiatives to establish ways of reducing methane emissions. Over the last 20 years, several feed additives, which limit rumen methane production, have been proposed, but few have enjoyed sustained success. The use of ionophores, known to promote propionate production in the rumen and thus reduce the amount of fermentation hydrogen available for methane production, are possibly the most successful. However, their use is being phased out in many countries and they are unlikely to gain long term approval within the EU. In Australia a research programme to develop a vaccine that would reduce or even remove all rumen methanogens (methane producing bacteria) has been ongoing for several years. After earlier claims of 100% elimination of methanogens, this has since been downsized to 20% and a recent study reported only a 7.7% reduction. It is unlikely that this approach will provide the improvements demanded. Even if it did, it is doubtful if such gains would result in any overall improvements in animal performance.

Bovine somatotrophin (BST) has been used regularly in the US over the last 8-10 years and has the potential to reduce methane levels indirectly. BST promotes milk yield and when the amount of methane produced as a result of animal maintenance and milk production is compared against the increased total yield of milk, the total methane burden is reduced per litre milk produced. BST is unlikely to be licensed for use within the EU, but the principle still applies. Higher yielding cows provide an important opportunity to control or reduce present day methane emissions.

On the basis of the data available for average yielding cows, an output of between 20 and 30 litres of methane per litre milk produced would be expected. In contrast Hattan (2003) measured higher yielding cows in early/mid lactation, and noted a mean value of 16.7 litres of methane per litre milk. Outputs increased progressively from 13.8 (week 6) to 19.5 (week 30) litres of methane per litre as milk yield declined and peak feed intake was achieved. An overall average increase in UK yields by 2000 litres per cow per annum would reduce methane output by almost 3 litres per litre of milk produced. Assuming this higher average yield, fewer cows would be required to produce the UK annual milk production quota of 14bn litres, resulting in an estimated reduction in methane production of 27,000 tonnes per annum, representing more than 10% of current estimates levels. Similarly, if such improvements in milk production were to occur across the main dairying countries of the EU, the predicted decline in methane output of 228,000 tonnes per annum would be equivalent to approximately 90% of current UK production. Clearly such improvements could make an important contribution to overall efforts to reduce total methane emissions from livestock. However it is rather perverse to note that such improvements would be achieved through intensification of production when most government agencies are anxious to encourage more extensive systems.

In a similar context, Garnsworthy (2003) examined the environmental impact of high cow replacement rates, which occurs in many herds due to poor fertility and early culling. He concluded that reductions in annual methane output could be achieved by a modest improvement in overall cow fertility through a direct reduction in the number of heifer replacements needed.

The situation with respect to nitrogen emissions is more complex. The amount of nitrogen excreted in faeces is related to overall feed digestibility in the whole tract, and microbial N digestibility in the small intestines. Urinary N excretion reflects inefficiencies in both rumen and host animal metabolism. The absorption of excess N from the rumen containing feed with high levels of readily available N has been known for some years. Better ration formulation focussing on the balance between ruminally available energy and nitrogen makes it possible to reduce this loss. On the other hand, many of the losses which occur during post-absorptive metabolism may be unavoidable especially in respect of normal turnover of body protein mass. Nevertheless, reducing the quantity of amino acids catabolised to produce glucose (by enhanced ruminal propionate production) would make an important contribution to reducing overall urinary nitrogen excretion.

Most dairy cow rations are designed to contain at least 17-18% total protein yet the proportion of this protein converted into milk protein is never likely to exceed 300-350g/kg (0.3-0.35%). This represents a major environmental load as well as a huge cost to the farmer and it is interesting to speculate why dietary protein levels are still so high when overall efficiency is so low. Supplying more dietary protein in supplementary feeds was considered one way of improving the voluntary intake of relatively wet grass silages, whilst there was a general misconception that feeding more protein would increase protein levels in the milk. In respect to grass silage, few very wet grass silages are now being fed to dairy cows whilst the overall forage base for dairy cows has changed dramatically with the introduction of maize and whole crop cereal silage. Equally there is considerable evidence that whilst feeding more protein will generally improve milk protein yield, few marked effects on milk protein content are seen (Keady, 2002) due to parallel increases in milk yield.

On the basis of current evidence it would appear that modest reductions in total ration protein levels could be achieved without any adverse effects on overall animal performance. Indeed it is suggested that high plasma urea levels generated as a consequence of high rumen or tissue losses of nitrogen may have an adverse effect on overall fertility, although this has yet to be confirmed, as well as milk processing qualities.

Reducing dietary protein levels may also improve animal health in terms of reduced laminitis. Recent research comparing high starch and high protein feeding to dairy cows concluded that increased levels of protein in early lactation stimulated body condition loss (Hattan, 2003).

Despite no improvement in measured ME intake, protein supplementation can significantly increase milk yield, with an associated improvement in milk fat yield, although the increase in milk protein yield is much less. As a consequence, cows fed high protein lose significantly higher levels of body tissue energy at weeks 6 and weeks 12 of measured lactation. This may be associated with reduced fertility.

Dairy cows will excrete phosphorus primarily in the faeces and thus the availability of dietary sources of phosphorus can have a major bearing on both faecal output and the amount of phosphorus required to meet the cow's actual requirements. Recent reviews have suggested that overall dietary levels of phosphorus could be reduced without any major effects on animal health and performance but until more is understood about how phosphorus may complex with other mineral ions in the gut and thus become unavailable for digestion, it is unlikely that any systematic reductions in total phosphorus excretions from dairy cows will be achieved.

Improved nutritional management

Whilst most herds contain a certain proportion of highly efficient and profitable cows, many cows in EU dairy herds fail to achieve their full potential. In a recent review of lifetime milk yields in Holland by the National Recording Scheme the 2003 average lifetime production of milk for all recorded cows was just over 27,000 litres. This compared with a total of 19,000 litres in 1988, demonstrating the impact of improved genetics and better feeding for milk yield over the intervening 15-year period. At the same time, average lactation number for all cows remained unchanged at 3.3, whilst calving interval increased by 2 days per year over the whole study. In the UK early records show that cows had an average lactation number of 3.0 in 1930. By 1940 this had increased to 3.4

and 4.0 by 1950, with the peak of 4.76 achieved around 1970. Currently it stands at 3.45 and, whilst better than the current average of 2.77 in the USA, this low lifespan represents considerable lost potential. If the cost of a downcalving heifer less cull cow price is assumed to be around EU800, then not until that animal has produced in excess of 30,000 litres milk in her lifetime will cow depreciation costs be less than 10% of current milk price. Most cows are capable of much higher yields and lifetime production should be a target for all dairy farmers.

Poor fertility is also a significant cost in dairy production. Many herds report first service conception rates of less than 50%, with overall required services per conception of between 2 and 2.5 and extended calving intervals with an annual replacement rate of over 30%. In reality first service conception rates of over 65% are achievable with not more than 1.5 services per conception, calving intervals of between 365 and 380 days and replacement rates of 20% in many herds. In reality some of the best-managed farms are achieving such targets.

Reasons for poor fertility are complex. Undoubtedly larger herds with less skilled staff devote less time to oestrus detection, which represents a major contributory factor and in this respect the use of pedometers may be an expensive but worthwhile investment. Cunningham (2004) indicated that there is clear evidence of significant inbreeding occurring within the Holstein breed and this may also be contributing to the overall decline in fertility due to reduced fitness. However it is the early and often severe loss of body condition that is a major contributory factor to poor fertility, with an increased number of these cows showing dysfunctional oestrus behaviour. The solution being proposed by some geneticists is to breed a robust cow and whilst it is accepted that some cow lines are less prone to poor reproductive performance, such initiatives are relatively long term and certainly do not provide the rapid solution required by farmers.

It remains the case that we must feed these cows better in order to control the extent and duration of body condition loss, or failing that, extend the calving interval. In high yielding cows, body energy loss in the first 10 weeks of lactation may amount to as much as 60 kg body fat (Beever, 2003). Reducing overall ration protein has been advanced as one possible means of reducing body tissue mobilisation. Avoiding excessive amounts of supplementary fat at this time, which usually promotes milk production, rather than increase body tissue repletion may help. Thereafter the options are relatively limited but highly important. Optimising rumen health in order to achieve high levels of feed intake is a top priority for all dairy farmers in the management of their cows. Rations containing adequate levels of physically effective fibre are an absolute prerequisite to getting cows to ruminate, the most effective indicator of good rumen health. Thereafter, relatively high levels of starch can be fed provided the sources are balanced according to rumen degradation rate, whilst it is advisable with higher yielding cows to avoid high levels of starchy concentrates in single meals offered at milking. In this context, feeding a significant part of the feed as a mixed ration is advantageous, and it is usual to see improvements in both body condition and milk yield when more feed is provided in this way.

This phenomenon, now being observed on an increasing number of farms, suggests a possible improvement in overall feed conversion efficiency. This can be determined as g milk solids (fat and protein) per kg feed DM consumed which is typical of data found in Australian literature or as litres milk, corrected to standard composition, per kg feed DM as proposed by Quinn *et al* (2003). The concept of FCE has been commonplace in the pig and poultry industry for many years and is acknowledged in the beef industry, but it is only now that its importance is being recognised in the dairy industry. The data of Quinn *et al* (2003) showed that by changing nutritional management with the introduction of mixed ration feeding, over 80% of the herds in the study recorded a significant improvement in FCE during the first 12 months following the change. In particular, the study showed substantial improvements across different countries including France, Germany, UK and Ireland, with the highest FCE levels being achieved in France. Sheehy & Quinn (2004) conducted a further study over 2 years and reported improvements in milk yield of 742kgs with increased fat and protein yields of 32 and 29kg respectively. By assuming an average genetic improvement in milk yield of 3% per annum, further analysis of this data concluded that between 60 and 80% of the overall improvement was attributable to improved feed management and utilisation. Overall, Beever (2004) concluded that a modest improvement in FCE from 1.1 to 1.3 kg milk per kg feed DM could reduce overall costs of milk production by as much as 1.3p (1.85 cents) per litre.

Conclusions

Dairying in the EU has experienced some poor returns for herd owners in terms of both their labour and financial investments. With milk prices unlikely to improve markedly in the next 5-10 years, farmers wishing to remain in dairying will need to improve production margins in order to remain financially viable. Adding value to milk by processing on the farm is certainly an option but not one that is available to all producers, leaving a more focussed control of costs as their only option. This paper has attempted to explore some of the issues that dairy farmers and those in supporting industries will need to face in the immediate future, drawing a number of important conclusions.

Of the choices available, enlarging herd size should only be considered once the current business is operating at maximum efficiency, a fact that may be surprising to those who have already invested heavily in extra quota and extra cows. Converting to spring and summer milk production has appealed to many farmers on the basis that grass is the cheapest form of nutrients, but the long term viability of such systems is questionable, given the penalties that increased seasonality of production are likely to incur. Finally, the importance of good nutrition is presented and through this it is possible to reduce some of the major costs of dairying, including poor fertility, poor milk composition and poor longevity. Many options remain for dairying farming in the EU to be profitable and to continue long into the future.

Acknowledgements

The author wishes to acknowledge the support provided by Professor David Colman, Farm Business Unit, School of Economic Studies, The University of Manchester, in the preparation of this paper.

References

Beever, D.E. (2003) Managing dairy cows for optimal performance.. Recent Advances in Animal Nutrition in Australia. 14, pp.33-41. University of New England, Australia.

Beever, D.E. (2004). Opportunities to improve the performance and profitability of dairy farms through better nutrition. 'Knowledge Agriculture, Perspectives towards a new model of milk production. Pp6-8. Richard Keenan & Co, Borris, Co Carlow.

Colman, D. (2004) Reducing the efficiency gap. 'Knowledge Agriculture, Perspectives towards a new model of milk production. Pp14-15. Richard Keenan & Co, Borris, Co Carlow.

Colman, D., Farrar, J & Zhuang, Y. (2004). Economics of milk production England and Wales 2002/03, Farm Business Unit, School of Economic Studies, The University of Manchester.

Cunningham, E.P. (2004). The genetic dimension. 'Knowledge

Agriculture, Perspectives towards a new model of milk production. Pp9-11. Richard Keenan & Co, Borris, Co Carlow.

Dairy Industry Association Limited (DIAL)/Federation of Milk Groups (FMG). Seasonality and the future of the UK dairy industry. Report of the DIAL/FMG seasonality working group, June 2004.

Garnsworthy, P.C. (2003). The impact of dairy cow fertility on methane emissions. European Association Animal Production, meeting no 54, p283. Wageningen Academic Publishers, The Netherlands.

Hattan, A.J. (2003). Energy utilisation in high yielding dairy cows. PhD, The University of Reading.

Hutjens, M.J. (2004). Meeting the educational needs of dairy clientele in 2020. In 'Nutritional Biotechnology in th Feed and Food Industries' (eds; T.P Lyons & K.A. Jacques). Pp 205-10. Proceedings Alltech 20th Annual Symposium, May 2004.

Keady, T.W.J., Mayne, C.S. & Fitzpatrick, D.A. (2000). The effects of concentrate energy source on milk composition of lactating dairy cattle offered grass silage. In 'Milk composition' (eds; R.E Agnew, K.W.Agnew & A.M.Fearon). pp 119-24. British Society Animal Science, Occasional Publication no 25.

Moorby, J.M., Miller, L.A., Evans,R.T., Scollan, N.D., Theodorou, M.K. & MacRae, J.C. (2001). Milk production and N partitioning in early lactation cows offered perennial ryegrass containing a high concentration of water soluble carbohydrate. Proceedings British Society Animal Science, 2001, p6.

Quinn, E., Purcell, C., Voss, M. & Downey, L. (2004). Quantifying the impact of TMR feeding on dairy and beef farms. DRC Dairylink, 1:16-19.

Sayers, H.J., Mayne, C.S & Bartram, C.C. (2003). The effect of level and type of supplement offered to grazing dairy cows on herbage intake, animal performance and rumen fermentation characteristics. Animal Science, 76, 439-54.

Sheehy, S. & Quinn, E. Establishing the economic value of the farm productivity gains derived from the Keenan Integrated Nutrition and Feed Delivery System. 'Knowledge Agriculture, Perspectives towards a new model of milk production. Pp12-13. Richard Keenan & Co, Borris, Co Carlow.

Williams, Y.J., Walker, G.P., Doyle, P.T., Egan, A.R & Stockdale, C.R. (2004) Rumen fermentation characteristics of dairy cows grazing different allowances of Persian clover- or perennial ryegrass- dominant swards in spring. Australian Journal Agricultural Research, (accepted for publication).

Index